Neonatal Ultrasound

Kushaljit Singh Sodhi
Editor

Neonatal Ultrasound

Springer

Editor
Kushaljit Singh Sodhi
Professor, Department of Radiodiagnosis
and Imaging
Post Graduate Institute of Medical
Education and Research
Chandigarh, India

Formerly: Professor, Mallinckrodt Institute
of Radiology, St. Louis Children's Hospital
Washington University in St. Louis School of Medicine
St. Louis, Missouri, USA

ISBN 978-981-97-8575-9 ISBN 978-981-97-8576-6 (eBook)
https://doi.org/10.1007/978-981-97-8576-6

This Springer imprint is published by the registered company Springer Nature Singapore Pte Ltd.
The registered company address is: 152 Beach Road, #21-01/04 Gateway East, Singapore 189721, Singapore

Foreword

It is with great pleasure that I write the Foreword for the textbook *Neonatal Ultrasound* which is intended to present a comprehensive text on the applications of ultrasonography in the evaluation of intra- and extracranial organs in neonates. Given the dramatic changes in sonographic technology, there is a need for an updated reference to help radiologists maximize the benefits of pediatric ultrasonography in their daily practices.

Historically, ultrasound has played a major role in pediatric imaging. Performing high-quality sonographic examinations in neonates requires meticulous attention to technique, knowledge of the spectrum of disease encountered in neonates, and understanding of normal and pathologic findings in this population. This book provides information on how to enhance the performance and interpretation of neonatal sonographic images and avoid technical and interpretative errors.

The text is organized into 12 anatomic chapters, including the brain, neck and orbit, lung and mediastinum, chest wall, liver and gallbladder, urinary track, adrenal gastrointestinal, musculoskeletal, and spine. In each chapter, organ-specific sonographic techniques, clinical applications, normal anatomy, and abnormal sonographic findings are described and illustrated. For completeness, relevant clinical information about a large number of disease processes is discussed. The material in the text is enriched with the highest quality images. It is further strengthened by tables that provide an overview of differential diagnoses. The authors are from multiple institutions and share their expertise in specific aspects of neonatal sonography.

Pediatric radiologists and general radiologists in practice, residents and fellows in training, and sonographers will find *Neonatal Ultrasound* of great value in expanding their knowledge or gaining new knowledge in this subspecialty area. Pediatricians who wish to understand the indications, limitations, and clinical applications of sonography will also gain value from this book.

In summary, this book strives to update the current knowledge on sonography in neonates. This textbook *Neonatal Sonography* will become a cornerstone in pediatric imaging and help radiologists and sonographers address the imaging needs in newborns.

Marilyn J. Siegel

Professor of Radiology and Pediatrics
Mallinckrodt Institute of Radiology
Washington University Medical School
St. Louis, MO, USA

Preface

The field of neonatal ultrasound has evolved dramatically over the recent years, becoming a cornerstone of modern neonatal care. As the demands of neonatal medicine grow, so does the need for precise, real-time imaging that can guide clinicians in the delicate and time-sensitive management of newborns. In this context, ultrasound serves as a vital tool, offering a noninvasive way to visualize the developing anatomy of neonates—from their tiniest vessels to their most complex organs.

Our goal in compiling this textbook was to create a ready reference that encompasses every aspect of neonatal ultrasound, from head to toe, although, it is not intended to be the most comprehensive source on this subject. Special emphasis is placed on both the foundational principles of ultrasound physics and the latest advancements in the field, ensuring that the content is meaningful to both newcomers and seasoned professionals. With numerous case studies, high-quality images, and step-by-step protocols, readers will find this book invaluable in their everyday practice, enhancing their ability to make informed decisions for their youngest patients.

This book, *Neonatal Ultrasound*, is a collaborative effort involving the expertise of some of the most distinguished radiologists from around the world. These authors bring decades of experience and deep insights into the application of ultrasound, across all aspects of neonatal care. Their contributions reflect the diversity and depth of knowledge that exists within the global medical community, making this book a truly international resource. It is through their dedication and commitment to excellence that we are able to offer a resource that is as rich in content as it is broad in scope.

I want to express my deepest gratitude to Prof. Marilyn Siegel for her invaluable support and for helping bring this vision to life. Her expertise and insights have been instrumental in shaping this project, and her thorough review has greatly enhanced the quality of the final product. It has been an honor to collaborate with her.

This book was started while I was at the Washington University in St. Louis and it gained momentum after that. I owe a deep debt of gratitude to my colleagues, both at the Post Graduate Institute of Medical education and Research (PGIMER), Chandigarh, India and Mallinckrodt Institute of Radiology, St. Louis Children's Hospital, Washington University in St. Louis School of Medicine, Missouri, USA, whose unwavering support, dedication to creating an environment that nurtures research, innovation, and scholarly collaboration and fostering a culture of academic excellence, made this book possible.

I would also like to express my gratitude to my wife, Shanujeet, whose unwavering support and understanding have been my anchor throughout this journey. I need to specifically mention my friend, Vivek Gupta, whose encouragement actually sparked the beginning of this book, and it has been on my subconscious mind for more than a decade.

I look forward to feedback from readers. We have just started this journey, and it shall be my sincere endeavor to improve this version in subsequent editions.

It is my hope that this book will serve as a trusted companion in neonatal units, radiology departments, and educational settings around the world. I believe that a deeper understanding of neonatal ultrasound, as presented in these pages, can directly contribute to improving outcomes for the most vulnerable patients—newborns who rely on our knowledge and skill.

May this book inspire and inform those who dedicate their lives to the care of neonates, and may it play a part in advancing the quality of care provided to newborns everywhere.

Chandigarh, India Kushaljit Singh Sodhi

Contents

Editors and Contributors

Editor

Dr. Kushaljit Singh Sodhi (MD, PhD, MAMS, FICR) Professor, Department of Radiodiagnosis, Post Graduate Institute of Medical Education and Research (PGIMER), Chandigarh, India and Formerly, Professor, Mallinckrodt Institute of Radiology, Washington University School of Medicine, St. Louis, MO, USA

Associate Editor

Dr. Marilyn J. Siegel, MD Professor of Radiology and Pediatrics, Mallinckrodt Institute of Radiology, Washington University Medical School, St. Louis, MO, USA

1 Cranial Ultrasound: Technique, Anatomy and Variants

Bernard F. Laya, Nathan David P. Concepcion, Joanna Marie D. Choa-Go, and Justin Luke D. Yap

1.1 Introduction

High-resolution cranial ultrasound (CUS) is a valuable imaging modality to evaluate normal anatomy and pathologic processes affecting the neonatal brain. Cranial ultrasound is portable and can be easily performed at bedside without the need to transfer the patient. The study is radiation-free, relatively less expensive compared to other modalities, and provides images in real time. Cranial ultrasound has played an important role in the evaluation of intracranial hemorrhage, hydrocephalus, ischemic changes, and intracranial infections. In addition, CUS provides information on major congenital and developmental abnormalities. High-frequency transducers further improved the detailed visualization of both superficial and deep cranial structures. Supplementary Doppler sonography, which is available in many ultrasound equipment, allows the evaluation of intracranial vascular anatomy, patency, flow velocities, as well as congenital or acquired vascular abnormalities.

Despite its advantages, CUS depends heavily on the operator's skill, knowledge, and experience in the performance and interpretation of the obtained ultrasound images. There are unique imaging findings in a child's developing brain that needs to be considered. It is important to recognize developmental variants and imaging artifacts for they could mimic true pathology. It is equally important to know that subtle or early abnormalities may not be readily apparent in an ultrasound study. If the patient remains symptomatic or if the clinical suspicion for an abnormality is heightened, a follow-up study utilizing ultrasound or another imaging modality may be warranted.

This chapter covers appropriate transducer selection and scanning techniques for performing cranial sonography. Normal brain anatomy with emphasis on pertinent sonographic landmarks will be presented. Developmental variants and scanning artifacts, which could mimic pathology will likewise be discussed.

B. F. Laya (✉)
St. Luke's Medical Center, Quezon City and Global City, Philippines

St. Luke's Medical Center College of Medicine—William H. Quasha Memorial, Quezon City, Philippines
e-mail: bflaya@stlukes.com.ph

N. D. P. Concepcion
St. Luke's Medical Center, Quezon City and Global City, Philippines

J. M. D. Choa-Go
The Doctors' Hospital Inc., Bacolod City, Negros Occidental, Philippines

J. L. D. Yap
Northern Mindanao Medical Center, Cagayan de Oro City, Philippines

K. S. Sodhi (ed.), *Neonatal Ultrasound*, https://doi.org/10.1007/978-981-97-8576-6_1

1.2 Ultrasound Equipment

1.2.1 Transducer Selection

Cranial ultrasound should be performed using transducers with a small footprint that can fit within the anterior fontanelle. The choice of transducer depends on the optimal frequency to attain the highest resolution with clinically appropriate beam penetration. Sector or curved linear array transducers with a frequency of 7.5 MHz (range of 7–10 MHz) are used in preterm and small-for-gestational-age term neonates, while those with a lower frequency of 5 MHz (range of 3.5–5 MHz) are utilized for larger and term babies as well as those with small or closing fontanelle. Higher frequencies (7.5–18 MHz) in linear array transducers are reserved for the evaluation of near-field superficial structures such as the cerebral cortices, extra-axial spaces, superior sagittal sinus and scalp [1–5]. If the anterior fontanelle is closed or very small, a lower frequency transducer may be used through an open suture or through the thin squamosal portion of the temporal bone [4].

The higher the frequency, the better the resolution but with less penetration. Low frequencies are utilized for better beam penetration when scanning deeper structures although with decreased resolution, whereas higher frequencies are used for the evaluation of more superficial structures [3–7].

1.3 Imaging Technique

1.3.1 Grayscale Imaging

A cranial ultrasound protocol should be standardized to optimize the quality of images, to ensure consistency of imaging between studies, and to achieve reproducibility of findings. However, it should also be flexible and adjusted depending on the specific indication for the examination. Infants are usually scanned at the bedside without necessary preparation.

The transducer pressure on the fontanelles should be kept at a minimum. Adequate gel, which may be warmed prior to and during the study, should be placed to ensure complete contact between the transducer faceplate and skin [4–7].

1.3.1.1 Anterior Fontanelle

Neonatal cranial ultrasound is performed most commonly through the anterior fontanelle [1, 2, 4, 5] in any position [6, 8] but preferably with the patient in the supine position [1]. The anterior fontanelle is the widest and most common acoustic window used in clinical practice to evaluate the supratentorial structures. It is the soft space located in the mid-anterosuperior aspect of the skull, at the junction of the coronal and sagittal sutures [1, 2, 7] (Fig. 1.1). The anterior fontanelle begins to close at approximately 9 months of age and is completely fused by the 15th–24th month of age. However, it may persist later in preterm infants, patients with chromosomal abnormalities (e.g., trisomies 13, 18, and 21), congenital hypothyroidism, increased intracranial pressure, and those with underlying bone conditions (e.g., achondroplasia, osteogenesis imperfecta, rickets, hypophosphatasia, or cleidocranial dysostosis) [1, 2, 9].

As much of the entire brain should be seen during the examination. A series of coronal and sagittal images are obtained through the center of the

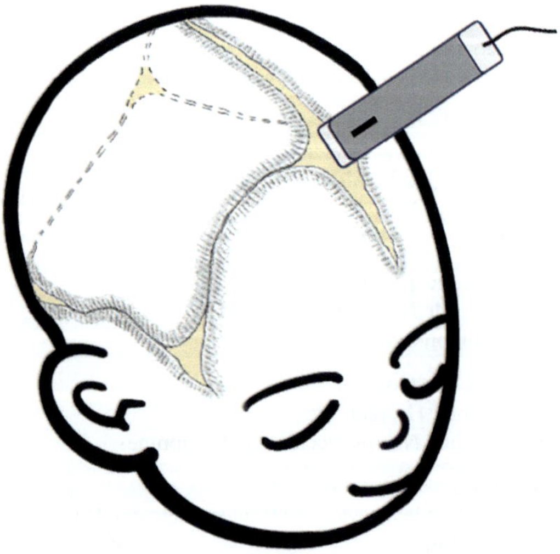

Fig. 1.1 Diagram of cranial ultrasound with the transducer at the anterior fontanelle. The anterior fontanelle is at the junction of the coronal and sagittal sutures

anterior fontanelle [1, 2]. As with other organs of the body, the right side of the brain on coronal images and the anterior aspect of the brain on sagittal images should be on the left side of the screen. On the coronal view, the right and left sides of the brain should be as symmetrical as possible although symmetry does not rule out pathology [1, 4, 5]. On the sagittal view, the probe is rotated 90° and the right and left sides should be properly and clearly labeled [3, 6, 7]. Any suspected finding should be imaged in both planes [4].

Evaluation of the brain on coronal views is done by angulation of the transducer from anterior to posterior, and on sagittal views through the midline and by angulation laterally to the right and to the left [1–4].

Standard representative stations in coronal view using the anterior fontanelle (Fig. 1.2) from anterior to posterior should include the following [1, 3]:

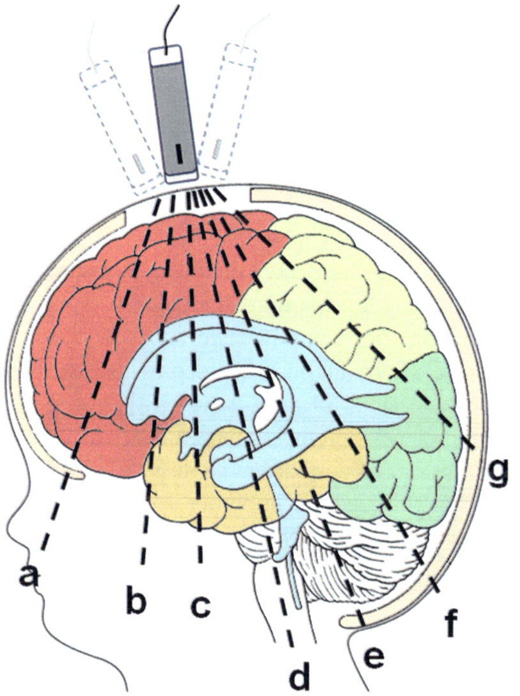

Fig. 1.2 Diagram that demonstrates scanning through the anterior fontanelle with coronal images: (**a**) through the frontal lobes, (**b**) through the frontal horns of the lateral ventricles, (**c**) through the foramina of Monro, (**d**) through the posterior third ventricle and brainstem, (**e**) through the quadrigeminal cistern, (**f**) through the atria of the lateral ventricles, and (**g**) through the parieto-occipital lobes

- Frontal lobes anterior to the frontal horns of the lateral ventricles (Fig. 1.3).
- Frontal horns of the lateral ventricles with the suprasellar cistern (Fig. 1.4).
- Bodies of the lateral ventricles at the level of the foramina of Monro including corpus cal-

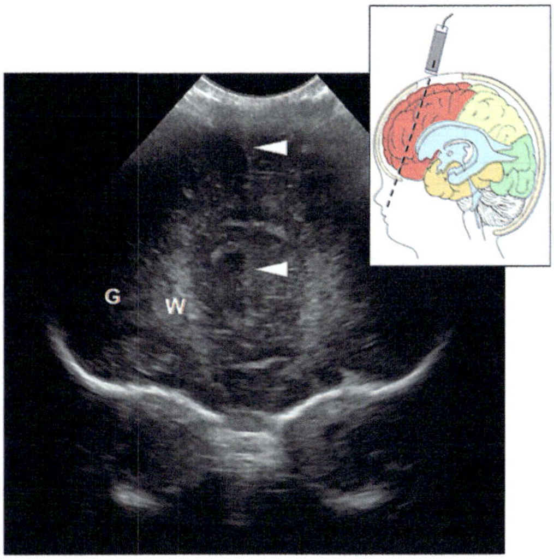

Fig. 1.3 Coronal image using the anterior fontanelle at the level of the frontal lobes including the interhemispheric fissure (arrowheads), gray (G) and white (W) matter. Inset: Diagram of the corresponding scan plane of the image

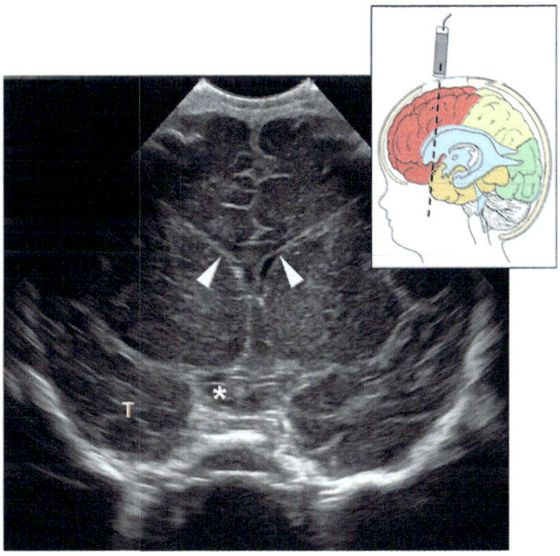

Fig. 1.4 Coronal image using the anterior fontanelle at the level of the frontal horns (arrowheads) including the sella (asterisk) and portion of the temporal lobe (T). Inset: Diagram of the corresponding scan plane of the image

losum, cavum septi pellucidi, caudate nuclei, putamina, globi pallidi, and Sylvian fissures (Fig. 1.5).
  - At this level, the anterior horn width, defined as the diagonal width of the anterior horn measured at its widest point, may be measured [10].
- Posterior third ventricle slightly posterior to the foramina of Monro including the brainstem, thalami, and caudothalamic grooves (Fig. 1.6)
  - The "three dot sign" is seen at this level representing the echogenic choroid plexus in the floor of the lateral ventricles and in the roof of the third ventricle [2].
- Quadrigeminal cistern and cerebellum with the cerebellar vermis (Fig. 1.7).
- Atria or trigones of the lateral ventricles containing echogenic glomi of the choroid plexuses (Fig. 1.8).

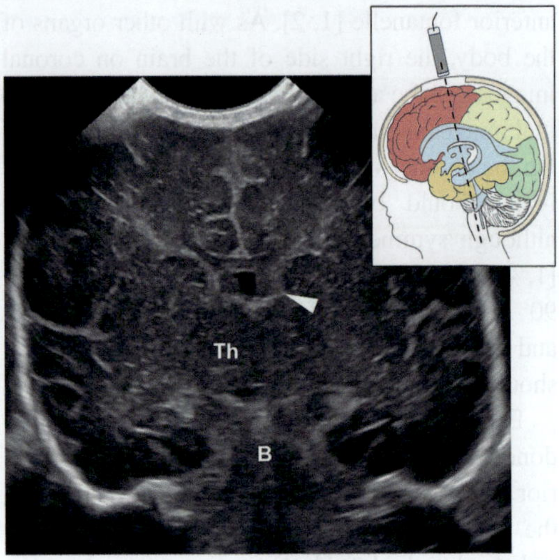

Fig. 1.6 Coronal image using the anterior fontanelle at the level of the posterior third ventricle including the brainstem (B), thalami (Th), and caudothalamic grooves (arrowhead). Inset: Diagram of the corresponding scan plane of the image

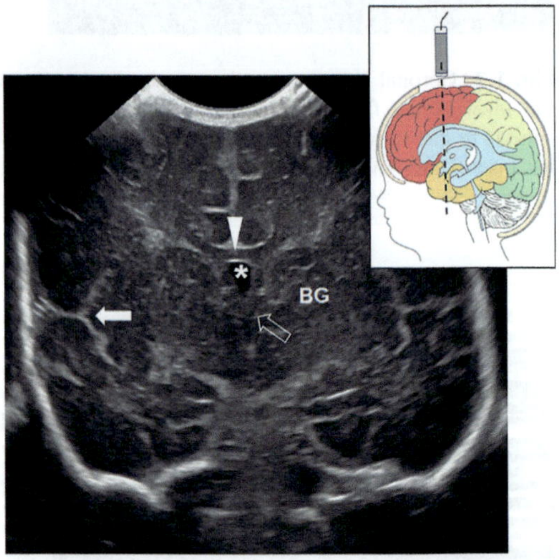

Fig. 1.5 Coronal image using the anterior fontanelle at the level of the foramen of Monro (open arrow) including the corpus callosum (arrowhead), cavum septum pellucidum (asterisk), Sylvian fissure (closed arrow) and basal ganglia (BG). Inset: Diagram of the corresponding scan plane of the image

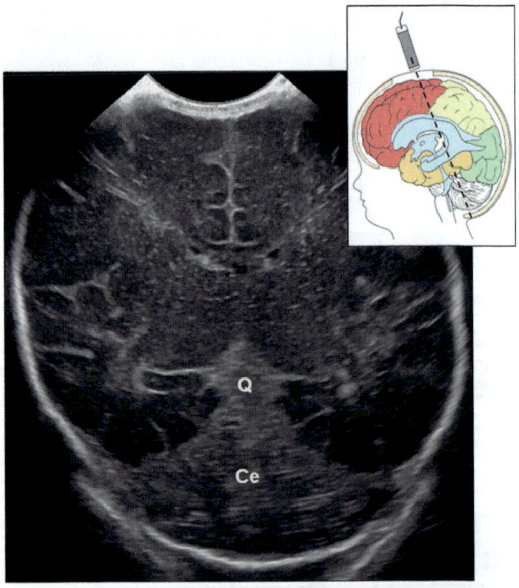

Fig. 1.7 Coronal image using the anterior fontanelle at the level of the star-shaped quadrigeminal cistern (Q) and cerebellum (Ce). Inset: Diagram of the relative scan plane of the image

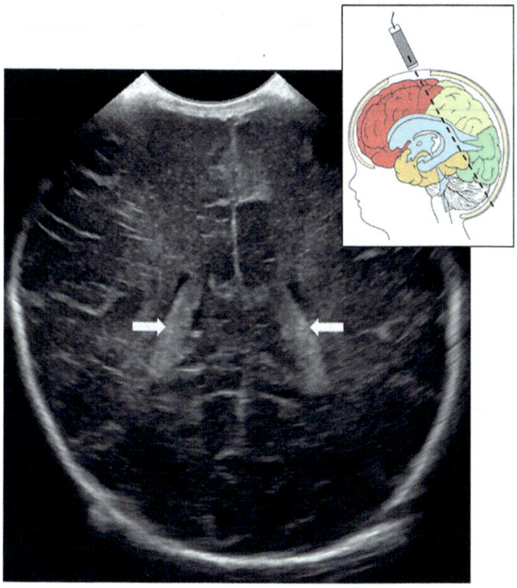

Fig. 1.8 Coronal image using the anterior fontanelle at the level of the atria of the lateral ventricles containing echogenic glomi of the choroid plexuses (arrows). Inset: Diagram of the corresponding scan plane of the image

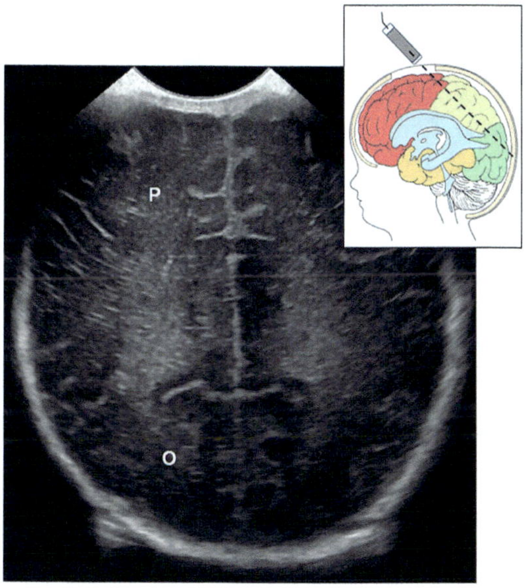

Fig. 1.9 Coronal image using the anterior fontanelle at the level of the parietal (P) and occipital (O) lobes. Inset: Diagram of the corresponding scan plane of the image

- Parieto-occipital lobes posterior to occipital horns of the lateral ventricles (Fig. 1.9).

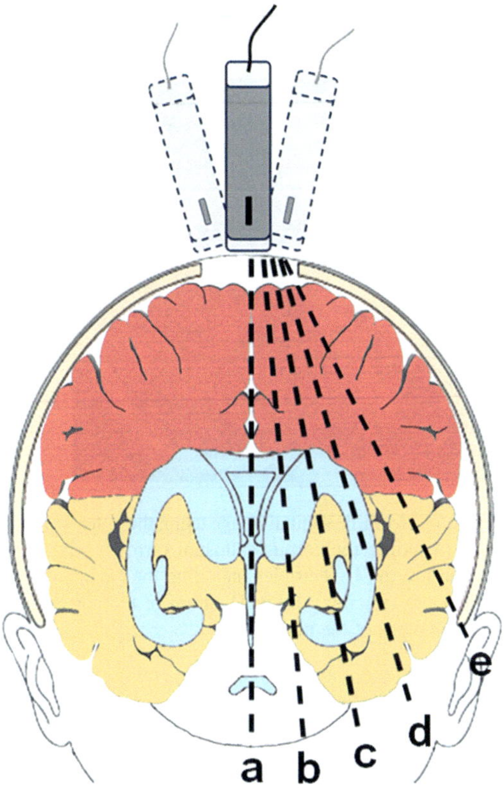

Fig. 1.10 Diagram that demonstrates scanning through the anterior fontanelle with sagittal images. (**a**) Through the midline including the corpus callosum, third and fourth ventricles, (**b**) through the caudothalamic junction, (**c**) through the atria of the lateral ventricles, (**d**) through the insula, and (**e**) through the frontotemporoparietal lobes

Standard sequential sagittal views from the midline to the periphery (Fig. 1.10) on each side should include the following [1, 3]:

- Midline sagittal views of the corpus callosum, third and fourth ventricles including the comma-shaped, fluid-filled cavum septum pellucidum, and aqueduct of Sylvius (Fig. 1.11).
- Parasagittal views of the lateral ventricles including the caudothalamic junction (Fig. 1.12)
  – The caudothalamic junction is a thin echogenic line where the caudate nucleus and thalamus meet at the floor of the lateral ventricle, and just anterior to it is where germinal matrix hemorrhage may occur. The caudate nucleus is slightly more echogenic than the thalamus.

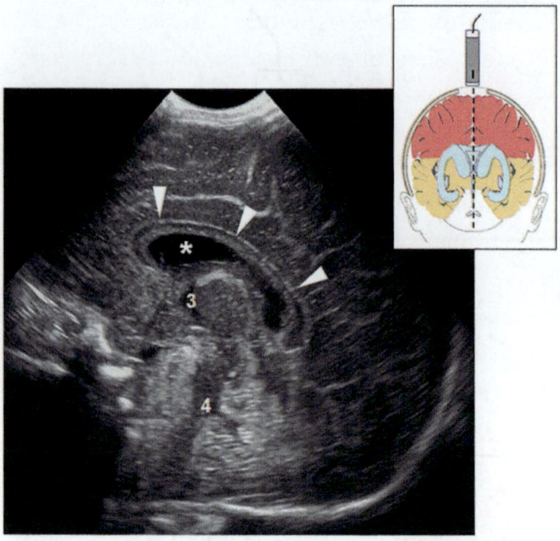

Fig. 1.11 Midline sagittal image using the anterior fontanelle including the corpus callosum (arrowheads), third (3) and fourth (4) ventricles including the cavum septum pellucidum (asterisk). Inset: Diagram of the corresponding scan plane of the image

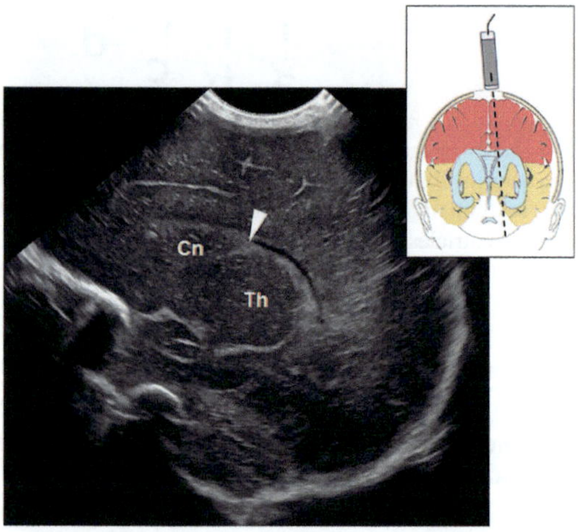

Fig. 1.12 Sagittal image using the anterior fontanelle at the level of the caudothalamic junction (arrowhead) between the caudate nucleus (Cn) and thalamus (Th). Inset: Diagram of the corresponding scan plane of the image

- Parasagittal views of the body and atria or trigones of the lateral ventricles with the glomi of the choroid plexus (Fig. 1.13)
  - At this level, the thalamo-occipital distance, defined as the distance between the outer edge of the thalamus and the tip of the occipital horn, may be measured [10].

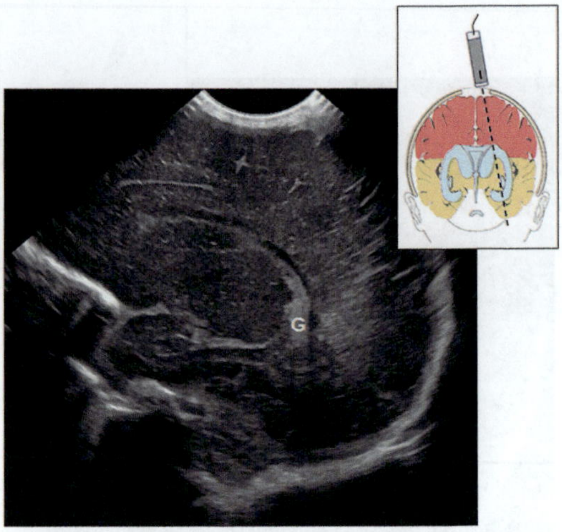

Fig. 1.13 Sagittal image using the anterior fontanelle at the level of the atria of the lateral ventricles with the glomi (G) of the choroid plexus. Inset: Diagram of the corresponding scan plane of the image

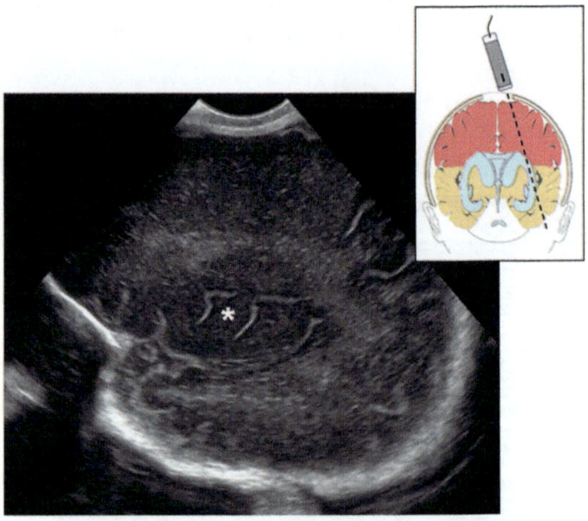

Fig. 1.14 Sagittal image using the anterior fontanelle at the level of the insula (asterisk). Inset: Diagram of the corresponding scan plane of the image

- Parasagittal to demonstrate the insula (Fig. 1.14).
- Parasagittal to demonstrate the frontotemporoparietal lobes with the Sylvian fissure (Fig. 1.15).

Near-field imaging using linear high-frequency transducers is performed to better evaluate the more superficial structures (Fig. 1.16) such as the superior sagittal sinus and extra-axial

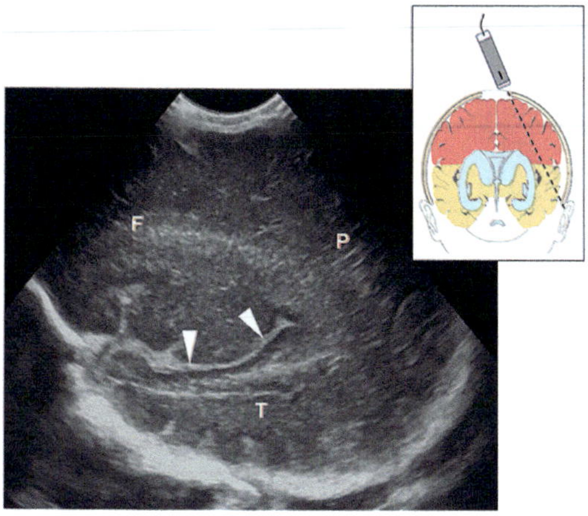

Fig. 1.15 Sagittal image using the anterior fontanelle at the level of the frontal (F), temporal (T) and parietal (P) lobes with the Sylvian fissure (arrowheads). Inset: Diagram of the corresponding scan plane of the image

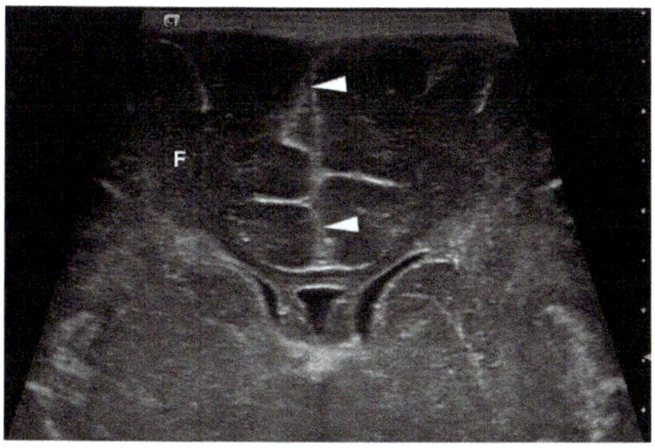

Fig. 1.16 Near-field imaging using a linear high-frequency transducer showing more superficial frontal (F) lobe at the interhemispheric fissure (arrowheads)

fluid spaces to measure the sinocortical distance, craniocortical distance, and width of the interhemispheric fissure, and to help differentiate between subarachnoid and subdural hemorrhage by identifying bridging cortical veins [3, 11].

Video or cine clips may also be recorded, in addition to standard static images, for questionable findings that may be further analyzed at a later time, especially when the study is performed at the bedside and in the neonatal intensive care unit or when the radiologist responsible for image interpretation may not be physically present at the time of scanning [1, 3, 12].

Additional views could likewise be taken through calvarial sutures, namely coronal, sagittal, lambdoid, squamosal, and metopic sutures in evaluating extracerebral fluid collections and in babies suspected of having craniosynostosis [3].

Single sweep volumetric data acquisition via three-dimensional ultrasound is also available in some machines that permit planar reconstruction to help further evaluate complicated pathology in the neonatal brain [1].

1.3.1.2 Other Supplemental Imaging Windows

Other acoustic windows in the head may also be utilized such as the posterior, temporal and mastoid fontanelles, and foramen magnum [1, 2].

Posterior Fontanelle

The posterior fontanelle is located at the junction of the lambdoid and sagittal sutures (Fig. 1.17a), which is just above the external occipital protuberance, and closes by about 2–3 months of age [1, 2, 4, 7]. The neonate is placed in the supine position [1, 4] with the head turned to one side [1, 2, 4] or in the lateral decubitus position [6]. Sagittal (Fig. 1.17b) and coronal views are also taken in this window when the occipital horns of the lateral ventricles, posterior periventricular halo, occipital lobes, and posterior fossa structures need to be evaluated further in patients suspected of having intraventricular extension of germinal matrix hemorrhage, posterior fossa malformations, posterior cerebral artery stroke, and the effects of severe hypoglycemia [1, 4].

Temporal Fontanelle

The temporal fontanelle is formed at the junction of the coronal and squamosal sutures (Fig. 1.18a) on each side, anterosuperior to the tragus of the ear or external auditory meatus [2, 4, 7]. The infant is scanned with the head turned either to the right or left, and the images are obtained in the axial or transverse plane [2, 4]. If the fontanelle is small, scanning through the thin squamosal part of the temporal bone may be performed using a low-frequency transducer [2, 3]. Scanning is done mainly in the transverse or axial plane

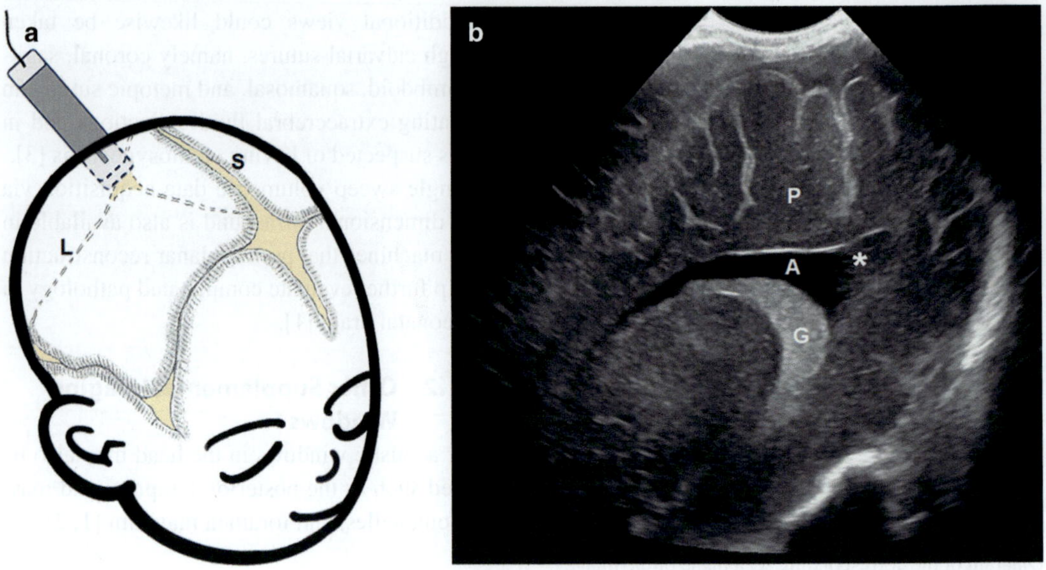

Fig. 1.17 (**a**, **b**) Cranial ultrasound diagram with the transducer at the posterior fontanelle in (**a**). The posterior fontanelle is at the junction of the lambdoid (L) and sagittal (S) sutures. Scanning through the posterior fontanelle in (**b**) shows the parietal (P) lobe, atria (A) and occipital horn (asterisk) of the lateral ventricle containing the glomus (G) of the choroid plexus

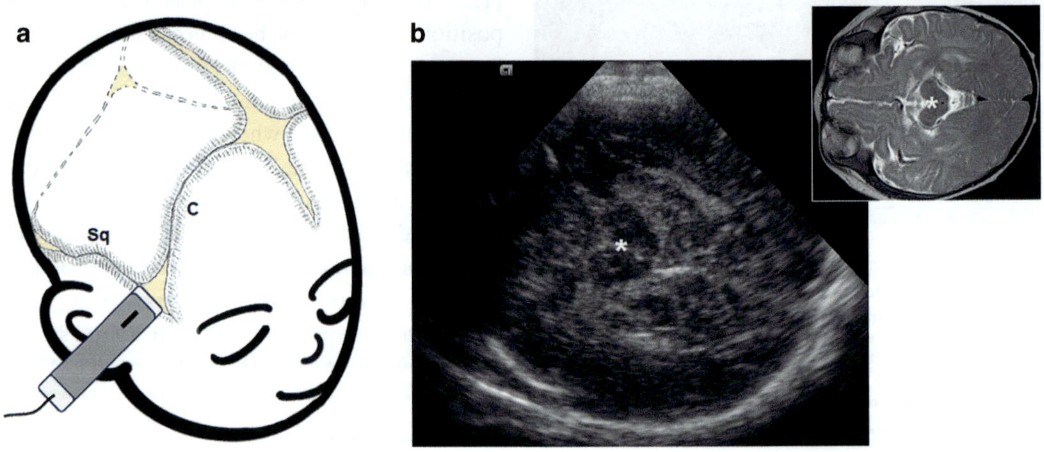

Fig. 1.18 (**a**, **b**) Cranial ultrasound diagram with the transducer at the temporal fontanelle in (**a**). The temporal fontanelle is at the junction of the coronal (C) and squamosal (Sq) sutures. Scanning through the temporal fontanelle in (**b**) shows the heart-shaped midbrain (asterisks) and perimesencephalic cistern around it. Inset: corresponding axial T2-weighted magnetic resonance image of the brain at the level of the midbrain

(Fig. 1.18b) to evaluate the thalami, midbrain, third ventricle, aqueduct of Sylvius, and perimesencephalic cistern [4, 6].

Mastoid Fontanelle

The mastoid fontanelle is retroauricular and located above the tragus of the ear at the junction of the temporal, parietal, and occipital bones [2, 4, 7, 13] (Fig. 1.19a). It closes at around 18–24 months of age [1, 2]. Scanning through either side with the infant's head turned to either right or left [4] or in the lateral decubitus position [6], better visualizes the posterior fossa (Fig. 1.19b) including the brainstem, cerebellar

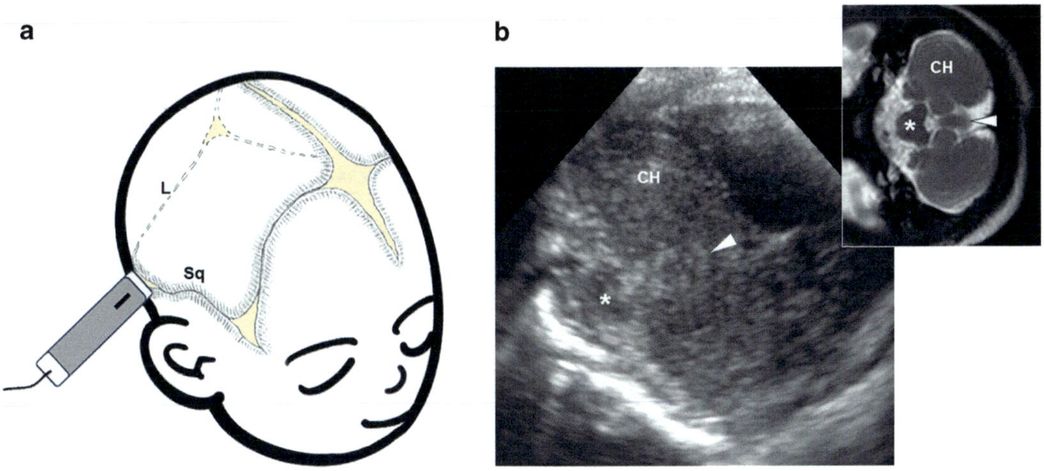

Fig. 1.19 (**a**, **b**) Cranial ultrasound diagram with the transducer at the mastoid fontanelle in (**a**). The mastoid fontanelle is at the junction of the lambdoid (L) and squamosal (Sq) sutures. Scanning through the mastoid fontanelle in (**b**) shows the brainstem (asterisks), cerebellar hemispheres (CH) and vermis (arrowheads). Inset: corresponding axial T2-weighted magnetic resonance image of the posterior fossa

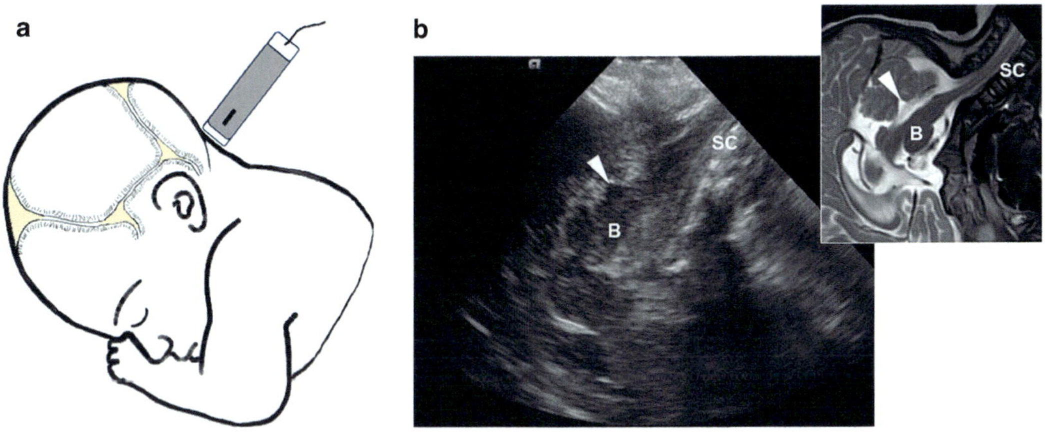

Fig. 1.20 (**a**, **b**) Cranial ultrasound with the transducer at the foramen magnum just below the external occipital protuberance in (**a**). Scanning through the foramen magnum in (**b**) shows the fourth ventricle (arrowheads), brainstem (B) and upper cervical spinal cord (SC). Inset: corresponding sagittal T2-weighted magnetic resonance image of the same structures

hemispheres and cerebellar vermis, fourth ventricle and cisterna magna [1–3, 5, 6, 13] for congenital and acquired abnormalities [1, 4, 14]. The posterior cerebral circulation [2] and the transverse and sigmoid sinuses [4] can be visualized in this window. Both transverse (axial) and coronal views are taken [4, 6].

Foramen Magnum

The foramen magnum just below the external occipital protuberance (Fig. 1.20a) may be utilized to evaluate the brainstem and upper cervical spine (Fig. 1.20b) particularly in patients with known or suspected Chiari 1 or 2 malformation and Dandy-Walker syndrome [2, 3]. Infants are placed in the lateral decubitus position with the neck flexed and the transducer angled cephalad [2, 4]. Scanning is performed in both the sagittal and transverse planes [4, 15].

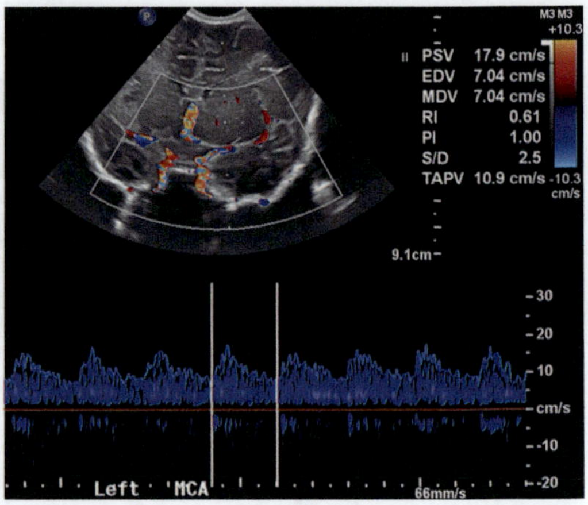

Fig. 1.21 Spectral Doppler imaging of a neonate interrogating the left middle cerebral artery (MCA) showing automatic calculation of the peak systolic velocity (PSV), end-diastolic velocity (EDV), resistive index (RI) and pulsatility index (PI). Case courtesy of Santiago Martinez-Correa, MD, Children's Hospital of Philadelphia, Philadelphia, Pennsylvania

1.3.2 Spectral and Color Doppler Imaging

Doppler ultrasound is used to evaluate the intracranial vasculature through a fontanelle or via a transcranial approach [3, 16]. There are three types: Pulsed or spectral Doppler imaging can specify the flow direction and measure velocity and vascular resistance. Color Doppler imaging differentiates whether the flow is antegrade or retrograde in relation to the transducer and the origin (artery or vein) of the Doppler signal. Power Doppler detects flow even if the velocity or amplitude is low [2].

Pulsed and color Doppler ultrasound may be done to evaluate the intracranial vasculature, cerebral blood flow, and congenital vascular anomalies [1, 2]. Power Doppler is utilized in cases where the presence of flow is more important than the flow direction [2]. In neonates suspected with sinus venous thrombosis, color or power Doppler may be performed, whereas in infants with hydrocephalus and hypoxic-ischemic brain injury, spectral Doppler may be helpful [3].

Cerebral blood flow velocities, resistive indices (RIs) and pulsatility indices (PIs) (Fig. 1.21) are variable and are affected by various factors such as age, body temperature, arterial carbon dioxide level, cerebral and systemic perfusion as well as state of patient arousal, mechanical ventilation and suctioning, presence of systemic shunts, cardiac disease, and/or anemia [16]. When performing serial studies, it is recommended to interrogate the same location of the same vessels [6].

For transcranial Doppler studies, the neonate is scanned in a supine position [1] and the patient should be quiet, calm, and awake except in patients being evaluated for brain death and for the detection of brain perfusion intra- or postoperatively [16]. Depending on the size of the fontanelle, the highest frequency transducer (5–15 MHz) that permits adequate cerebrovascular interrogation is recommended [17]. Doppler power output should be as low as reasonably achievable (ALARA) [3, 16]. Depending on which vessel the operator wants to evaluate, any open fontanelle or suture may be used.

1.3.2.1 Imaging Approaches

Anterior Fontanelle Approach

The anterior fontanelle may be used to evaluate abnormalities of the major intracranial arteries and branches, including the anterior, middle cerebral, and distal internal carotid arteries (Fig. 1.22) although the transtemporal approach may be better for the middle cerebral artery (MCA) [16, 18]. The vein of Galen and straight sinus may also be interrogated. A high-resolution linear array transducer as with grayscale imaging is used for more superficial vessels including dural sinuses [2] (Fig. 1.23). The superior sagittal sinus can also be assessed through an open sagittal suture [16].

Interrogation of the pericallosal branch of the anterior cerebral artery may be done for basic assessment of global cerebral arterial flow and spectral waveform analysis as well as for infants with elevated intracranial pressure [16].

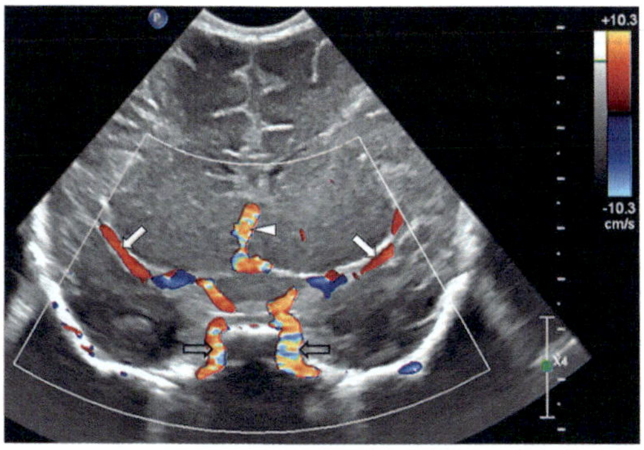

Fig. 1.22 Normal color Doppler study of the circle of Willis of a 10-day-old girl diagnosed to have Tetralogy of Fallot complicated by cardiac arrest. A coronal scan obtained through the anterior fontanelle shows patent middle cerebral arteries (white arrows), A1 segment of the anterior cerebral artery (arrowhead) and distal internal carotid arteries (black open arrows). Case courtesy of Santiago Martinez-Correa, MD, Children's Hospital of Philadelphia, Philadelphia, Pennsylvania

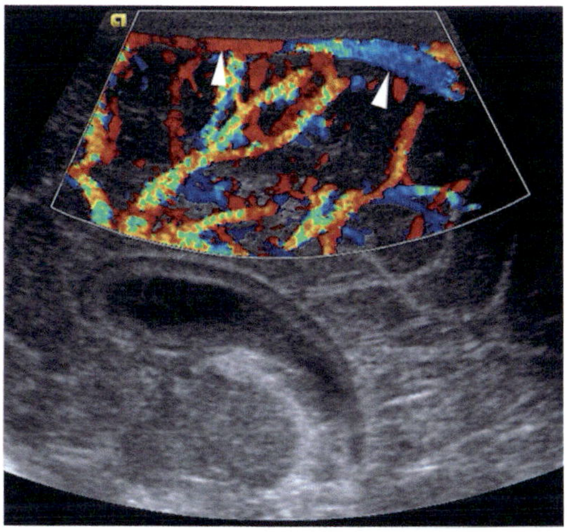

Fig. 1.23 Color Doppler imaging using a linear high-frequency transducer on the anterior fontanelle showing the superior sagittal sinus (SSS, arrowheads). The red color of the SSS reflects blood flow towards the transducer and the blue color reflects blood flow away from the transducer

Temporal Fontanelle/Bone Approach

Scanning through the temporal fontanelle or through the thinnest part of the temporal bone is performed to interrogate the major branches of the circle of Willis [2, 3, 7] using both color and spectral Doppler [16]. The temporal approach is more sensitive than the anterior fontanelle approach for evaluating the middle cerebral artery because of a more favorable Doppler angle [2]. The flow of cerebrospinal fluid through the aqueduct of Sylvius can also be visualized [4]. The landmark for the circle of Willis is the hypoechoic, heart-shaped cerebral peduncles and echogenic, star-shaped interpeduncular and suprasellar cisterns [16].

The transducer is angled upward and anteriorly. The middle cerebral artery is identified on color Doppler imaging. Multiple spectral waveforms are acquired bilaterally at 2-mm intervals in the proximal, mid and distal middle cerebral artery. A single waveform is obtained bilaterally in the anterior cerebral artery, posterior cerebral artery, and terminal portion of the internal carotid artery. The ultrasound probe is orientated posteriorly to interrogate the posterior cerebral artery and internal carotid artery. The normal spectral waveform shows a sharp systolic upstroke and gradual deceleration with antegrade end-diastolic flow (Fig. 1.24a–c). The flow measurements automatically recorded are the time averaged mean of the maximal velocities (TAMAX), end-diastolic (ED), and peak systolic (PS) velocities [2].

Posterior Fontanelle Approach

The posterior fontanelle can be used to evaluate the interpeduncular, quadrigeminal, and distal segments of the posterior cerebral arteries as well as the most distal parts of the vein of Galen and the straight sinus [18].

Mastoid Fontanelle Approach

The mastoid or posterolateral fontanelle can be utilized to study the posterior arterial circulation [16, 19] and venous sinuses, namely the sigmoid and transverse sinuses [6].

Foramen Magnum Approach

The foramen magnum can be used to interrogate the vertebrobasilar arteries. The basilar and V-shaped vertebral arteries are visualized with the hypoechoic medulla as the landmark [15, 16].

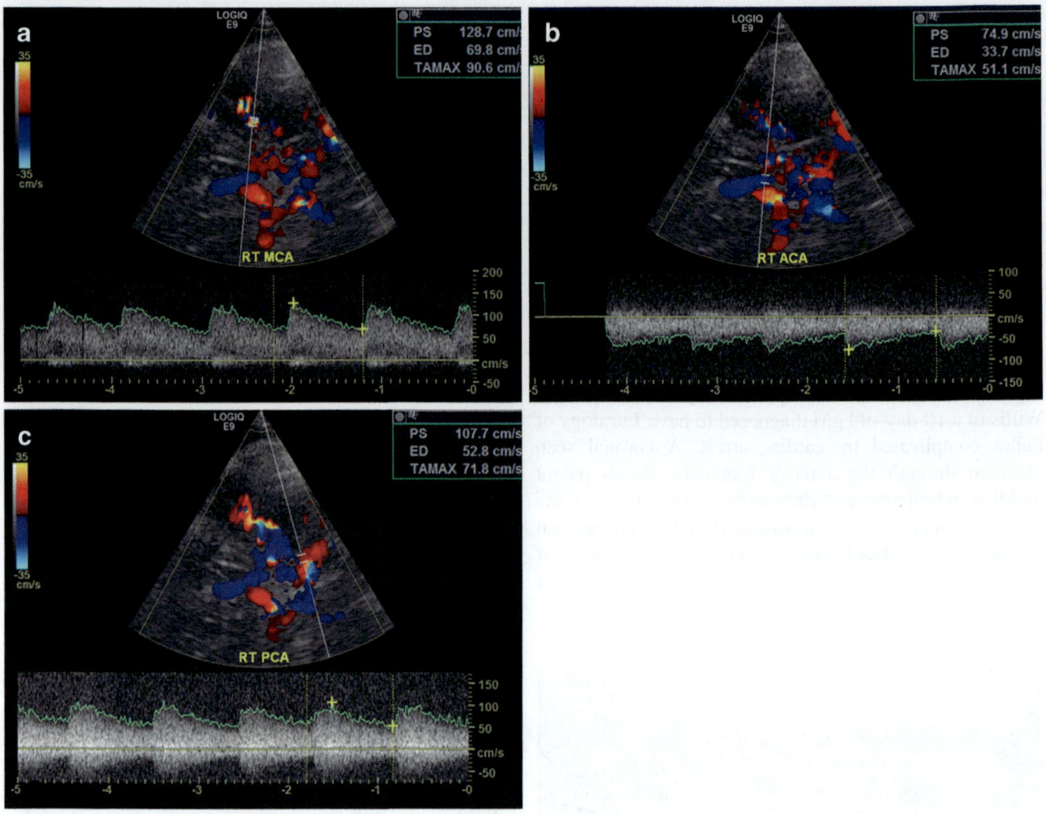

Fig. 1.24 (**a**–**c**) Normal spectral waveform. Transcranial Doppler interrogation of the right middle cerebral artery (RT MCA) in (**a**), right anterior cerebral artery (RT ACA) in (**b**), and right posterior cerebral artery (RT PCA) in (**c**) show a sharp systolic upstroke and gradual deceleration with antegrade end-diastolic flow. Images courtesy of Prof. Marilyn J. Siegel of the Edward Mallinckrodt Institute of Radiology, Washington University School of Medicine, St. Louis, Missouri

1.3.2.2 Normal Arterial Blood Flow Patterns

Flow velocity and resistive index (RI) can be calculated using spectral Doppler imaging automatically depending on the ultrasound machine or manually using the following formula: peak systolic velocity (PSV) minus minimum end-diastolic velocity [EDV] divided by PSV (PSV-EDV/PSV) [2].

Flow velocities in the anterior, middle, and posterior cerebral arteries as well as internal carotid and basilar arteries increase as the postnatal age and birth weight increase due to changes in cerebrovascular resistance [2, 13, 20]. In very premature infants (<1500 g), PSVs range between 26.3 and 37.0 cm/s and EDVs range between 6.5 and 8.3 cm/s. In term infants, PSVs range between 48.8 and 57.5 cm/s and EDVs range between 13.0 and 15.9 cm/s [2, 20]. The normal spectral waveform should demonstrate a sharp systolic upstroke and a gradual deceleration with antegrade end-diastolic flow [2] (Fig. 1.24a–c).

Resistive indices, however, do not significantly vary even with increasing gestational age or birth weight [2, 20]. In the larger cerebral arteries, the normal RI can approximately range from 0.71 to 0.80 for both term and preterm infants [2, 20–22], and can be lower in smaller arteries (e.g., striatal branches) [2, 22]. Gentle transducer pressure on the anterior fontanelle is also important because an increase in the pressure can also increase the RI by a mean of 5.2% [2].

1.3.2.3 Normal Venous Blood Flow Patterns

Doppler imaging can also be used to interrogate the vein of Galen, straight sinus behind the cerebellum, internal cerebral vein behind the third ventricle, and terminal/subependymal veins at the level of the caudate nuclei, as well as the superior sagittal sinus and superficial cortical veins in the sagittal plane via the anterior fontanelle. There are two types of waveforms: (a) Sinusoidal waveforms are high-velocity, low-amplitude pulsations that are typical of larger central veins such as the vein of Galen and straight or sagittal sinus. (b) Monophasic (continuous) low-velocity patterns are observed in smaller internal cerebral and terminal veins. Unlike in the arteries, venous flow velocities do not significantly vary with increasing gestational age or birth weight [2, 20].

The neonate should be calm and quiet because fluctuations can occur during forceful crying as a result of rapid changes in intrathoracic pressure and with motion of the infant's head [2].

1.3.3 Contrast-Enhanced Ultrasound of the Neonatal Brain

Doppler ultrasound is the first-line imaging study in evaluating flow dynamics in the neonatal brain. However, it only measures macrovascular flow. Contrast-enhanced ultrasound (CEUS) of the brain is an adjunct not only to Doppler US but also to magnetic resonance imaging (MRI) [23, 24] in the dynamic visualization of microvascular perfusion in neonates especially for preterm, low-birth weight, and/or critically ill infants who require imaging of the brain at bedside [24]. Based on the study of Squires and colleagues, the overall sensitivity of CEUS when compared with MRI for any abnormality is 93.3% (95% CI 80.7–100), and specificity is 100% (95% CI 100–100) [25].

CEUS involves intravenous injection of ultrasound contrast agents (UCA), the most common of which is sulfur hexafluoride lipid-type A microbubbles. Unlike iodinated and gadolinium-based contrast agents, which are excreted by the kidneys, the internal inert gas, and its lipoprotein shell are eliminated via respiratory and hepatobiliary excretion, respectively. This makes UCAs very suitable for neonates who have an immature renal function [24]. Currently, however, the United States Food and Drug Administration (FDA) has only approved the use of these microspheres for intravenous use for focal liver lesions and during echocardiography in pediatric patients, making UCAs in cranial sonography as an off-label use [23, 24, 26].

1.3.3.1 Scanning Technique Before and During Contrast Administration

The mechanical index or acoustic power should be below 0.3 to ensure the stability of the microbubbles. The depth should cover the entire brain. The focal zone is set deeper to the region of interest to prevent premature destruction of microbubbles in the field of view. The gain is also adjusted to minimize background noise prior to contrast administration [23].

UCA is administered at a dose of 0.03 mL/kg [23–26] followed by a 3-mL saline flush [24, 25]. Bolus injection may be done twice with the image acquisition in cine mode. Initial injection is performed while scanning through the anterior fontanelle in coronal view at the third station (i.e., at the level of the foramen of Monro and basal ganglia) (Fig. 1.25a, b) until maximum contrast enhancement is reached [23, 26], followed by an anterior-to-posterior scan of the entire brain. The second injection is performed after complete clearance of the first dose, which based on preliminary studies, is about 6–8 min in normal subjects [26]. This second sweep is done through the brain during peak enhancement to reproduce and validate the findings from the first injection or re-evaluate the rest of the brain [23, 26, 27].

1.3.3.2 Clinical Applications

CEUS has been reported to be of added value in the following scenarios: (a) evaluation of hypoxic-ischemic encephalopathy [23, 24, 26]; (b) delineation of the hemorrhagic core and the extent of cerebral perfusion compromise in

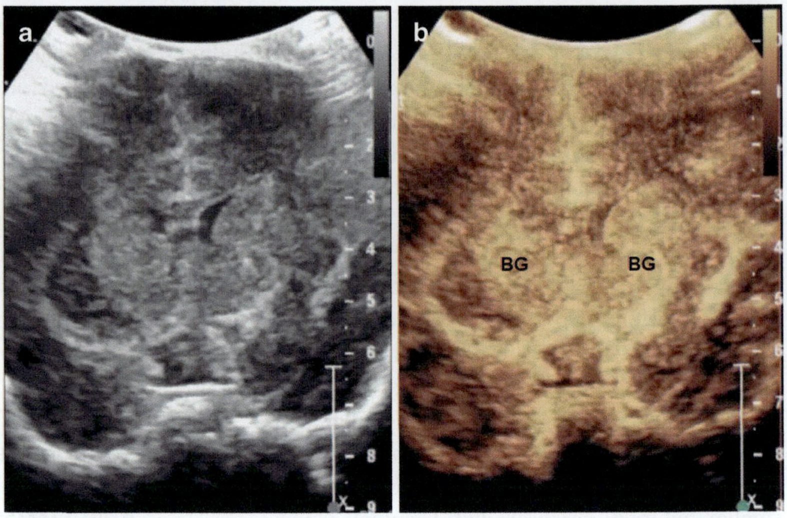

Fig. 1.25 (**a**, **b**) Midcoronal pre-contrast grayscale ultrasound scan through the brain of a normal subject (**a**). After 15 s post-injection of contrast, there is relatively more avid enhancement to the basal ganglia (BG) with respect to the remainder of the brain (**b**). Adapted with permission from [26].

patients with high-grade intracranial hemorrhage as well as in post-hemorrhagic hydrocephalus; (c) brain tumors [23, 24, 26]; (d) monitoring brain perfusion in infants undergoing surgery for congenital heart disease [23, 24] or for neurovascular disease [23]; and (e) in diagnosing brain death [24].

1.4 Brain Anatomy

1.4.1 Cerebral Cortex

The cortex and the development of the sulci correlate well with brain maturity. Extremely preterm infants have a smooth, featureless cerebral cortex termed as "lissencephalic appearance" (Fig. 1.26). As early as 26 weeks, echogenic curvilinear structures known as sulci begin to develop, forming shallow grooves and separating the relatively hypoechoic gyri, a process called primary sulcation (Fig. 1.27), which would be evident at the insula when it is covered by the Sylvian fissure at 27 weeks (Fig. 1.28). The sulci's echogenic appearance is attributed to the pia mater's interface of collagen and blood vessels with the underlying predominantly water-containing brain parenchyma [1]. White matter has loosely packed echoes with distributed, more hyperechoic, punctate foci producing a low-level granular echo pattern, while gray matter is even more hypoechoic, almost anechoic even, compared to white matter [28]. By 28 weeks onwards, the cingulate sulcus is well visualized on midline sagittal and parasagittal planes (Fig. 1.29) with its secondary sulcations appearing at around 31–33 weeks (Fig. 1.30 and 1.31). Upon reaching the eighth and ninth month of gestation, the cortical sulcations become more intricate, bending and branching to form the remaining secondary and most of the tertiary sulci (Fig. 1.32 and 1.33) [2]. By full-term gestational age, the sulci become more serpiginous with a cobblestone configuration best appreciated at the cingulate region (Fig. 1.34) [2, 29]. Subcortical white matter myelination proceeds in the postnatal period seen to be more hyperechoic relative to other less myelinated regions such as the deep gray nuclei and thalamus [30, 31]. However, by this time, these are now appropriately assessed with MRI.

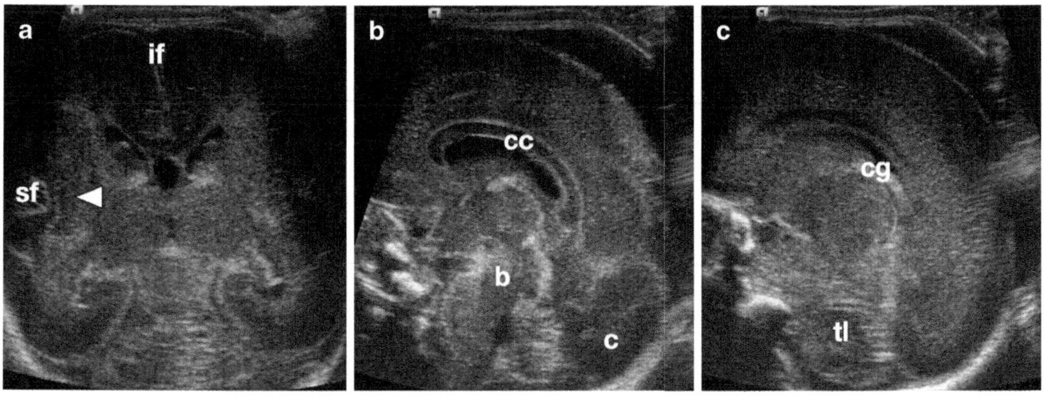

Fig. 1.26 Images taken through the anterior fontanelle in coronal (**a**), midline sagittal (**b**), and parasagittal (**c**) planes demonstrate the expected appearance of the brain from 24 weeks until 27 weeks gestational age. (**a**–**c**) The neonatal brain at 24–25-weeks gestational age shows the typical smooth brain appearance. Open Sylvian fissure with exposed insula (arrowhead) is depicted, brainstem (b), cerebellum (c), corpus callosum (cc), caudothalamic groove (cg), interhemispheric fissure (if), sylvian fissure (sf), temporal lobe (tl)

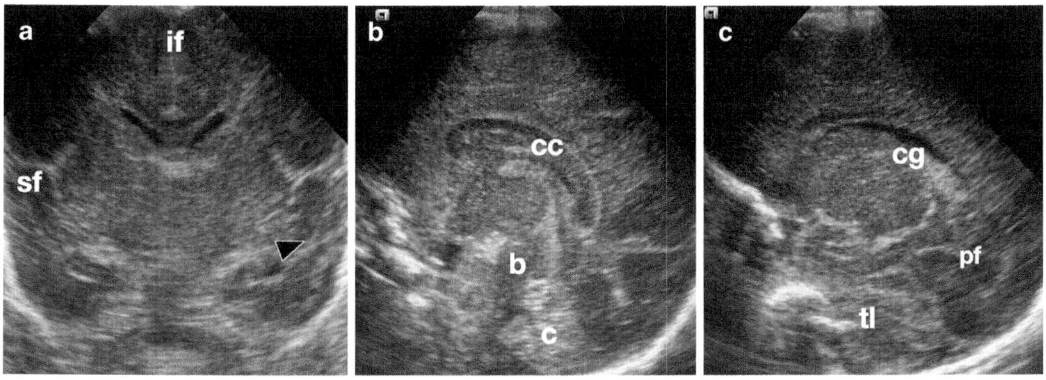

Fig. 1.27 (**a**–**c**) By 26 weeks, primary gyration (black arrowhead) is now obvious. The parieto-occipital fissure (pf) is visualized on parasagittal views, brainstem (b), cerebellum (c), corpus callosum (cc), caudothalamic groove (cg), interhemispheric fissure (if), sylvian fissure (sf), temporal lobe (tl)

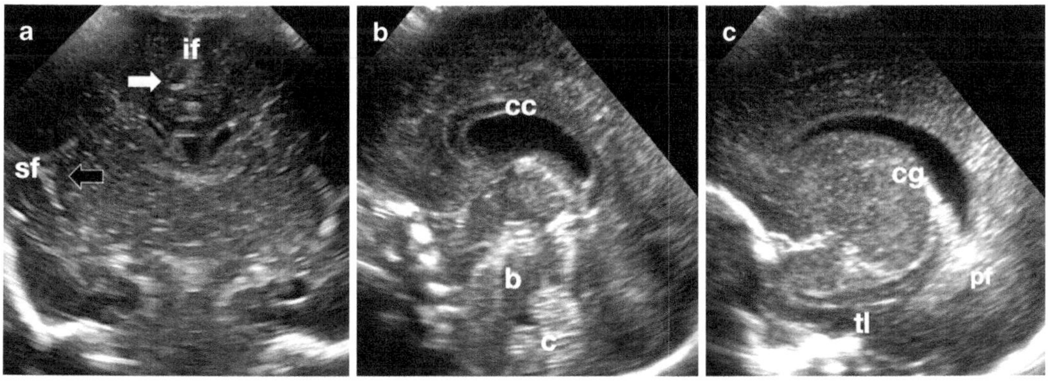

Fig. 1.28 (**a**–**c**) At 27 weeks, the insula (black arrow) is now covered by the Sylvian fissure. Primary branching of the interhemispheric fissure begins (white arrow), brainstem (b), cerebellum (c), corpus callosum (cc), caudothalamic groove (cg), interhemispheric fissure (if), parieto-occipital fissure (pf), sylvian fissure (sf), temporal lobe (tl)

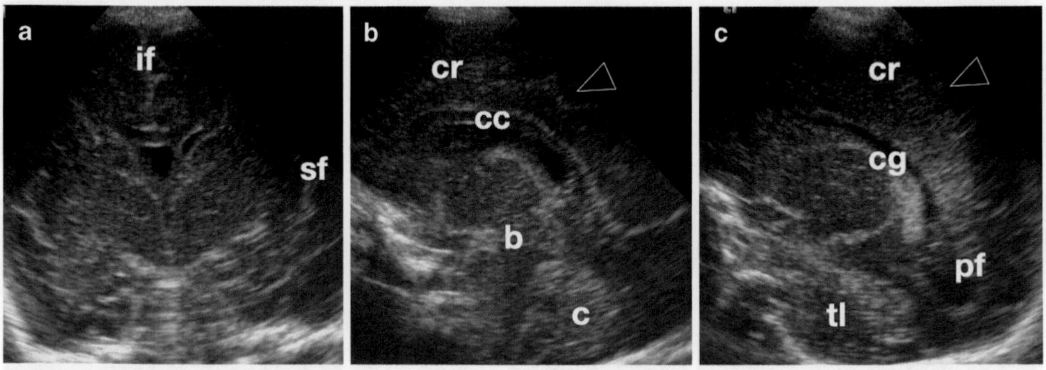

Fig. 1.29 Images taken through the anterior fontanelle in coronal (**a**), midline sagittal (**b**), and parasagittal (**c**) planes demonstrate the expected appearance of the brain from 28 weeks until 33 weeks gestational age. (**a–c**) The neonatal brain at 28- to 29-week gestational age shows the cingulate sulcus on both midsagittal and parasagittal planes (black arrowheads), a key finding at this age, brainstem (b), cerebellum (c), corpus callosum (cc), caudothalamic groove (cg), cingulate region (cr), interhemispheric fissure (if), parieto-occipital fissure (pf), sylvian fissure (sf), temporal lobe (tl)

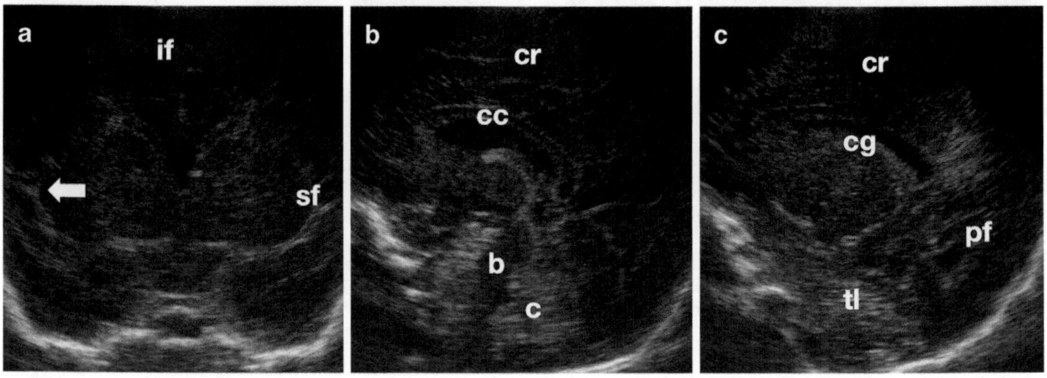

Fig. 1.30 (**a–c**) At 30- to 31-week gestational age, complete coverage of the insula (white arrow) by the closed Sylvian fissure was observed in 100% of neonates, brainstem (b), cerebellum (c), corpus callosum (cc), caudothalamic groove (cg), cingulate region (cr), interhemispheric fissure (if), parieto-occipital fissure (pf), sylvian fissure (sf), temporal lobe (tl)

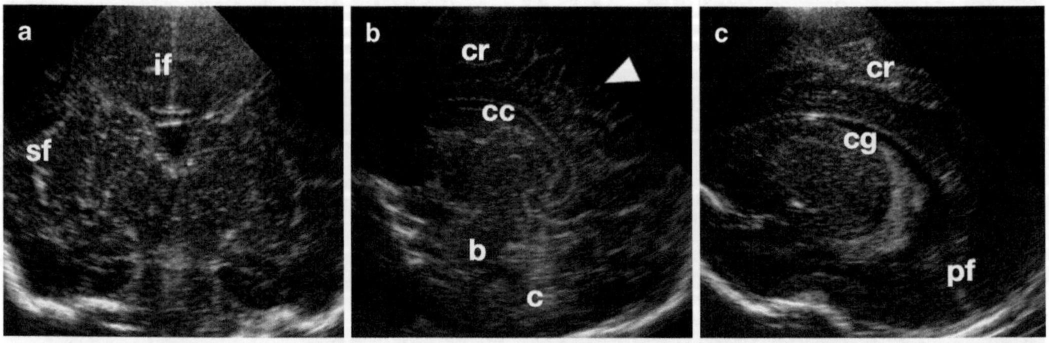

Fig. 1.31 (**a–c**) By 32- to 33-week gestational age, multiple branching of the cingulate sulcus (white arrowhead), brainstem (b), cerebellum (c), corpus callosum (cc), caudothalamic groove (cg), cingulate region (cr), interhemispheric fissure (if), parieto-occipital fissure (pf), sylvian fissure (sf), temporal lobe (tl)

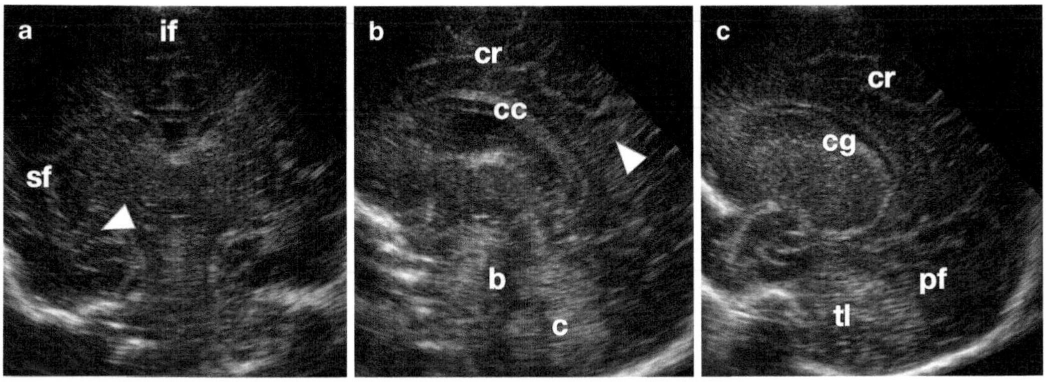

Fig. 1.32 Images taken through the anterior fontanelle in coronal (**a**), midline sagittal (**b**), and parasagittal (**c**) planes demonstrate the expected appearance of the brain from 34 weeks until term. (**a**–**c**) The neonatal brain at 34- to 35-week gestational age depicts the secondary cortical sulcation (white arrowheads) at the insular (**a**) and cingulate regions (**b**), brainstem (b), cerebellum (c), corpus callosum (cc), caudothalamic groove (cg), cingulate region (cr), interhemispheric fissure (if), parieto-occipital fissure (pf), sylvian fissure (sf), temporal lobe (tl)

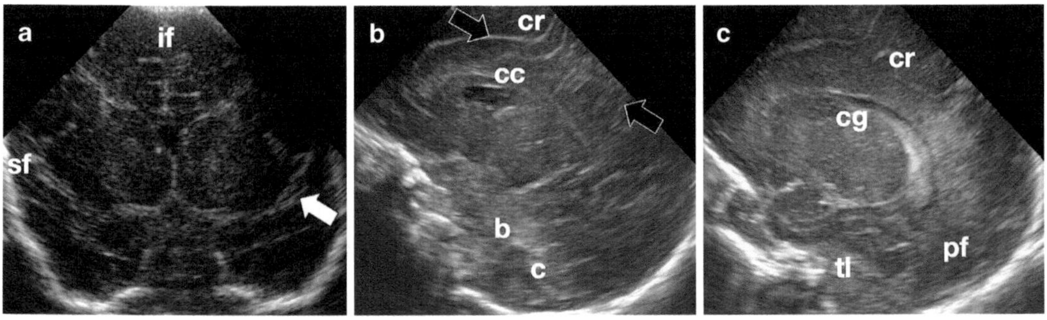

Fig. 1.33 (**a**–**c**) At 36- to 37-week gestational age, tertiary cortical sulcations are now seen (black arrows). Insular sulci (white arrow) are visible, brainstem (b), cerebellum (c), corpus callosum (cc), caudothalamic groove (cg), cingulate region (cr), interhemispheric fissure (if), parieto-occipital fissure (pf), sylvian fissure (sf), temporal lobe (tl)

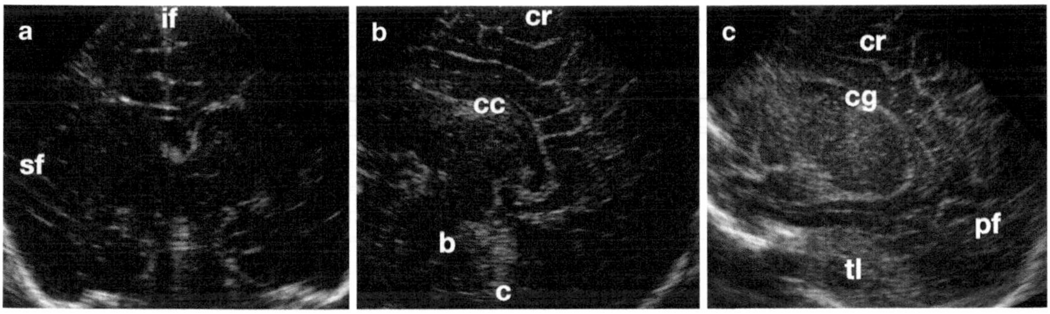

Fig. 1.34 (**a**–**c**) By term range of 38- to 42-week gestational age, the typical "cobblestone" pattern of the cingulate region is well appreciated on midline sagittal (b) and parasagittal planes (c), brainstem (b), cerebellum (c), corpus callosum (cc), caudothalamic groove (cg), cingulate region (cr), interhemispheric fissure (if), parieto-occipital fissure (pf), sylvian fissure (sf), temporal lobe (tl)

1.4.2 Basal Ganglia and Thalami

The basal ganglia is composed of a group of subcortical nuclei. It comprises the caudate, putamen, and globus pallidus in the cerebral hemispheres, the substantia nigra in the midbrain, and the subthalamic nucleus in the diencephalon. The caudate, putamen, globus pallidus, and thalami are well depicted on ultrasound in a full-term healthy neonate (Figs. 1.5 and 1.12). The basal ganglia and thalami appear isoechoic relative to the cortical gray matter and hypoechoic to the subcortical white matter. They are homogeneous and hyperechoic relative to the adjacent white matter prior to 32 weeks gestational age [1]. An echogenic appearance of the basal ganglia and thalami stems from the relative difference in echogenicities between the immature deep gray matter and white matter arising from contrasting water content, myelination extent, or both. This has also been ascribed to prematurity-related maturation [32].

1.4.3 Ventricles

The ventricles are anechoic cavities channeling the flow of cerebrospinal fluid. They decrease in size as the neonate nears term and are expectedly larger in preterm infants [33]. The largest and most visible lateral ventricles have regions extending to the frontal, temporal, and occipital lobes. On each side, it abuts the caudate nuclei, thalami, and cerebral peduncles [1]. Ventricular size may change with scanning position such as in a decubitus position where the ventricle on the dependent side is relatively smaller [2]. The third ventricle is seen as a rhomboid-shaped cavity at midline on the third coronal scanning plane, while the fourth ventricle appears as a triangular cavity posterior to the brainstem at midline sagittal plane. The distinct borders allow for the lateral ventricles to be easily measured with a consensus normal value of <10 mm taken at the posterior margin of the choroid plexus glomus on the axial plane through the thalami [1, 34, 35]. US and MRI measurements are highly concordant when measured in the coronal plane [34]. Other commonly used measurements of significance with good inter-observer and intra-observer agreement include the following [4, 7]:

1. Ventricular index (VI, Levene index) (Fig. 1.35a): This is measured between the falx cerebri and lateral wall of the lateral ventricles in the midcoronal plane at the level of

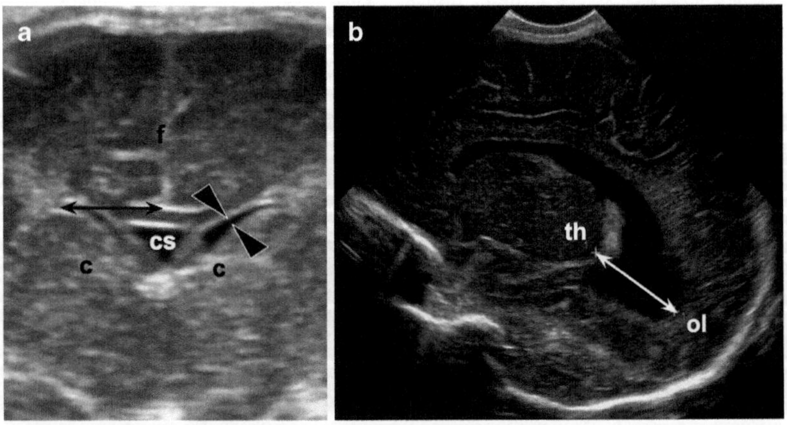

Fig. 1.35 Coronal image using the anterior fontanelle at the level of the foramen of Monro (**a**) demonstrates the ventricular index (horizontal black line) and anterior horn width (arrowheads). Parasagittal image using the anterior fontanelle demonstrates (**b**), demonstrates the thalamo-occipital distance measured as the widest distance depicted by the white line are measured. Falx (f), cavum septum pellucidum (cs), caudate (c), thalamus (th), occipital lobe (ol)

the foramen of Monro. Reference range for each gestational age is available with values 7.8–15.4 mm (<97th centile) considered to be normal [36].

2. Anterior horn width (Fig. 1.35a): Also taken in the mid coronal plane at the level of the foramen of Monro wherein the diagonal width of the frontal horns is measured. Prior studies covering normal preterm to term neonates showed a range of 1.27–3.34 mm [36]. Values of 6–10 mm are classified as moderate ventriculomegaly and more than 10 mm are categorized as severe [7].
3. Thalamo-occipital distance (Fig. 1.35b): Distance measured from the thalamus to the distal tip of the occipital horn measured in the appropriate sagittal plane. Its value lies in the fact that mild lateral ventricular dilatation is first detected in the occipital horns. Various studies show the normal range for all gestational age to fall between 15.0 and 20.5 mm [36].

The choroid plexus is closely related to the posterior horns of the lateral ventricles and is of sonographic imaging importance. It is highly echogenic due to the multiple interfaces of liquid and solid structures in the villus crypts as well due to being highly vascularized [37]. It becomes an important reference point for several pathologies that usually appear more hyperechoic compared to it.

1.4.4 Corpus Callosum

The corpus callosum (CC) is the largest telencephalic white matter commissure seen as a sonolucent curved and elongated structure seen along the midline sagittal plane (Fig. 1.11) with well-defined contours overlying the laminae of the septum pellucidum [13, 34, 37]. It is responsible for interhemispheric sensory, motor, and higher order brain communication [37]. Its identification is crucial since CC anomalies may hint towards other related pathologies [7]. A decrease in its volume may suggest white matter damage [38]. Indirect signs of callosal development are helpful in cases wherein direct and complete visualization of the CC proves difficult. Absence of the cavum septum pellucidum (CSP), dilated ventricles (atria and occipital horns), and inferiorly oriented medial hemispheric sulci are findings that could raise the possibility of callosal abnormalities [34].

1.4.5 Brainstem and Cerebellum

The mastoid fontanelle and foramen magnum (FM) provides a better window in evaluating the posterior fossa structures that are typically farthest when scanning from an anterior fontanelle (AF) approach [1–3, 39]. The cerebellar hemispheres, vermis, brainstem as well as the cisterna magna and fourth ventricle (Figs. 1.19 and 1.20) can be properly identified helping to detect large and obvious pathologies [40]. Assessing the size of its components show no significant differences when taken from either the AF or FM approach. Cerebellar growth velocity has shown to be associated with abnormal neurobehavioral outcomes, particularly in preterm newborns [39]. It appears as a dumbbell-shaped structure showing symmetrical lobes with the central vermis being more echogenic than the lateral hemispheres. Measuring the widest diameter across the cerebellum perpendicular to the falx correlates with the gestational age in millimeters until 20 weeks (Fig. 1.36). Therefore, a trans-cerebellar diameter measuring 2 mm less than gestational age warrants investigation [41].

1.4.6 Cisterna Magna

The cisterna magna is an arachnoid-lined, anechoic structure that communicates with the fourth ventricle and is located inferior to the vermis. Normal values have been long established with its height at the midsagittal plane ranging from 3 to 8 mm measured from the posterior lip of the foramen magnum to the caudal margin of the inferior vermis [42]. Below normal raises the suspicion of an Arnold-Chiari malformation while greater than normal values suggest a mega

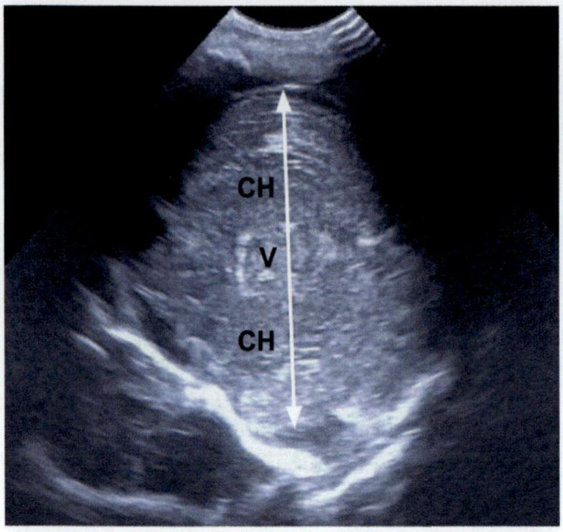

Fig. 1.36 Cerebellar diameter measured through an image acquired via the mastoid fontanelle. Widest diameter (double-sided arrow) taken perpendicular to the falx with values that should correspond to gestational age in millimeters until 20 weeks and not fall more than 2 mm less for age in weeks, cerebellar hemisphere (CH), vermis (V)

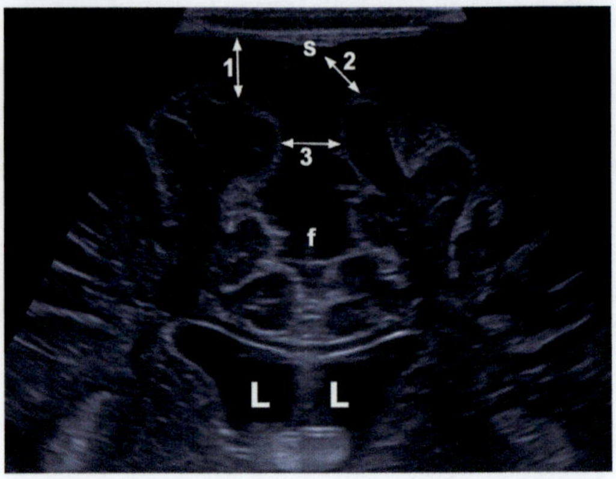

Fig. 1.37 Near-field imaging in the coronal view using a linear transducer shows corresponding markers to measure craniocortical (*1*), sinocortical (*2*), and interhemispheric widths (*3*), superior sagittal sinus (s), falx (f), lateral ventricles (L)

cisterna magna, arachnoid cyst, or even a Dandy-Walker abnormality [2].

1.4.7 Extra-Axial Spaces

The CSF spaces between the brain and the skull are bounded by the leptomeninges and traversed by blood vessels. The anterior, posterior, and lateral regions of the extra-axial fluid spaces are known limitations of ultrasound, thereby evaluation is confined to the midline extra-axial spaces, which are best evaluated using a high-frequency linear transducer (12 MHz). The craniocortical space is the shortest vertical measurement from the calvarium to the cortical surface with upper limits of normal ranging from 3.3 to 5 mm in neonates while values >10 mm are considered significantly widened and is true across all modalities. The sinocortical space is the shortest distance between the lateral wall of the triangular sagittal sinus and adjacent cortical surface with a reported upper limit set at 4 mm. Meanwhile, the interhemispheric subarachnoid space represents the widest horizontal distance between the cerebral hemispheres with normal values falling below the 95th percentile measuring <6 mm (Fig. 1.37). Although no imaging criteria and established cut-off values exist for BESS, age-compatible craniocortical, sinocortical and interhemispheric widths above the 95th percentile are classified abnormal. Other features leaning towards BESS include fluid that does not cause mass effect upon the brain as well as no flattened cortical outlines, no midline shift, no unusual hyperechoic areas within the CSF and no visible arachnoid membrane [11, 43, 44]. Cortical veins can also be visualized with the help of Color Doppler, which extends from the brain surface to the skull [1].

1.5 Developmental Variants and Scanning Artifacts

This section presents some of the more common developmental variants and scanning artifacts which can be seen on cranial ultrasound (Table 1.1). Familiarity with these structures and their corresponding sonographic manifestations are important as they can mimic an abnormality.

Table 1.1 Summary of developmental variants and scanning artifacts

Ventricular and periventricular area	Connatal cysts Asymmetric lateral ventricles Slit-like ventricles
Extra-axial spaces	Mega cisterna magna Benign enlargement of the subarachnoid space (BESS)
Pseudolesions	Calcar Avis Pseudolesion Parenchymal pseudolesion/hyperechoic white matter pseudolesion Periventricular halo/peritrigonal white matter echogenicity Thalamic pseudolesion
Choroid plexus variants	Lobular choroid plexus Double choroid Choroid cysts
Persistent Fetal fluid-filled spaces	Cavum septi pellucidi and cavum vergae Cavum veli interpositi
Others	Lenticulostriate hyperechogenicity/vasculopathy

1.5.1 Ventricular and Periventricular Lesions

1.5.1.1 Connatal Cysts

Also known as coarctation of the lateral ventricles or subfrontal or frontal horn cysts, this entity refers to focal approximation of the walls of the lateral ventricles near the external angles thereby producing a rounded configuration and mimicking a cyst [2, 45]. This is hypothesized to be a result of incomplete coaptation of the fetal ventricles [46] and is considered normal, ependymal-lined, neurodevelopmental variant [45]. It is important to note that this occurs at the external angle of the frontal horns anterior to the foramen of Monro as compared to germinal matrix hemorrhages, which are seen posterior to the foramen of Monro at the subependymal area [47] (Fig. 1.38). In addition, this should not be seen above the frontal horns, as seen in cases of cystic periventricular leukomalacia. On the sagittal view, multiple cysts may appear as a string of pearls. This entity is rare and is seen only in up to 1.05% of premature or low-birth weight infants [2]. No treatment is necessary as this may resolve spontaneously.

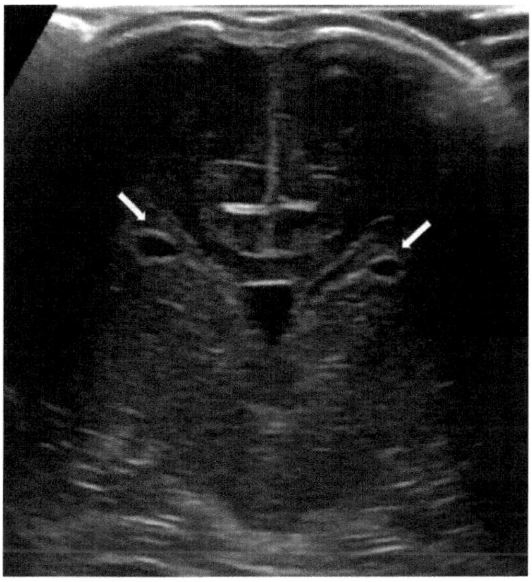

Fig. 1.38 Connatal cysts. Coronal view of the brain of a 33-week-old neonate through the anterior fontanelle approach shows a cyst-like structure inferolateral to the frontal horns of the lateral ventricle (white arrows)

1.5.1.2 Asymmetric Lateral Ventricles

Normal ventricular size measures <10 mm in widest transverse diameter [45] (Fig. 1.39). As the name implies, this pertains to unequal sizes of the ventricles, wherein one size or portion is larger than the other (Fig. 1.40). This is a common instance and can be seen in up to two thirds of normal neonates. The usual variance is that the left lateral ventricle is larger than the right or the occipital horn is larger than the frontal horn [2]. There may also be a corresponding larger size of the choroid plexus at the larger ventricle [47].

1.5.1.3 Slit-like Ventricles

Slit-like or closed ventricles refers to ventricles measuring <2 mm in diameter. This may be nor-

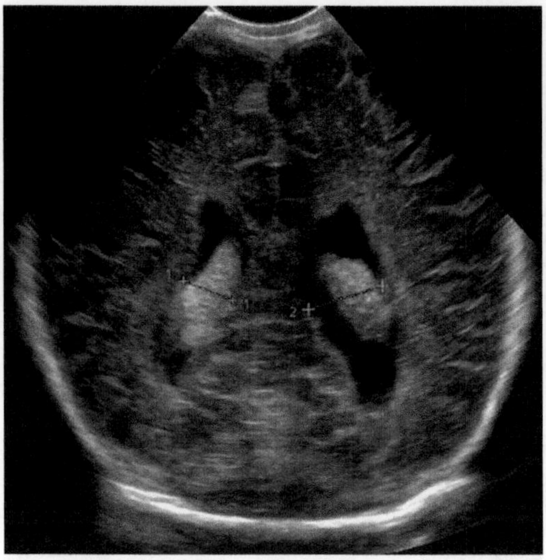

Fig. 1.39 Measurement of lateral ventricular diameter. On coronal view, the widest lateral ventricular diameter is measured as seen on the caliper. The lateral ventricular diameter must not be more than 10 mm

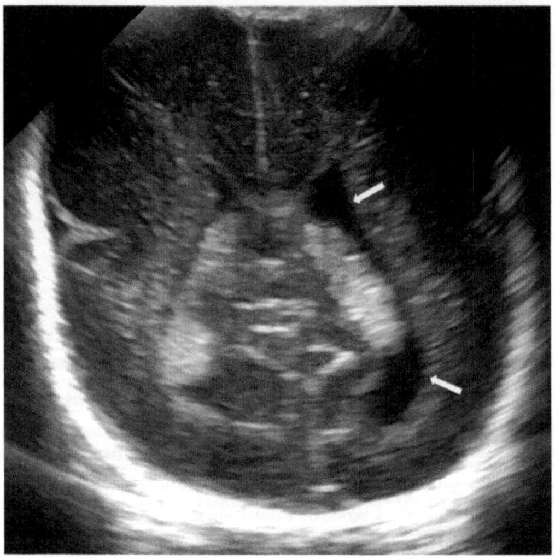

Fig. 1.40 Asymmetric lateral ventricles. Coronal view of the brain of a 25-week-old neonate through the anterior fontanelle approach shows asymmetry of the lateral ventricles, with the left (white arrows) appearing larger than the right, which is a common occurrence

mally appreciated in about 80% of term infants and 30% of premature infants [1, 2] (Fig. 1.41). Developmentally, the size of the lateral ventricle decreases with increasing fetal age, i.e., meaning premature infants have larger ventricles, especially the frontal horns, compared to term infants.

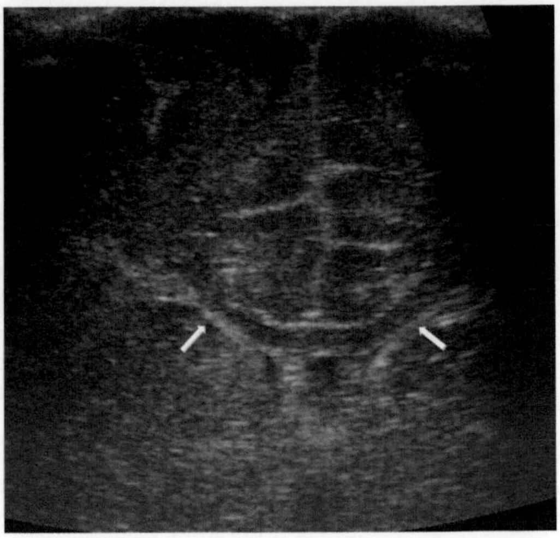

Fig. 1.41 Slit-like or closed ventricles. Coronal view of the brain of a 27-week-old neonate through the anterior fontanelle approach shows the lateral ventricles to be closed or "slit-like," as the name implies (white arrows). This is more commonly encountered in term infants

After birth, these ventricles may eventually open after about 1.5–3 days (average of 2.5 days) [2]. It has been reported that patient position may also affect ventricular size wherein the dependent side may appear smaller than the one on the non-dependent side [45, 46]. Pathologically, this can also be seen in cases of cerebral edema particularly if coupled with other findings such as increased parenchymal echogenicity, poor definition of the sulci and gyri, and decreased vascular pulsation [1, 2].

1.5.2 Extra-Axial Spaces

1.5.2.1 Mega Cisterna Magna

Mega cisterna magna refers to a cistern that is more than 8–10 mm in diameter on axial and midsagittal planes but with no mass effect or scalloping of the adjacent calvarium [2, 5] (Fig. 1.42). The cisterna magna is an arachnoid-lined, anechoic structure between the posterior lip of the foramen magnum to the inferior vermis and communicates with the fourth ventricle. There should also be a normal-appearing cerebellar vermis to differentiate it from Dandy-Walker malformation.

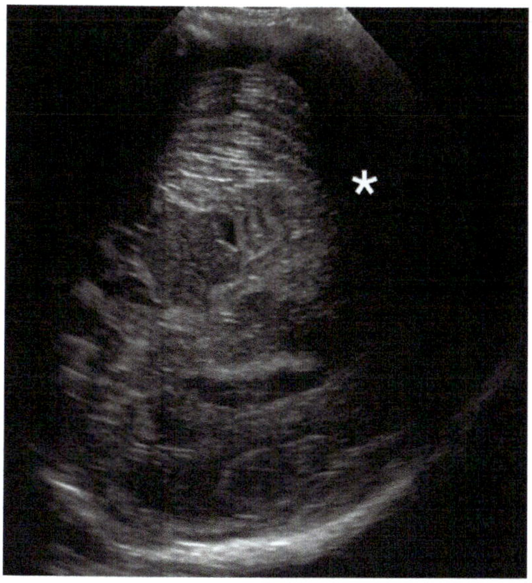

Fig. 1.42 Mega cisterna magna. Axial or transverse view of the brain of a term neonate through the mastoid approach showing the posterior fossa structures exhibiting a large, fluid collection at the retrocerebellar region (white asterisk) with no associated significant mass effect on the adjacent cerebellum

1.5.2.2 Benign Enlargement of the Subarachnoid Space (BESS)

Common among infants aged 2–7 months and in males more than females, benign enlargement of the extra-axial spaces (BESS) is considered to be due to inadequate absorption of CSF by immature arachnoid villi [2]. It is also known as benign macrocrania of infancy, benign hydrocephalus-megalocephaly, and benign extraventricular obstructive hydrocephalus. A family history of macrocephaly is often elicited. Infants usually present with an enlarged head (head circumference above the 95th percentile) but with normal neurologic function. In sonography, there are bilateral, symmetric, anechoic subarachnoid fluid collections along the frontal and parietal regions with normal brain parenchyma as well as normal to minimally enlarged lateral and third ventricles (Fig. 1.43). As mentioned in the previous section, due to the lack of imaging consensus regarding the appropriate cut-off values for BESS, values

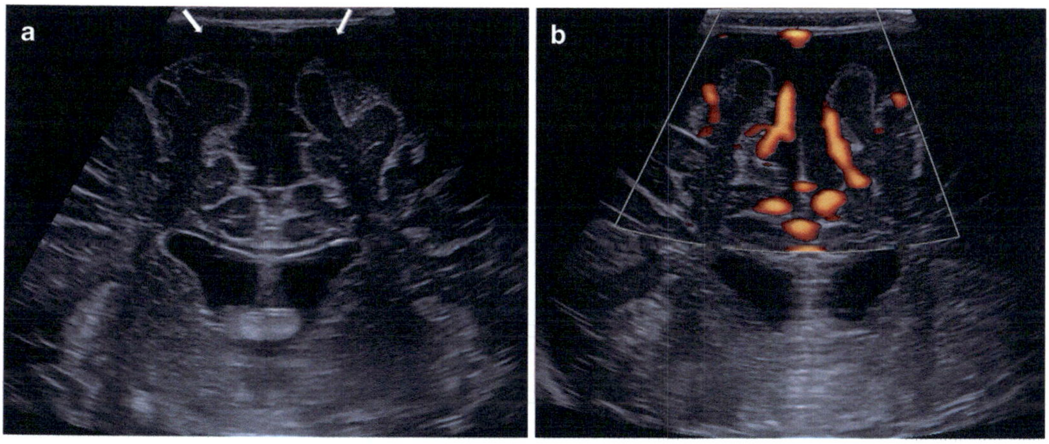

Fig. 1.43 (**a**, **b**) Benign enlargement of the subarachnoid spaces (BESS). Coronal view of the brain of a 6-month-old infant through the anterior fontanelle approach (**a**), due to macrocephaly, shows the enlarged subarachnoid spaces anterior to the frontal lobes (white arrow). The brain parenchyma shows normal sulcation and gyration with no significant volume loss. Power Doppler imaging (**b**) may show crossing veins along the subarachnoid space draining into the superior sagittal sinus

that are above the 95th percentile for age are usually considered abnormal. For neonates, the normal craniocortical width range may be from 3.3 to 5 mm while infants that are <1 year of age may have values ranging from 4 to 10 mm. Therefore, regardless of imaging modality utilized, values that are above 5 mm are considered enlarged and more than 10 mm are significantly widened [44]. The width of the interhemispheric extra-axial space should measure 5–10 mm [5]. Color Doppler imaging may show crossing veins along the subarachnoid space that may appear elongated but not displaced as they enter the superior sagittal sinus, which differentiates it from subdural collection. There is often resolution of this condition by the second year of life without neurologic sequelae in most of the patients while some may exhibit psychomotor delay [2].

1.5.3 Pseudolesions

1.5.3.1 Calcar Avis Pseudolesion

The Calcar Avis is an anatomic variant wherein there is protrusion of white matter (calcarine gyrus) on the medial wall of the occipital horn of the lateral ventricle. When viewed from the posterior fontanelle view, it projects over the occipital horns and mimics an intraventricular hemorrhage [2]. This artifact is created when the occipital horn is imaged slightly off center and the adjacent brain is averaged with the ventricle. Therefore, angling or positioning the transducer more laterally will eliminate the tissue averaging. This protrusion likewise continues with the calcarine gyrus and is seen at its characteristic location with a central echogenic sulcus [8] (Fig. 1.44). Doppler study also shows perfusion of the calcar avis as compared to a non-vascular hemorrhage/clot.

1.5.3.2 Parenchymal Pseudolesion/Hyperechoic White Matter Pseudolesion

Parenchymal pseudolesion happens when a normal sulcus is imaged tangentially, as it goes around a gyrus, producing a more hyperechoic area relative to the adjacent parenchyma [2] (Fig. 1.45). This usually occurs during imaging at coronal view. Therefore, rotating the transducer to an orthogonal plane will be able to confirm that the involved brain parenchyma is normal.

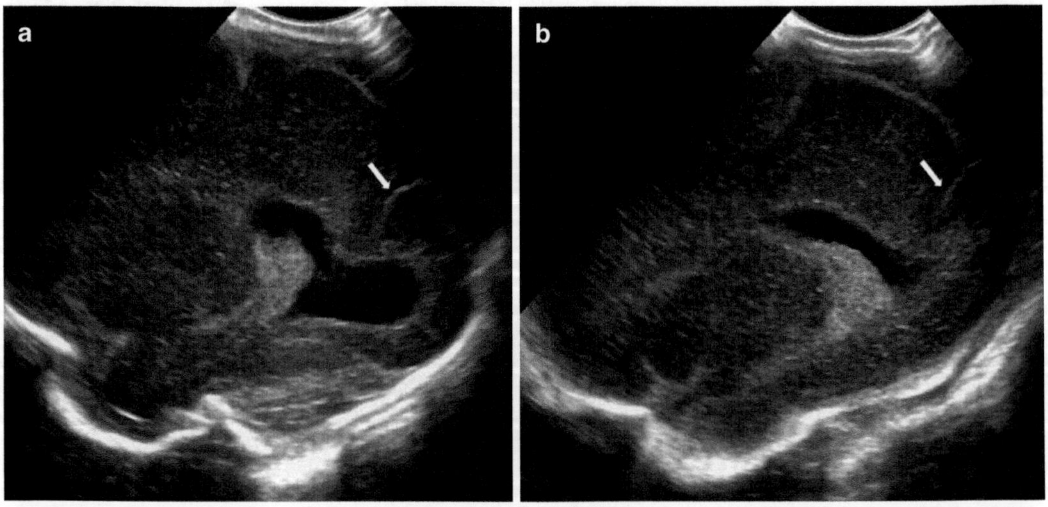

Fig. 1.44 (**a**, **b**) Calcar avis pseudolesion. Sagittal view (**a**) through the posterior fontanelle of a 26-week-old neonate shows indentation of the calcarine gyrus (white arrow) at the occipital horn of the right lateral ventricle, which exhibits a central echogenic sulcus. This is a scanning artifact, which can be eliminated by angling or positioning the transducer more laterally, as in image (**b**)

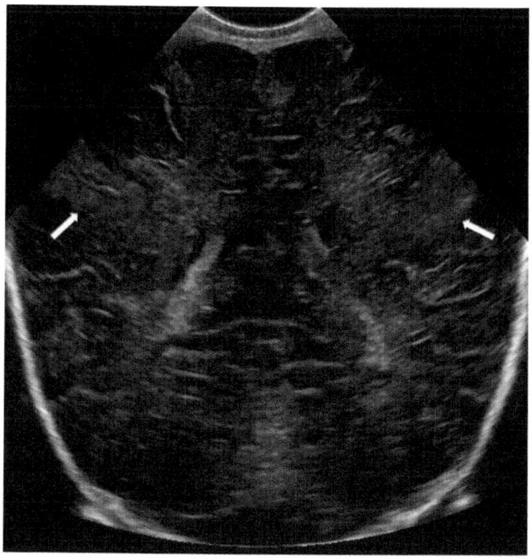

Fig. 1.45 Parenchymal pseudolesion/hyperechoic white matter pseudolesion. Coronal view of the brain of a term infant shows ill-defined, hyperechogenic areas at the bilateral frontal lobes, representing pseudolesions, which were not seen in another orthogonal view

This entity is also frequently seen in preterm infants and resolves during the first month of life [5]. Few other differentiating qualities are no mass effect exerted and are adjacent to normal sulci.

1.5.3.3 Periventricular Halo/ Peritrigonal White Matter Echogenicity

Similar to the parenchymal pseudolesion, peritrigonal hyperechogenicity occurs when ultrasound waves come into contact with nerve fibers and vessels in the peritrigonal areas almost perpendicularly on anterior fontanelle view, creating multiple interfaces [2, 47]. This creates a homogeneous, poorly defined, flame-shaped, or brush-like area of periventricular echogenicity commonly referred to as "halo or blush" sign at the external angles of the peritrigonal region [47] (Fig. 1.46). Its appearance is very similar to cerebral hemorrhage or leukomalacia. Therefore, one

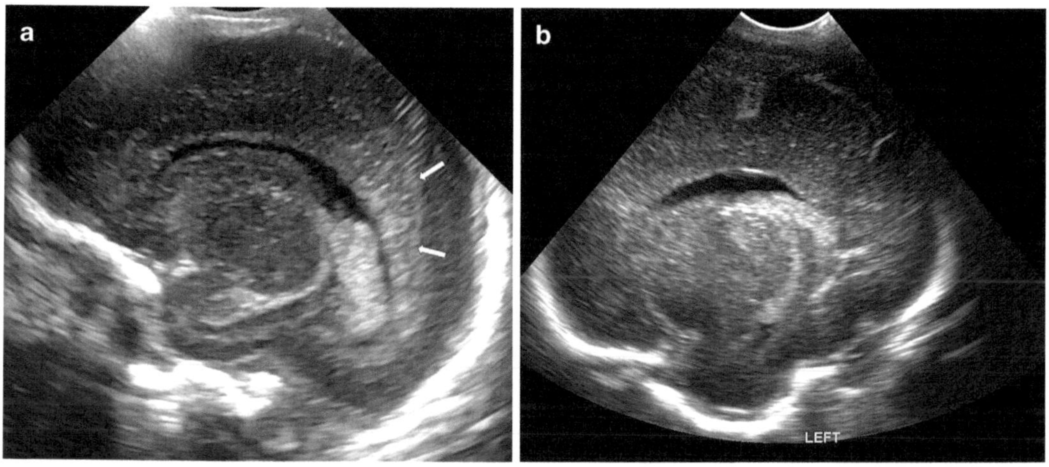

Fig. 1.46 (a, b) Peritrigonal white matter echogenicity/ periventricular halo. Sagittal view of the brain of a 25-week-old neonate through the anterior fontanelle approach (a) shows a brush-like area or halo of periventricular echogenicity at the peritrigonal region (white arrows), mimicking leukomalacia. Additional view of the same region through the posterior fontanelle approach (b) does not show these periventricular echogenicities

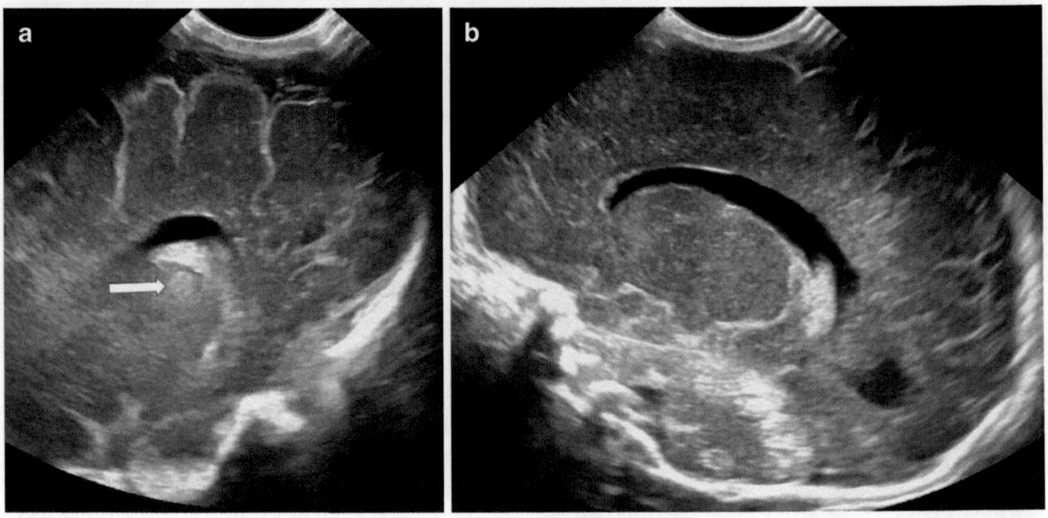

Fig. 1.47 (**a**, **b**) Thalamic pseudolesion. Sagittal view through the posterior fontanelle of a 37-week-old neonate (**a**) shows a small echogenic focus at the region of the thalamus (white arrow). Scanning through the anterior fontanelle (**b**), no longer demonstrates this finding, which represents a scanning artifact

should inspect the echogenicity of this halo or blush. Periventricular halo should appear symmetric, homogeneous, and less than that of the choroid plexus. There should also be less evident or even disappearance of the blush on the posterior fontanelle view as the ultrasound waves are now parallel with the nerve fibers and vessels [45]. This occurrence is more common among premature infants and fades with age.

1.5.3.4 Thalamic Pseudolesion

Thalamic pseudolesion is another artifact secondary to anisotropic scanning effect [47]. The thalamus shows a rounded hyperechoic structure when ultrasound waves come into contact with multiple parallel fibers of the thalamus perpendicularly on posterior fontanelle view [2, 47] (Fig. 1.47). This artifact can be easily mistaken for a bleed or infarct [45]. As with other similar artifacts, this pseudolesion should resolve on another tangential view (e.g., anterior fontanelle view).

1.5.4 Choroid Plexus Variants

1.5.4.1 Lobular Choroid Plexus

This refers to the lobulated and bulbous appearance of the glomus of the choroid plexus, particularly at the ventricular atria and lateral ventricles [45, 48], which is a common and normal variant (Fig. 1.48). Due to its shape, it can be mistaken as hemorrhage. Color Doppler study can help differentiate this entity from a non-vascular hemorrhagic clot. Likewise, stability of its appearance, as compared to a resolving or developing hemorrhage, will help set them apart.

1.5.4.2 Double/Bifid Choroid

Double or bifid choroid plexus is defined as a choroid plexus having a body divided into two arms that are located in different areas. The division can be as mild as a small cleavage or as large as dividing the corpus into two separate segments, with two reported orientations of the arms—either cranio-caudal or latero-lateral [49]

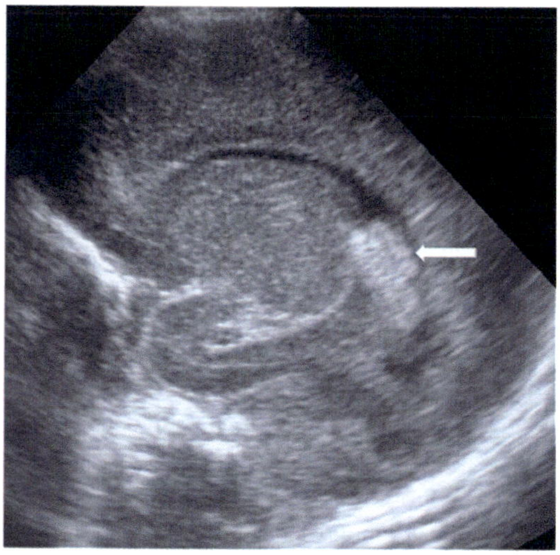

Fig. 1.48 Lobular choroid plexus. Sagittal view of the brain of a 26-week-old neonate through the anterior fontanelle approach shows lobulated or bulbous appearance of the choroid plexus (white arrow). This should be differentiated from a resolving hemorrhage or clot due to the presence of vascularity as well as its stability over time

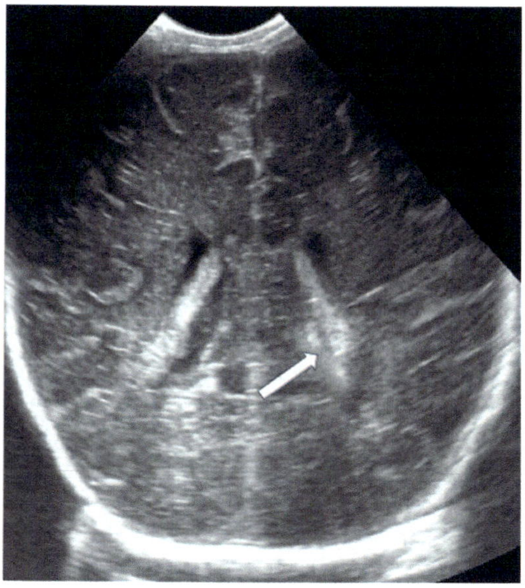

Fig. 1.49 Double/bifid choroid. Coronal view of the brain of a term neonate through the anterior fontanelle approach shows another arm of the corpus of the left choroid plexus located medial to it (white arrow)

(Fig. 1.49) Although majority of bifid choroid plexus is considered a variant, few cases have shown that in particular when bilateral, is related to certain chromosomal abnormalities such as trisomy 9, other brain (corpus callosum, cisterna magna, gyration), and extracranial structural malformations [49, 50]. One study also showed that there is a direct relationship between the presence of bifid choroid plexus and increased ventricular diameter due to increased CSF production [49].

1.5.4.3 Split-Choroid and Truncated Choroid

Split-choroid implies having a central cleft at the glomus of the chronic plexus, giving the appearance of a cut or double choroid pattern, and is a common variant [2, 47]. Its appearance, however, can mimic a choroid or intraventricular hemorrhage. Being a highly vascular structure, color Doppler study can thus help distinguish split-choroid from avascular hemorrhage. Truncated choroid, on the other hand, means flattening of the usual rounded appearance of the lower portion of the choroid plexus, giving it a solid-fluid level [47] (Fig. 1.50). This is more common on the left side.

1.5.4.4 Choroid Plexus Cysts

Choroid plexus cysts are small anechoic foci at the glomus of the choroid plexus measuring

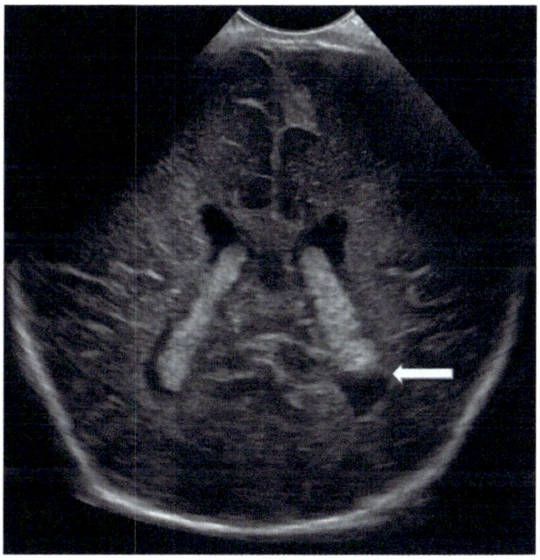

Fig. 1.50 Split-choroid or truncated choroid. Coronal view of the brain of a term neonate through the anterior fontanelle shows flattening of the lower portion of the left choroid plexus (white arrow) producing a solid-fluid level

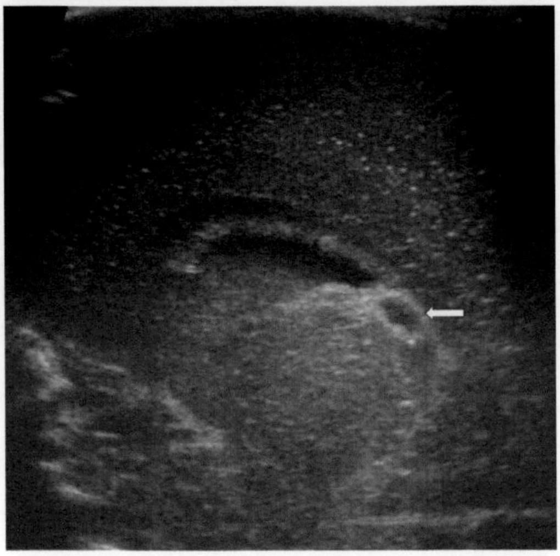

Fig. 1.51 Choroid plexus cysts. Sagittal view of the brain of a 26-week-old neonate through the anterior fontanelle approach shows small (<1 cm) cystic foci at the left choroid plexus (white arrows)

<1 cm in diameter [2] (Fig. 1.51). They are usually unilateral and clinically insignificant in an otherwise healthy infant with no structural abnormality [45]. However, the presence of multiple, bilateral, or larger sizes (>1 cm) have been associated with trisomy 18 and 21 as well as Aicardi syndrome [2].

1.5.5 Persistent Fetal Fluid-Filled Spaces

1.5.5.1 Cavum Septi Pellucidi and Cavum Vergae

These are midline, continuous, fluid-filled spaces that are located between the lateral ventricles, which do not communicate with the ventricular or subarachnoid spaces. The cavum septi pellucidi is seen between the anterior horns of the lateral ventricles, anterior to the foramen of Monro. The cavum vergae, on the other hand, lies between the bodies of the lateral ventricles and is posterior to the foramen of Monro (Fig. 1.52). These spaces form at around the third month of gestation and close from posterior to anterior starting at around the third month of gestation [5]. Thus, the first to close at around 6 months of gestation is the cavum vergae while the cavum septi pellucidi closes just before the end of gestation. In nearly all term infants at birth, the cavum vergae is no longer identified while the cavum septi pellucidi may often still be observed up to about 2–6 months after birth [2]. Some may even persist into adulthood with no neurologic sequelae. Normal measurement of these spaces is from 2 mm to 10 mm in width, as measured in coronal views [2]. There may also be linear echoes, representing septal veins, at the cavum septum pellucidum.

1.5.5.2 Cavum Veli Interpositi

Cavum veli interpositi is not as common as the above two entities but may still be encountered in routine sonography of patients <2 years of age [48]. This is a comma-shaped, anechoic, potential space identified between the roof of the third ventricle and the inferior surfaces of the lateral ventricles. Its apex is located anteriorly at the level of the foramen of Monro and its base posteriorly at the suprapineal recess [2] (Fig. 1.53). This may mimic a cyst at the pineal region on sagittal view. However, its lack of mass effect differentiates it from cystic lesions at this region, such as arachnoid cysts. Utilizing Doppler study is also important in the investigation of fluid-filled spaces at this region as vascular entities, such as vein of Galen malformations, also occupy the same area.

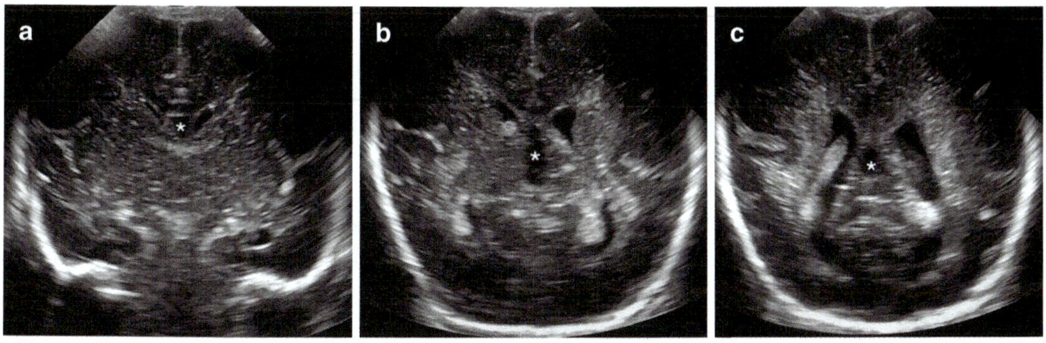

Fig. 1.52 (**a**–**c**) Cavum septum pellucidum and cavum vergae. Contiguous coronal views of the brain of a term neonate through the anterior fontanelle approach (**a**–**c**) show a fluid-filled space (white asterisks) between the anterior horns and the bodies of the lateral ventricles with a width of <10 mm

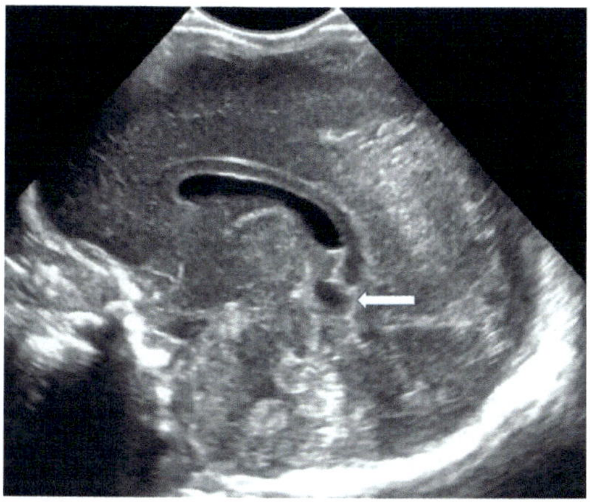

Fig. 1.53 Cavum veli interpositi. Sagittal view of the brain of a 28-week-old neonate shows an anechoic space between the lateral and third ventricles (white arrow) mimicking a cyst

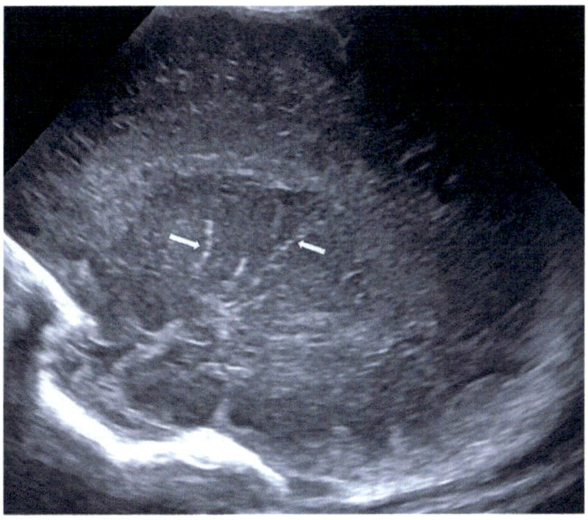

Fig. 1.54 Lenticulostriate hyperechogenicity/vasculopathy. Sagittal view of the brain of a 32-week neonate through the anterior fontanelle shows several branching, echogenic foci (white arrow) suggestive of lenticulostriate vasculopathy

1.6 Others

1.6.1 Lenticulostriate Hyperechogenicity/Vasculopathy (LSV)

Lenticulostriate hyperechogenicity or lenticulostriate vasculopathy (LSV) refers to increased homogenous echogenicity (>90%) or punctate or linear branching echogenic foci (~20%) in the basal ganglia and within the thalami, which can be unilateral or bilateral [2, 51]) (Fig. 1.54). It is hypothesized to be caused by benign vasculitis of the lenticulostriate vessels and thickening and mineralization (deposition of amorphous basophilic material, iron, and calcium) of the arterial wall [45, 46, 51]. This can be commonly seen among healthy preterm neonates of <32 weeks gestation and is transient, with gradual regression as gestation age increases. Lenticulostriate vasculopathy is now divided into low grade (one or two fine striations) and high grade (three or more striations) [5]. Due to higher capabilities of modern ultrasound machines, low-grade LSV is more commonly seen and is considered a variant [5]. High-grade LSV, on the other hand, may be associated with hypoxic-ischemic events and infections. It is thus important to correlate this entity with clinical history and laboratory findings to exclude ischemic injury, infection (e.g., TORCH), metabolic disorders, and chromosomal abnormalities (e.g., Patau syndrome) as the cause [46, 48, 51]. There are no reported significant adverse short-term outcomes for isolated LSV. However, long-term consequences may include attention-deficit/hyperactivity disorders and tics [45].

References

1. Kim HHR, Kim WG, Lee EY, Phillips GS. Brain. In: Paltiel HJ, Lee EY, editors. Pediatric ultrasound. Switzerland AG: Springer Nature; 2021.
2. Siegel MJ. Brain. In: Siegel MJ, editor. Pediatric sonography. 5th ed. Philadelphia, PA: Wolters Kluwer; 2019. p. 40–42–53–58.
3. American College of Radiology. ACR–AIUM–SPR–SRU practice parameter for the performance of neurosonography in neonates and infants, revised 2019. Available at: https://www.acr.org/-/media/ACR/Files/Practice-Parameters/Neurosonog. Accessed September 23, 2023.
4. Dudink J, Steggerda SJ, Horsch S, eurUS.Brain group. State-of-the-art neonatal cerebral ultrasound: technique and reporting. Pediatr Res. 2020;87:3–12. https://doi.org/10.1038/s41390-020-0776-y.
5. Caro-Domínguez P, Lecacheux C, Hernandez-Herrera C, Llorens-Salvador R. Cranial ultrasound for beginners. Transl Pediatr. 2021;10(4):1117–37. https://doi.org/10.21037/tp-20-399.
6. Ecury-Goossen GM, Camfferman FA, Leijser LM, Govaert P, Dudink J. State of the art cranial ultrasound imaging in neonates. J Vis Exp. 2015;96:e52238. https://doi.org/10.3791/52238.
7. James AC. Practical guide to neonatal cranial ultrasound (CrUS): basics. Paediatr Child Health. 2018;28(9):424–30. https://doi.org/10.1016/j.paed.2018.07.003.
8. Di Salvo DN. A new view of the neonatal brain: clinical utility of supplemental neurologic US imaging windows. Radiographics. 2001;21(4):943–55. https://doi.org/10.1148/radiographics.21.4.g01jl14943.
9. D'Antoni AV, Donaldson OI, Schmidt C, Macchi V, De Caro R, Oskouian RJ, l. A comprehensive review of the anterior Fontanelle: embryology, anatomy, and clinical considerations. Childs Nerv Syst. 2017;33(6):909–14. https://doi.org/10.1007/s00381-017-3406-1.
10. Brouwer MJ, de Vries LS, Groenendaal F, Koopman C, Pistorius LR, Mulder EJH, et al. New reference values for the neonatal cerebral ventricles. Radiology. 2012;262:224–33. https://doi.org/10.1148/radiol.11110334.
11. Frankel DA, Fessell DP, Wolfson WP. High resolution sonographic determination of the normal dimensions of the intracranial extraaxial compartment in the newborn infant. J Ultrasound Med. 1998;17:411–5. https://doi.org/10.7863/jum.1998.17.7.411.
12. O'Dell MC, Cassady C, Logsdon G, Varich L. Cinegraphic versus combined static and Cinegraphic imaging for initial cranial ultrasound screening in premature infants. Pediatr Radiol. 2015;45:1706–11. https://doi.org/10.1007/s00247-015-3382-0.
13. Franco A, Lewis KN. Neonatal cranial ultrasound: current perspectives. Rep Med Imaging. 2013;6:93–103. https://doi.org/10.2147/RMI.S46473.
14. Steggerda SJ, de Bruïne FT, Smits-Wintjens VE, Verbon P, Walther FJ, van Wezel-Meijler G, et al. Posterior fossa abnormalities in high-risk term infants: comparison of ultrasound and MRI. Eur Radiol. 2015;25:2575–83. https://doi.org/10.1007/s00330-015-3665-8.
15. Brennan CM, Taylor GA. Sonographic imaging of the posterior fossa utilizing the foramen magnum. Pediatr Radiol. 2010;40:1411–6. https://doi.org/10.1007/s00247-010-1635-5.
16. American College of Radiology. ACR–AIUM–SPR–SRU practice parameter for the performance of transcranial doppler ultrasound, revised 2022. Available at: https://www.acr.org/-/media/ACR/Files/Practice-Parameters/US-Transcranial. Accessed September 23, 2023.
17. Bulas D. Transcranial Doppler: applications in neonates and children. Ultrasound Clin. 2009;4:533–51. https://doi.org/10.1016/j.cult.2009.11.001.
18. Siegel MJ. Brain. In: Siegel MJ, editor. Pediatric sonography. 4th ed. Philadelphia, PA: Wolters Kluwer; 2011. p. 43–60.
19. Buckley KM, Taylor GA, Estroff JA, Barnewolt CE, Share JC, Paltiel HJ. Use of the mastoid Fontanelle for improved sonographic visualization of the neonatal midbrain and posterior fossa. AJR Am J Roentgenol. 1997;168:1021–5. https://doi.org/10.2214/ajr.168.4.9124108.
20. D'Orey C, Mateus M, Guimaraes H, Ramos I, Melo MJ, Silva J, et al. Neonatal cerebral Doppler: arterial and venous flow velocity measurements using color and pulsed Doppler system. J Perinat Med. 1999;27:352–61. https://doi.org/10.1515/jpm.1999.048.
21. Allison JW, Faddis LA, Kinder DL, Roberson PK, Glasier CM, Seibert JJ. Intracranial resistive index (RI) values in normal term infants during the first day of life. Pediatr Radiol. 2000;30:618–20. https://doi.org/10.1007/s002470000286.
22. Ecury-Goossen GM, Raets MMA, Camfferman FA, Vos RHJ, van Rosmalen J, Reiss IKM, et al. Resistive indices of cerebral arteries in very preterm infants: values throughout stay in the neonatal intensive care

unit and impact of patent ductus arteriosus. Pediatr Radiol. 2016;46:1291–300. https://doi.org/10.1007/s00247-016-3615-x.
23. Hwang M, Barnewolt CE, Jüngert J, Prada F, Sridharan A, Didier RA. Contrast-enhanced ultrasound of the pediatric brain. Pediatr Radio. 2021;51(12):2270–83. https://doi.org/10.1007/s00247-021-04974-4.
24. Gumus M, Oommen KC, Squires JH. Contrast-enhanced ultrasound of the neonatal brain. Pediatr Radiol. 2022;52(4):837–46. https://doi.org/10.1007/s00247-021-05157-x.
25. Squires JH, Beluk NH, Lee VK, Yanowitz TD, Gumus S, Subramanian S, Panigrahy A. Feasibility and safety of contrast-enhanced ultrasound of the neonatal brain: a prospective study using MRI as the reference standard. AJR Am J Roentgenol. 2022;218:152–62. https://doi.org/10.2214/ajr.21.26274.
26. Hwang M. Introduction to contrast-enhanced ultrasound of the brain in neonates and infants: current understanding and future potential. Pediatr Radiol. 2019;49(2):54–262. https://doi.org/10.1007/s00247-018-4270-1.
27. Stiles J, Jernigan TL. The basics of brain development. Neuropsychol Rev. 2010;20(4):327–48. https://doi.org/10.1007/s11065-010-9148-4.
28. Daneman A, Epelman M, Blaser S, Jarrin JR. Imaging of the brain in full-term neonates: does sonography still play a role? Pediatric Radiol. 2006;36(7):636–46. https://doi.org/10.1007/s00247-006-0201-7.
29. Yap JL, Concepcion NDP. Normal sulcation and gyration in neonatal cranial sonography from 24 weeks gestational age until term: a pictorial essay. Pediatric Radiol. 2023;53(11):2281–90. https://doi.org/10.1007/s00247-023-05732-4.
30. Rutherford MA, Pennock JM, Counsell SJ, Mercuri E, Cowan FM, Dubowitz LM, et al. Abnormal magnetic resonance signal in the internal capsule predicts poor neurodevelopmental outcome in infants with hypoxic-ischemic encephalopathy. Pediatrics. 1998;102(2 Pt 1):323–8. https://doi.org/10.1542/peds.102.2.323.
31. Friede RL. Gross and microscopic development of the central nervous system. In: Developmental neuropathology. 2nd ed. Berlin, Heidelberg: Springer-Verlag; 1989. p. 2–20.
32. van Wezel-Meijler G, Leijser LM, Wiggers-de FT, Steggerda SJ, van, Walther FJ. Diffuse hyperechogenicity of basal ganglia and thalami in preterm neonates: a physiologic finding? Radiology. 2011;258(3):944–50. https://doi.org/10.1148/radiol.10101086.
33. Zhan J, Dinov ID, Li J, Zhang Z, Hobel S, Shi Y, et al. Spatial–temporal atlas of human fetal brain development during the early second trimester. NeuroImage. 2013;82:115–26. https://doi.org/10.1016/j.neuroimage.2013.05.063.
34. Glenn OA. MR imaging of the fetal brain. Pediatric Radiol. 2009;40(1):68–81. https://doi.org/10.1007/s00247-009-1459-3.
35. Grossman R, Hoffman C, Mardor Y, Biegon A. Quantitative MRI measurements of human fetal brain development in utero. NeuroImage. 2006;33(2):463–70. https://doi.org/10.1016/j.neuroimage.2006.07.005.
36. Brouwer MJ, de Vries LS, Pistorius L, Rademaker KJ, Groenendaal F, Benders MJNL. Ultrasound measurements of the lateral ventricles in neonates: why, how and when? A systematic review. Acta Paediatr. 2010;99(9):1298–306. https://doi.org/10.1111/j.1651-2227.2010.01830.x.
37. Gonçalves FG, Hwang M. Superficial anatomy of the neonatal cerebrum—an ultrasonographic roadmap. Pediatric Radiol. 2020;51(3):353–70. https://doi.org/10.1007/s00247-020-04794-y.
38. Veyrac C, Couture A, Saguintaah M, Baud C. Brain ultrasonography in the premature infant. Pediatr Radiol. 2006;36(7):626–35. https://doi.org/10.1007/s00247-006-0202-6.
39. Chen SJ, Hu CF, Tien CH, Chen CY. Sonographic measurement of brainstem through the foramen magnum in premature neonates can predict neurodevelopment outcome? Front Neurol. 2021;12:770908. https://doi.org/10.3389/fneur.2021.770908.
40. Fumagalli M, Parodi A, Ramenghi L, Limperopoulos C, Steggerda S. Ultrasound of acquired posterior fossa abnormalities in the newborn. Pediatric Res. 2020;87:25–36. https://doi.org/10.1038/s41390-020-0778-9.
41. Bethune M, Alibrahim E, Davies B, Yong E. A pictorial guide for the second trimester ultrasound. Australas J Ultrasound Med. 2013;16(3):98–113. https://doi.org/10.1002/j.2205-0140.2013.tb00106.x.
42. Goodwin L, Quisling RG. The neonatal cisterna magna: ultrasonic evaluation. Radiology. 1983;149:691–5. https://doi.org/10.1148/radiology.149.3.6647845.
43. Libicher M, Tröger J. US measurement of the subarachnoid space in infants: normal values. Radiology. 1992;184:749–51. https://doi.org/10.1148/radiology.184.3.1509061.
44. Raissaki M, Adamsbaum C, Argyropoulou MI, Choudry AK, et al. Benign enlargement of the subarachnoid spaces and subdural collections. Pediatr Radiol. 2023;53:752–67.
45. North K, Lowe LH. Modern head ultrasound: normal anatomy, variants, and pitfalls that may simulate disease. Ultrasound Clin. 2009;4(4):497–512.
46. Lowe LH, Bailey Z. State-of-the-art cranial sonography: Part 2, pitfalls and variants. Am J Roentgenol. 2011;196(5):1034–9. https://doi.org/10.2214/ajr.10.6203.
47. Enríquez G, Correa F, Lucaya J, Piqueras J, Aso C, Ortega A. Potential pitfalls in cranial sonography. Pediatric Radiol. 2003;33:110–7.
48. Gupta P, Sodhi KS, Saxena AK, Khandelwal N, Singhi P. Neonatal cranial sonography: a concise review for clinicians. J Pediatr Neurosci. 2016;11(1):7.

49. Centini G, Imperatore A, Morelli M, Rosignoli L, Passamonti U, Caprioli F, Lituania M. Bifid choroid plexus: always a normal fetal brain structure variant? Congenit Anom (Kyoto). 2013;53(2):73–7.
50. Tonni G, Grisolia G. Ultrasound diagnosis of central nervous system anomalies (bifid choroid plexus, ventriculomegaly, Dandy Walker malformation) associated with multicystic dysplastic kidney disease in a trisomy 9 fetus: case report with literature review. J Clin Ultrasound. 2013;41(7):441–7.
51. Meijler G, de Vries L, Güleryüz H. In: Beek E, van Rijn RR, editors. Diagnostic pediatric ultrasound. New York: Thieme; 2016. p. 31.

2 Cranial Ultrasound: Applications

Poonam Sherwani, Ajay Taranath, and Manisha Jana

2.1 Introduction

Cranial Ultrasound (CUS) is an essential and beneficial tool in the diagnosis of various pathologies. It offers several benefits, being affordable, portable, safe (no anesthesia required, no ionizing radiation), can be easily performed, and repeatable as often as needed. CUS is the initial diagnostic as well as screening modality in neonates. In addition to the anterior fontanelle, several other windows aid in the visualization of the brain parenchyma, and, therefore, aid in the identification of a variety of abnormalities. Doppler sonography is becoming a standard component of CUS and helps detect sinus thrombosis and arterial patency [1]. CUS is the preferred imaging modality in several conditions such as hypoxic ischemic encephalopathy (HIE), germinal matrix hemorrhage, hydrocephalus, and congenital abnormality [2]. Various limitations include subjectivity, dependence on the radiologists' expertise in the field, and narrow fontanelles with insufficient windows in older infants.

P. Sherwani
Department of Diagnostic and intervention Radiology, All India Institute of Medical Sciences, Rishikesh, Uttarakhand, India

A. Taranath
Women's and Children's Hospital, University of Adelaide, Adelaide, SA, Australia

M. Jana (✉)
Department of Radiodiagnosis and Interventional Radiology, All India Institute of Medical Sciences, New Delhi, India

2.2 Indications

Various indications of CUS include the following:

1. Increase in head size.
2. Suspected hypoxic ischemic encephalopathy (Preterm and Term).
3. Intracranial hemorrhage.
4. Intracranial infection (congenital and acquired)—diagnosis and to look for various complications.
5. Hydrocephalus.
6. Congenital disorders.
7. Symptoms or signs suggestive of cranial pathology (seizures, macrocephaly, positive neurocutaneous disorder, etc.)
8. Vascular anomalies/sinus thrombosis.
9. Neonates on hypothermia or extracorporeal membrane oxygenation or any other medical support.
10. As a part of screening in syndromic babies.

Causes are adapted from Ref. [2] (Adapted from ("AIUM Practice Parameter for the Performance of Neurosonography in Neonates and Infants," 2020)).

K. S. Sodhi (ed.), *Neonatal Ultrasound*, https://doi.org/10.1007/978-981-97-8576-6_2

2.3 Increase in Head Size

Causes of increased head size (macrocephaly/macrocrania) in infants can be multifactorial. Common causes include hydrocephalus, extra-axial fluid collection, primary macrocephaly, or rarely intracranial tumors. For primary evaluation of an increased head size in a neonate, CUS remains the first imaging modality of choice. The measurement of ventricular size should be done in both coronal and oblique parasagittal planes (Fig. 2.1).

2.3.1 Ventriculomegaly

The size of ventricles varies depending on the gestational age of the newborn. Three parameters are usually taken into consideration: lateral ventricle frontal horn width, ventricular index (distance from the midline falx till the lateral end of the frontal horn of lateral ventricle), and thalamic-occipital diameter (distance from the posterior margin of thalamus till the posterior margin of the occipital horn). While the ventricular index tends to increase with an increasing gestational age (approx. 12 mm near term), the other two parameters do not show a strictly linear relationship with gestational age. While a single measurement is helpful in the diagnosis of ventriculomegaly; serial measurement of the same parameters is more useful [3]. Along with grayscale measurements, serial measurement of resistive index (RI) of the cerebral vasculature can be a guide to the need for intervention [3]. The causes of neonatal ventriculomegaly with an increased head size can be either obstructive (congenital and acquired), or non-obstructive (choroid plexus papilloma) [4]. The mechanism and imaging findings are discussed in Table 2.1.

2.3.2 Extra-Axial Fluid Collections

Extra-axial fluid collections resulting in an increased head size can develop either after intracranial infections, trauma, or bleeding disorders, and rarely, after abusive head trauma. CUS helps in differentiating a subdural fluid collection from an enlarged subarachnoid space (which is a benign finding). While the latter shows the presence of traversing vessels on Doppler imaging,

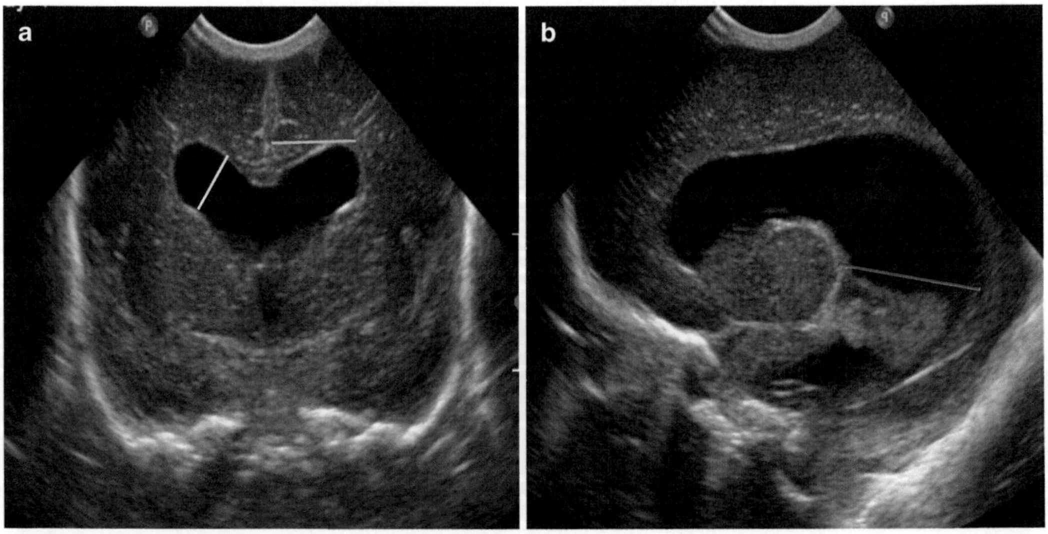

Fig. 2.1 Coronal Ultrasound image (**a**) at the level of the foramen of Monro – Width of frontal horn of the lateral ventricle obtained perpendicular to the axis of the frontal horn (yellow line) and Ventricular Index at the same plane (green line). Oblique parasagittal image (**b**) – Thalamo-occipital distance from posterior thalamus to occipital horn (pink line)

Table 2.1 Causes of ventriculomegaly with increased head size in neonates

		CUS findings
Obstructive ventriculomegaly		
• Congenital	Aqueductal stenosis (Fig. 2.2)	Dilated lateral and third ventricle Normal sized fourth ventricle
• Post-hemorrhagic hydrocephalus	Secondary to intraventricular hemorrhage (IVH) (Fig. 2.3)	All ventricles dilated Markers of previous IVH • Germinal matrix echogenicity • Germinolytic cyst • Echogenic foci along ventricular walls • Enlarged/asymmetric choroid plexus • Echogenic-dependent fluid-fluid level through transmastoid Fontanelle approach • Periventricular hemorrhagic infarct
Oversecretion of CSF	Choroid plexus papilloma (rare)	Intraventricular echogenic mass with vascularity

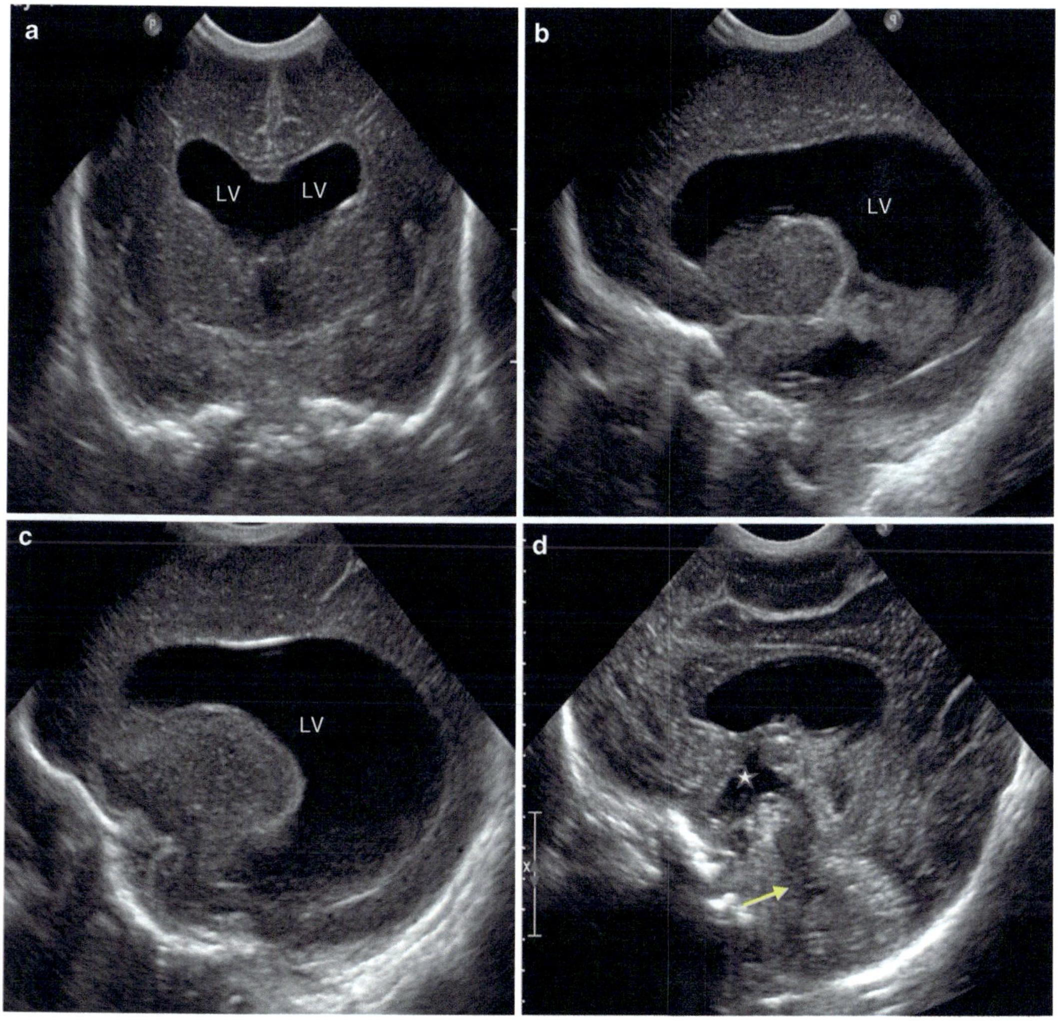

Fig. 2.2 (**a**–**d**) Coronal (**a**), right (**b**) and left (**c**) parasagittal images show dilated lateral ventricles (LV). Midline sagittal image (**d**) showing dilated 3rd ventricle (asterisk), and a normal size 4th ventricle (arrow)

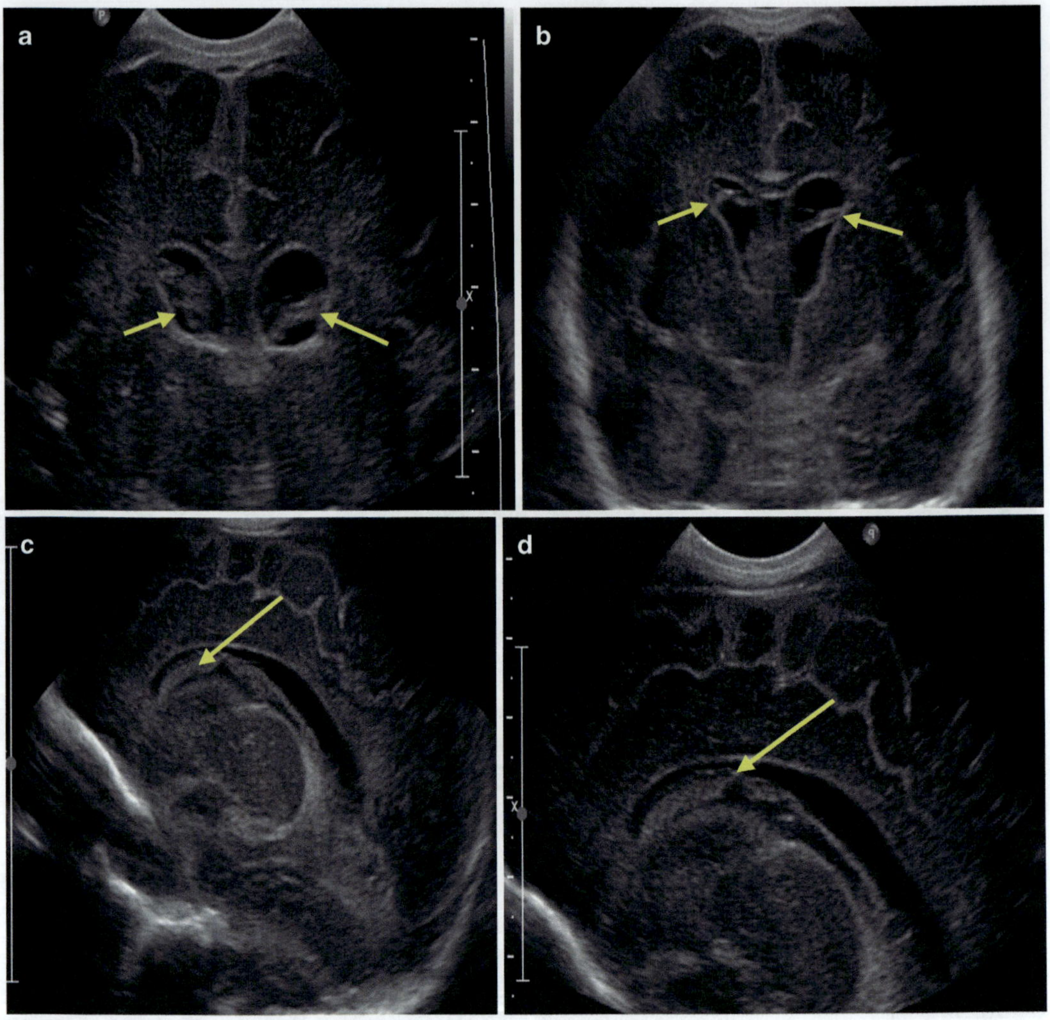

Fig. 2.3 (**a**–**d**) Post-hemorrhagic hydrocephalus. Coronal (**a**, **b**), right (**c**) and left (**d**) parasagittal images show dilated lateral ventricles with synechiae (arrows)

the former shows a displacement of the vessels towards the cortex. Detecting the nature of the fluid collection may not be possible on CUS alone, but it can be an important tool in follow-up.

2.3.3 Intracranial Hemorrhage

Intracranial hemorrhage (ICH) can cause obstruction to the CSF flow at both intraventricular and extra-ventricular levels. Secondary to ICH and IVH, the hemosiderin deposition can hamper CSF drainage at the arachnoid villi level [4]. The stages of IVH are discussed in detail later in this chapter.

2.3.4 Intracranial Neoplasms

Rare cause of ventricular enlargement in neonatal period, discussed above.

2.3.5 Megalencephaly/Hemimegalencephaly

Enlargement of brain parenchyma with associated enlarged ventricles in megalencephaly/hemimegalencephaly can be associated with variable neuronal migration anomalies. CUS is useful in measurement of ventricular dimensions and excluding associated congenital malformations; it is not sensitive for detection of migration/gyrational abnormalities [5].

2.4 Hypoxic Ischemic Encephalopathy (HIE) in Preterm and Term Neonates

Imaging findings of HIE in preterm differs from term due to presence of a germinal matrix along the ventricular system in preterm babies; which undergoes involution in term neonates.

2.4.1 Preterm Neonates

Germinal matrix (GM) is a highly vascular structure that is prone to bleeding when there is haemodynamic instability [4]. It comprises neurons that will migrate to the cortex. It is located along the ventricular walls in preterm neonates. The caudothalamic groove is the last location of the GM in the process of it's involution.

2.4.1.1 Germinal Matrix Hemorrhage (GMH)

Germinal matrix hemorrhage (GMH) is seen predominantly in premature infants under 30 weeks neonates or birth weight <1500 g or both [6]. As in 90% of neonates, GMH occurs within 7 days and rarely within 24 h; therefore, screening ultrasound is done within 72 h. Appropriate time for CUS in neonates at risk is 7–10 days of age and follow-up ultrasound at 4–6 weeks of age [7].

Germinal matrix hemorrhage (GMH) is classified into four stages depending on the location and the extension into the ventricular system and parenchyma by Papile and colleagues [8]. The staging is based on the continuum of the hemorrhage from the caudothalamic groove to the ventricular system and the involvement of cerebral [8] parenchyma. Parenchymal involvement is the infarction of the brain parenchyma rather than the extension of the ventricular bleed.

2.4.1.2 Sonographic Findings

Grade 1: During the first week of life, Grade I hemorrhage is seen as a subependymal echogenic region next to the caudothalamic groove. Though it has a distinct structure and is more echogenic than typical choroid plexus, GMH might be mistaken for the choroid plexus. The choroid plexus is thin anteriorly, fills the space around the foramen of Monro, and is thickened posteriorly. It is absent in the frontal and occipital horn. Carefully examining the coronal and parasagittal views is necessary to make the diagnosis confidently. Therefore, coronal and parasagittal views should be viewed carefully. Echogenic area which develops late in the neonatal period suggests hyperechoic germinolysis instead of GMH [9] (Fig. 2.4).

Grade II and III: Grades II and III hemorrhage occurs due to minimal or extensive rupture of the ependymal layer into the ventricular system with resultant ventricular dilatation due to obstruction by a blood clot [7]. Grade II GMH is ventricular dilatation caused by blood that occupies <50% of the ventricular lumen in the sagittal view, and Grade III GMH is caused by blood that occupies more than 50% of the ventricular lumen (Fig. 2.5).

Grade IV GMH: This is characterised by a fan-shaped echogenicity, which is not initially attached to the ventricular wall but eventually merges with the ventricular wall and appears as a single hyperechoic lesion (Fig. 2.6). The GMH need not necessarily follow a sequential progression from Grade I through Grade II, III to Grade IV. A Grade I GMH could co exist with Grade IV

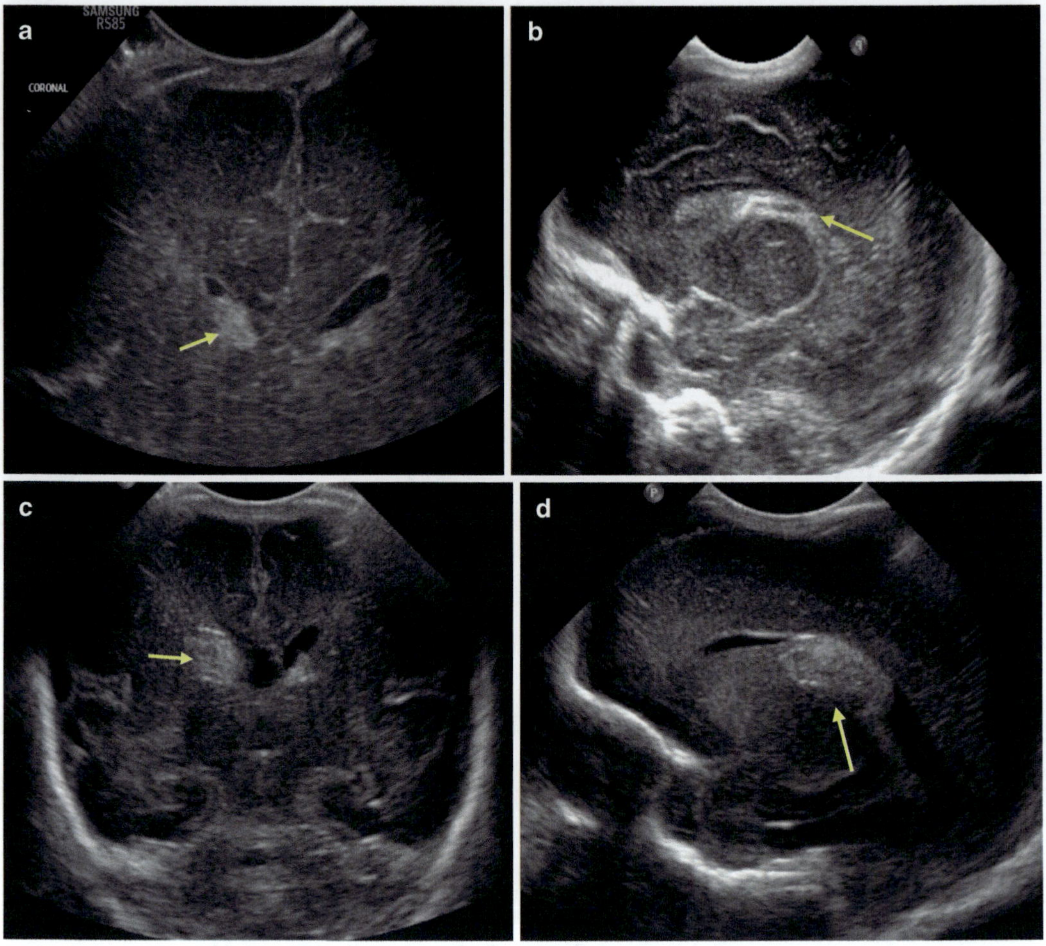

Fig. 2.4 (**a–d**) Grade 1 germinal matrix hemorrhage (GMH) in 2 neonates. (**a**, **b**) Right grade 1 GMH in the caudothalamic groove (arrows). (**c**, **d**) Right posterior subependymal hemorrhage

GMH. Similalrly, the neonate could present with a Grade IV GMH.

Follow-up ultrasound also shows a reduction of the intraparenchymal component as there is a decrease in the congestion surrounding the bleed. Finally, the bleed resolves into cavitation and, subsequently, porencephalic cyst, which is a single large, asymmetric and persistent, while the cysts of PVL are multiple and located in the posterior distribution and regress within a few weeks.

Follow-up ultrasound should be done in all the stages of GMH and is important for Grade III and Grade IV to look for post-hemorrhagic ventricular dilatation (PHVD) which results from the imbalance of production, absorption, and circulation of CSF [10]. PHVD is seen till term age equivalent or, in rare cases, after term equivalent. Depending on the obstruction site, ventricular dilation is seen. Obstruction at the foramen of Monro leads to dilatation of the lateral ventricle, while obstruction at the aqueduct causes lateral and third ventricle ventricular dilation. Dilatation of the entire ventricular system, also known as communicating hydrocephalus, occurs due to obstruction in the absorption in the subarachnoid spaces. In rare cases, isolated dilatation of the fourth ventricle occurs due to obstruction at the aqueduct and foramen of Magendie and Luschka. No role of Doppler has been identified so far. The sonographic findings are enlisted in Table 2.2.

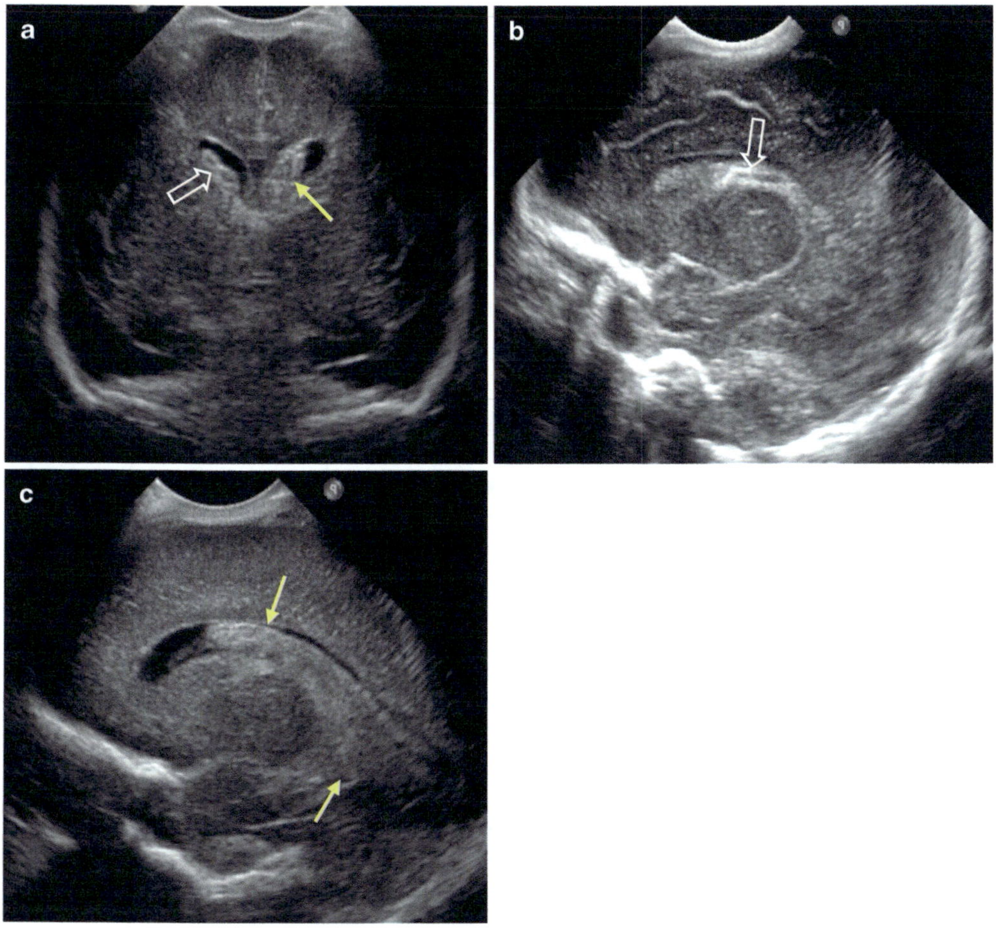

Fig. 2.5 (**a**–**c**) Grade 2 and 3 GMH. Coronal (**a**), right sagittal (**b**) and left sagittal (**c**) US images showing right sided grade 2 (open arrow) and left grade 3 (yellow arrow) GMH

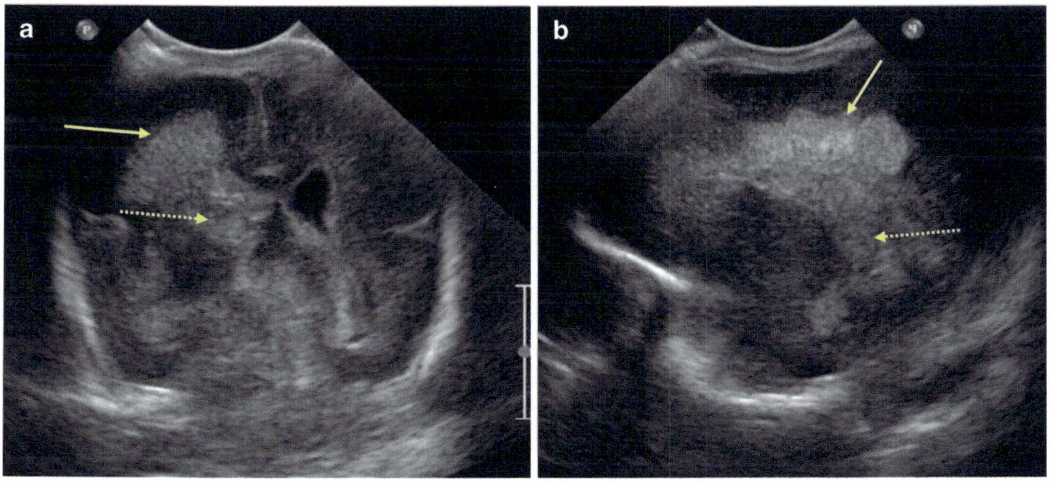

Fig. 2.6 (**a**, **b**) Grade 4 GMH/periventricular hemorrhagic infarct coronal (**a**) and right parasagittal (**b**) images showing large right periventricular echogenic area (arrow) with extensive intraventricular hemorrhage (dotted arrow)

Table 2.2 Grades of germinal matrix hemorrhage and their sonographic findings (Figs. 2.4, 2.5, 2.6 and 2.7)

Grade	CUS in acute/early stage	CUS in late stage
I	Echogenic focus in caudothalamic groove Asymmetric enlargement of the choroid plexus (no vascularity)	Cyst in caudothalamic groove
II	Asymmetric enlargement of choroid plexus with echogenic layering of contents in occipital horn (through mastoid Fontanelle approach)	Echogenic wall of ventricles/lobular echogenic foci in ventricular wall Ventriculomegaly might be present
III	As above + ventriculomegaly caused by blood products. If this criterion is not satisafied, consider a diagnosis of Post-haemorrhagic ventricular dilatation	Echogenic wall of ventricles/lobular echogenic foci in ventricular wall Ventriculomegaly
IV	IVH+ echogenic/heterogeneous area in periventricular cerebral parenchyma	Cystic changes in periventricular white matter, ventriculomegaly

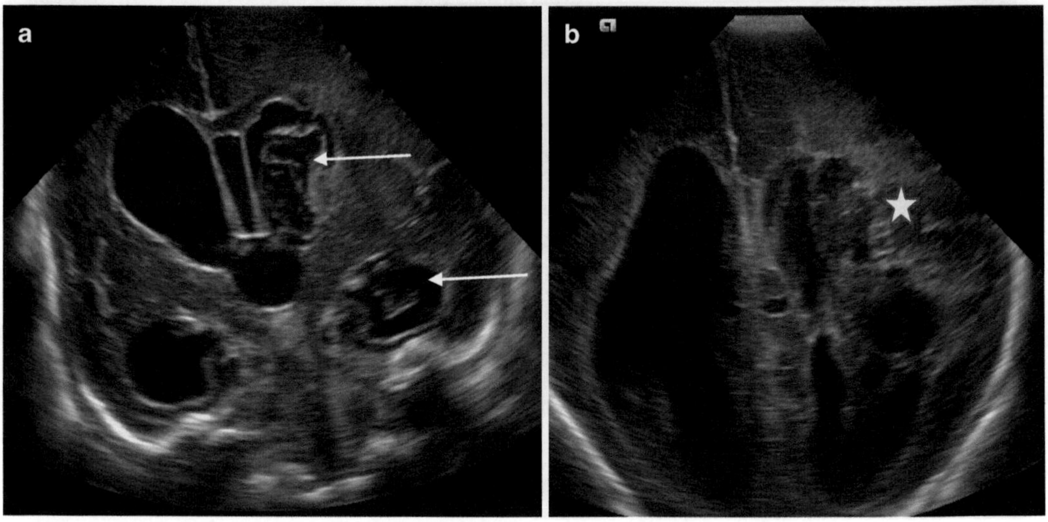

Fig. 2.7 (**a**, **b**) Grade 4 GMH/periventricular hemorrhagic infarct with cystic changes. (**a**, **b**) Coronal images showing ventriculomegaly, intraventricular bleed in left lateral ventricle (arrows) and periventricular parenchymal echogenic area (asterisk) having internal cystic changes

2.4.1.3 Premature White Matter Injury/ PVL

PVL is another manifestation of HIE in preterm neonates and is the result of hypoxia and reduced perfusion. Perinatal asphyxia, sepsis, circulatory compromise, recurrent apnea, sepsis, maternal chorioamnionitis, and severe respiratory distress are among the risk factors. As the name indicates, there is white matter injury resulting in infarction leading to necrosis with sparing of gray matter, which on CUS is seen as a bilateral asymmetric heterogeneous area of hyperechogenicity adjacent to the frontal and atrium of lateral ventricles. These echogenicities eventually develop into cysts, volume loss, and corpus callosum thinning as a result of white matter necrosis and a reduction in the number of crossing fibers. CUS findings of PVL have to be differentiated from periventricular blush and flare.

Periventricular Blush: Typically detected in early scans, bilateral symmetrical moderately hyperechoic regions in the white matter are most likely a normal maturational feature.

Periventricular Flare: Areas of increased echogenicity in the periventricular white matter which are considered normal till 7 days of life [11].

Depending on the extent of involvement, the grading system is described by De Vries [12].

Grade 0: Transient periventricular echogenicities (>7 days).
Grade 1: Periventricular echogenicities with cysts.
Grade 2: Extensive cysts in frontoparietal and occipital white matter (Cystic PVL).
Grade 3: Grade 2 with subcortical cysts (Cystic subcortical leukomalacia).

Various limitations in interpreting the PVL findings exist particularly Grade 0. There are a lot of subjective variations in the interpretation of periventricular echogenicities. Periventricular echogenicity is considered pathological provided its echogenicity is more than the choroid plexus, patchy and asymmetrical, and inhomogeneous. However, in the case of very premature neonates, the choroid plexus is enlarged and very echogenic so comparison becomes challenging. Depending on the duration of periventricular echogenicity, the grading system was proposed by Damman and Leviton as mild (1–6 days), intermediate (7–13 days), or prolonged (14 days or more) [11].

A sequential ultrasound is recommended to look for the resolution or progression of echogenicity to cysts (Figs. 2.8 and 2.9) which have

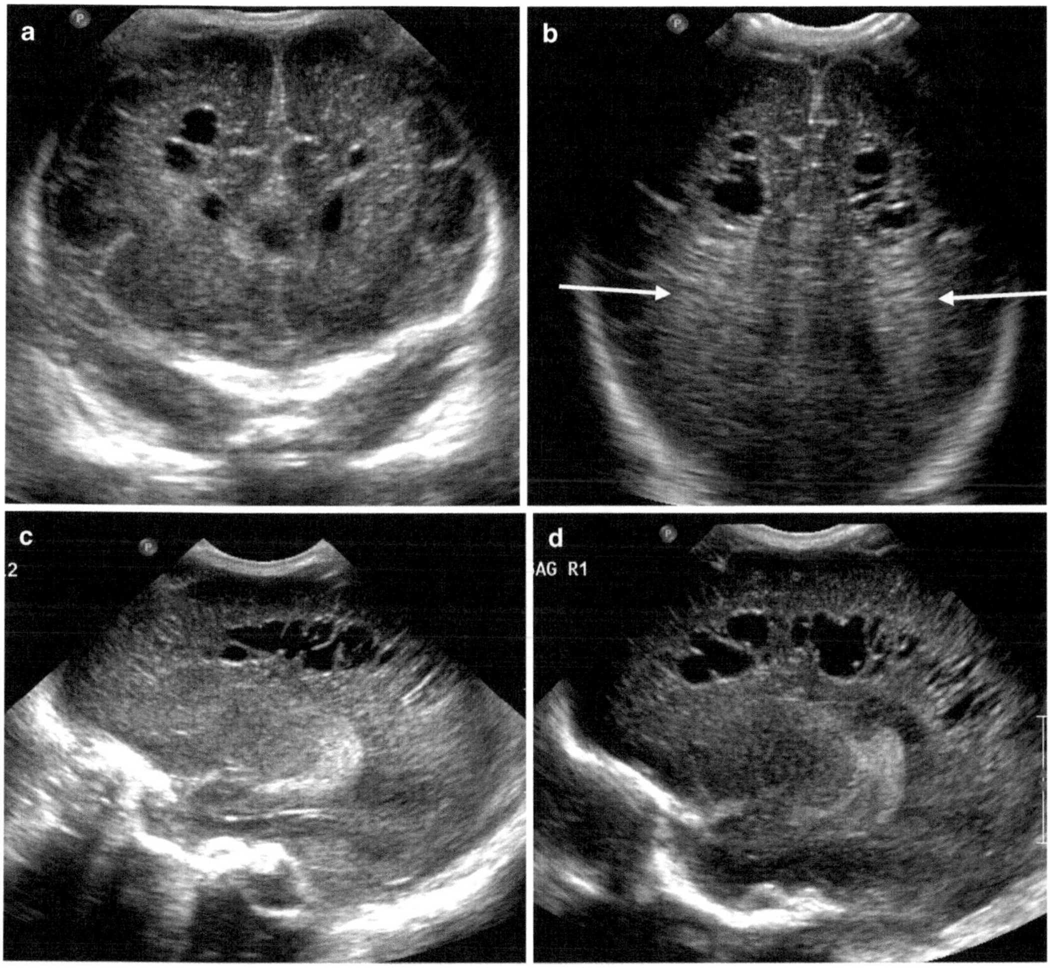

Fig. 2.8 (**a**–**d**) Cystic periventricular leukomalacia. Coronal (**a**, **b**), left (**c**) and right (**d**) parasagittal US images showing increased echogenicity of the periventricular white matter (arrows), with cystic changes

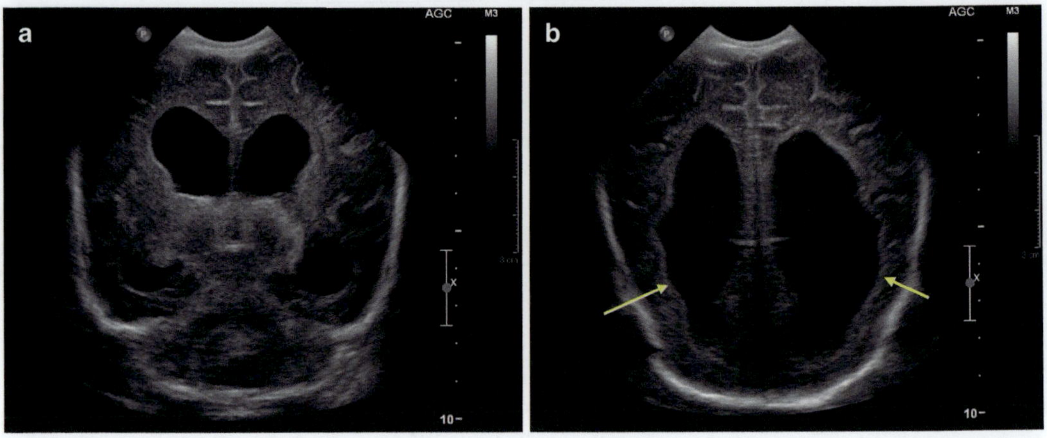

Fig. 2.9 (**a**, **b**) Periventricular leukomalacia (PVL). Coronal anterior (**a**) and posterior (**b**) images showing ventriculomegaly, and undulating margins of the lateral ventricles (arrows)

to be differentiated from germinolytic cysts or porencephalic cysts secondary to Grade IV Germinal matrix hemorrhage or chronic arterial infarction. Clinical symptoms depend on the location of involvement. The cyst, which is located in the central groove, causes spastic cerebral palsy (CP), while the cysts in the frontal region do not cause CP. These cysts can resolve due to the resorption of the cysts in the surrounding brain parenchyma with subsequent gliosis.

There is eventually white matter atrophy leading to dilatation of the lateral ventricles with undulating margins, widened interhemispheric fissure, and subarachnoid spaces.

2.4.2 Term Neonates

In contrast to preterm neonates where there is the involvement of periventricular white matter, involvement of watershed areas between the anterior cerebral artery, middle cerebral artery, and posterior cerebral artery are more commonly seen in term neonates. The reason for periventricular involvement in the preterm neonates is due to immature premyelinating oligodendrocytes and the watershed areas which are located in the periventricular area.

The involvement of watershed areas occurs when there is a significant disruption in blood flow [13]. Watershed areas are impacted by mild to moderate injury, but severe hypoxia affects the central gray matter, which includes the thalamus and basal ganglia. These areas are crucial for survival and have a bad neurological prognosis [14].

Based on the severity and pattern of involvement, CUS findings can be divided into central and peripheral patterns.

2.4.2.1 Central Gray Matter Involvement

As the central areas are metabolically active these areas are spared in mild to moderate insult due to shunting of blood; however in severe injury, there is involvement of thalamus and basal ganglia. On coronal ultrasound, thalami and basal ganglia appear echogenic and ventrolateral thalami are more echogenic than ventromedial one (Fig. 2.10). Normally thalami are of intermediate echotexture in term neonates while in preterm neonates (<32 weeks) thalami and basal ganglia are normally echogenic [15]. The involvement of thalami and basal ganglia can be either symmetrical or asymmetrical. The enhanced echogenicity of thalami and basal ganglia is the cause of the enhanced accentuation of the internal capsule. Normally anterior limb of

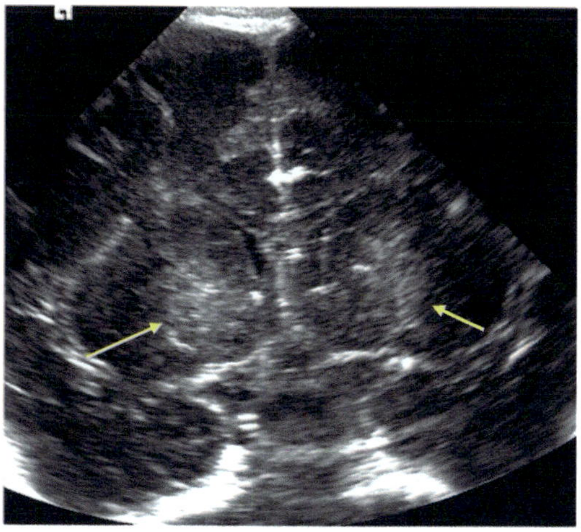

Fig. 2.10 Central grey matter injury in term HIE. Coronal images show echogenic basal ganglia. Note that the ventrolateral thalami (yellow arrows) are more echogenic than ventromedial part. This is a poor prognostic marker

the internal capsule is more echogenic than the posterior limb due to the perpendicular and parallel orientation of the white matter tracts, respectively [16]. Therefore, the anterior limb is accentuated in case of increased echogenicity of basal ganglia while the discrimination between the thalamus and posterior limb increases. Therefore, knowledge of the deep gray and white matters normal echogenicity is a crucial precondition for identifying hypoxic ischemic injury affecting the central gray matter.

2.4.2.2 Peripheral Injury

In mild to moderate injury, insult is seen in the peripheral areas in the watershed areas due to which there is either accentuation or loss of gray white matter distinction [17]. In the anterior-most coronal scan, peripheral white matter appears echogenic, and the periventricular white matter appears echogenic, however, in the midcoronal scan the subcortical areas are not hypoechoic. In hypoxia, these subcortical areas become echogenic. Normal periventricular halo which is seen in the sagittal plane is relatively echogenic which is due to anisotropy and is seen through the anterior fontanelle and disappears through the posterior fontanelle. While in HIE, due to the involvement of subcortical white matter either due to ischemia or edema appears echogenic and the periventricular halo becomes indistinct. The perirolandic area also appears echogenic which can be visualized through anterior fontanelle with posterior angulation [18]. In the peripheral insult, central areas are also looked for central injury.

Various critical ultrasound findings which can be seen in very severe ischemia include intraventricular hemorrhage, parenchymal hamorrhage, reversal of gray white matter echogenicity, and cerebral edema. As described earlier, gray matter is hypoechoic compared to subcortical white matter, however in severe ischemia, there is increased echogenicity of the gray matter causing the reversal of gray white matter differentiation. Cerebral edema is seen as effacement of sulcal spaces with slit ventricular system. Finally, the brain damage leads to gliosis, cystic encephalomalacia with ex vacuo dilatation and porencephalic cyst formation [19].

2.5 Intracranial Hemorrhage

2.5.1 Parenchymal Hemorrhage

Parenchymal hemorrhage in acute phase is manifested as echogenic focal lesion (Fig. 2.11a). In subacute/chronic phase, it can be seen as a less echogenic area with or without cystic areas within [4].

2.5.2 Extra-Axial Hemorrhage

Extra-axial hemorrhage can be either in the form of IVH, subpial, subdural, and subarachnoid hemorrhage (Fig. 2.11b–d) [4]. IVH has been discussed earlier in this chapter.

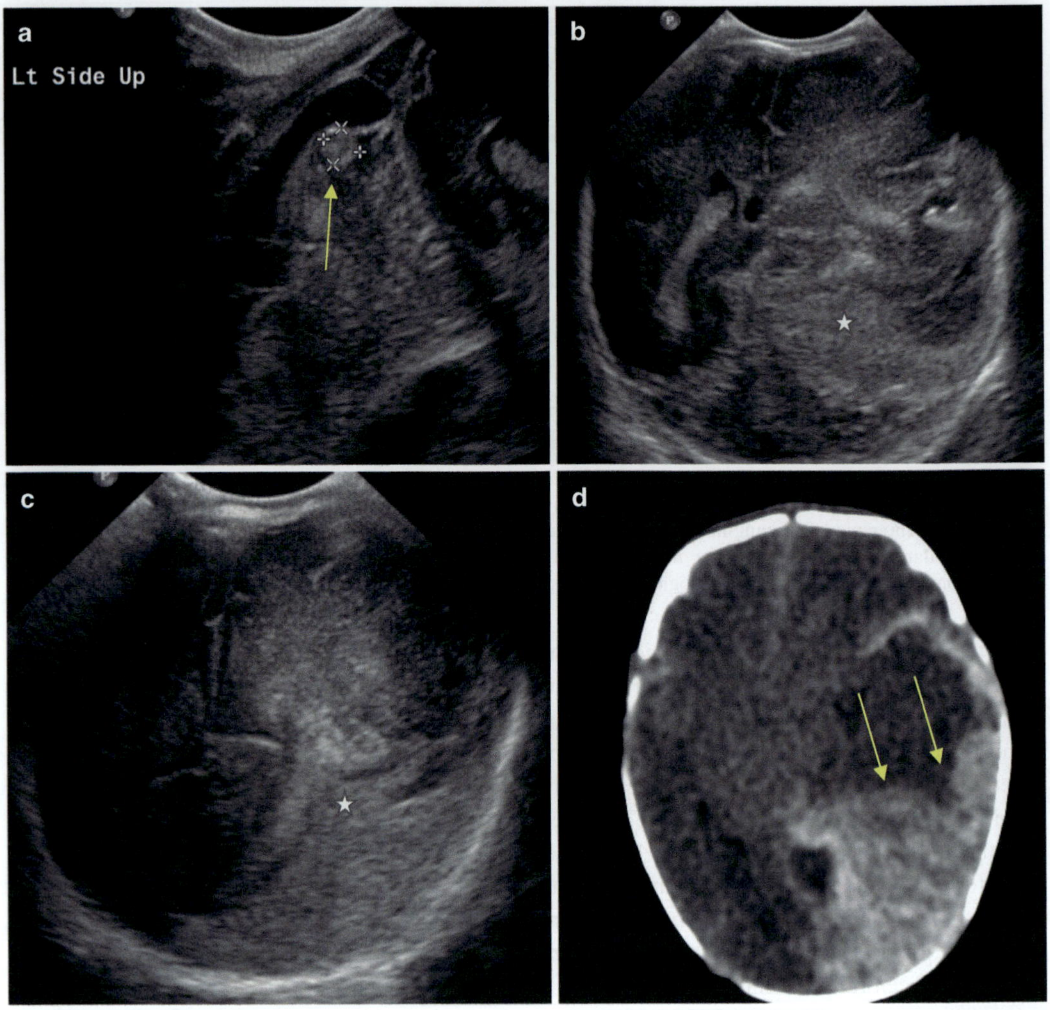

Fig. 2.11 (**a**–**d**) Intracranial hemorrhage. (**a**) Axial US image through mastoid fontanelle showing a small intraparenchymal hematoma (arrow). (**b**, **c**) Coronal US images show left occipital subpial hemorrhage (asterisk). (**d**) Hyperdense subpial hematoma (arrows)

2.6 Venous Sinus Thrombosis

Cranial US can be used for diagnosis and follow-up in venous sinus thrombosis in neonates [20]. While anterior approach provides a suitable window for a large part of the superior sagittal sinus, mastoid approach is ideal for the evaluation of the transverse and sigmoid sinuses. Normal venous sinuses are seen as anechoic triangular area, showing color flow on Doppler. In cases of sinus thrombosis, the sinuses become echogenic and Doppler signal is absent (Fig. 2.12).

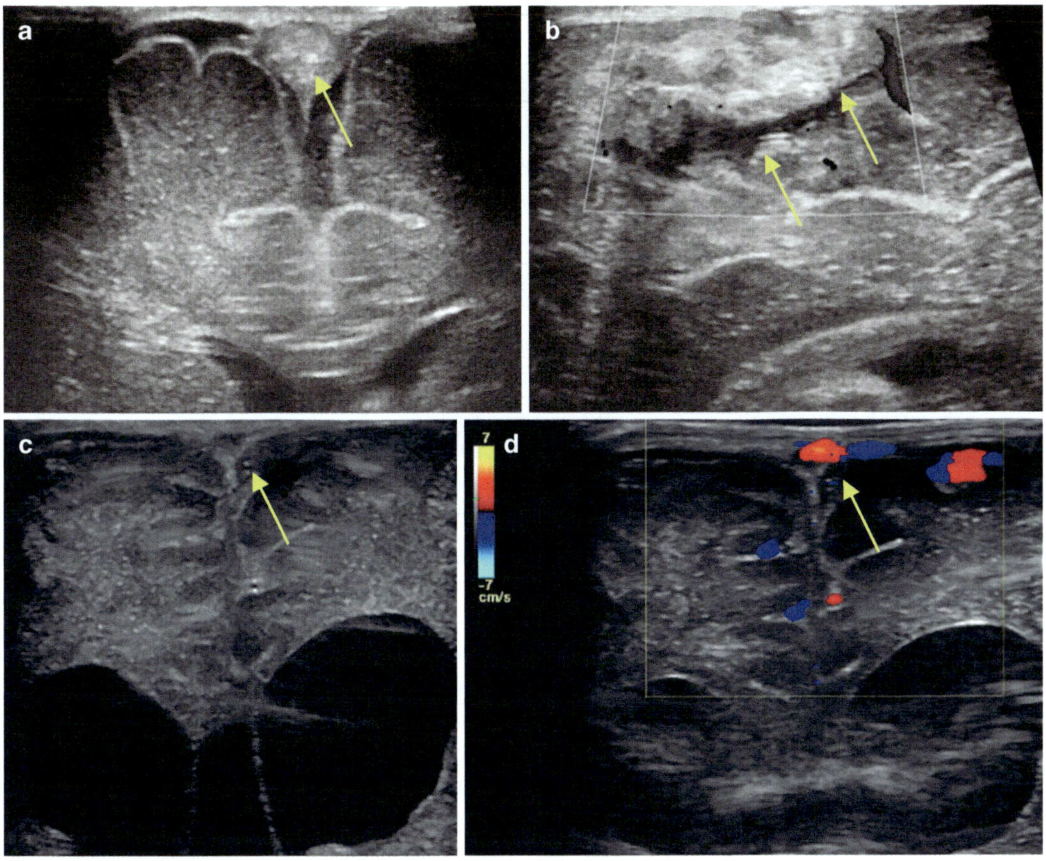

Fig. 2.12 (**a**–**d**) Coronal and parasagittal views of cranial ultrasound of an unresponsive neonate reveals an eccentric echogenic thrombus (arrows in **a**, **b**) causing luminal expansion in the superior sagittal sinus evident on limited color Doppler imaging. Coronal greyscale (**c**) and Doppler (**d**) images on follow-up of the same neonate post anticoagulant treatment reveals near complete resolution of echogenic thrombus in the superior sagittal sinus (arrow in **c**) with partial recanalization evident on color doppler imaging (arrow in **d**)

2.7 Lenticulostriate Vasculopathy

Lenticulostriate Vasculopathy (LSV) refers to echogenic vessels in the basal ganglia region. There is thickening of the corresponding walls on histopathology. On CUS, it is seen as a linear/strip-like or branching echogenicity in the basal ganglia (Fig. 2.13). It can be seen in association with various conditions such as neonatal cytomegalovirus infections, congenital anomalies, chromosomal abnormalities, hypoxic ischemic insult, fetal alcohol or drug exposure, neonatal lupus erythematosus, twin-to-twin transfusion or diabetic fetopathy, etc. The prognostic implications of LSV are unclear [21].

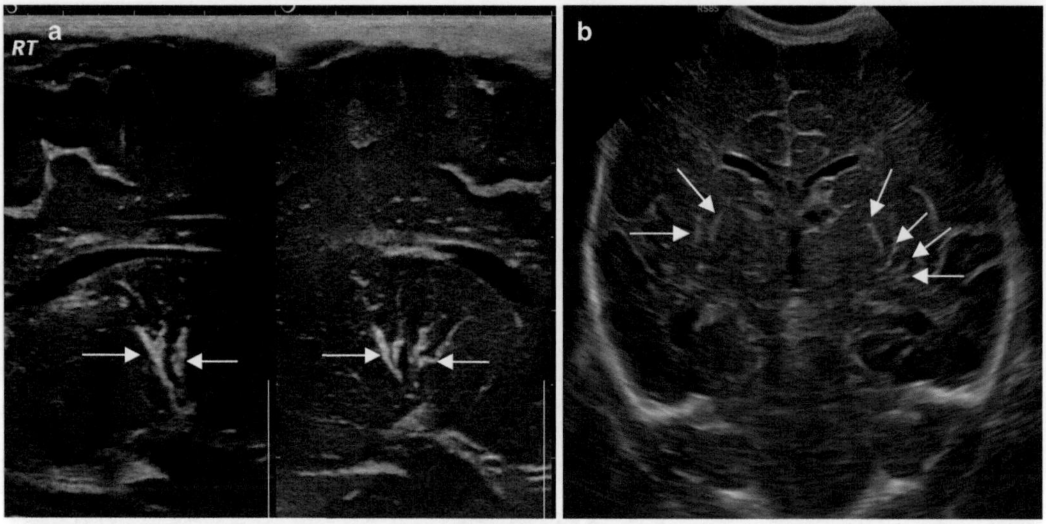

Fig. 2.13 Lenticulostriate vasculopathy (LSV). Parasagittal (**a**) and coronal (**b**) ultrasound images showing echogenic linear radiating pattern of the vessels (arrows) in basal ganglia

2.8 Intracranial Infections

2.8.1 Congenital Infections

Congenital infections such as cytomegalovirus may manifest as microcephaly, sensorineural hearing loss, and cataract. CUS features include periventricular/basal ganglia calcification, abnormal gyral pattern, extra-axial fluid collection, and LSV.

2.8.2 Neonatal Infections

CT and MRI remain the choice of investigation in suspected intracranial infections. However, CUS serves as a good screening tool in suspected ventriculitis or following up a known case of intracerebral focal lesion. On CUS, ventriculitis can be manifested as echogenic debris inside the ventricles and increased echogenicity of the walls [22]. However, Doppler ultrasound may not be very sensitive in detecting the inflammation along the ventricular wall. Contrast-enhanced ultrasound (CEUS) might have an additional role in detecting ventriculitis/ependymitis [23]. Meningitis is manifested as increased echogenicity of the pial lining of the parenchyma (Fig. 2.14). Ventricular adhesion and debris may result in ventriculomegaly on follow-up (Fig. 2.15). Intracranial focal lesions (focal cerebritis/abscess) can be detected and followed up on USG [22].

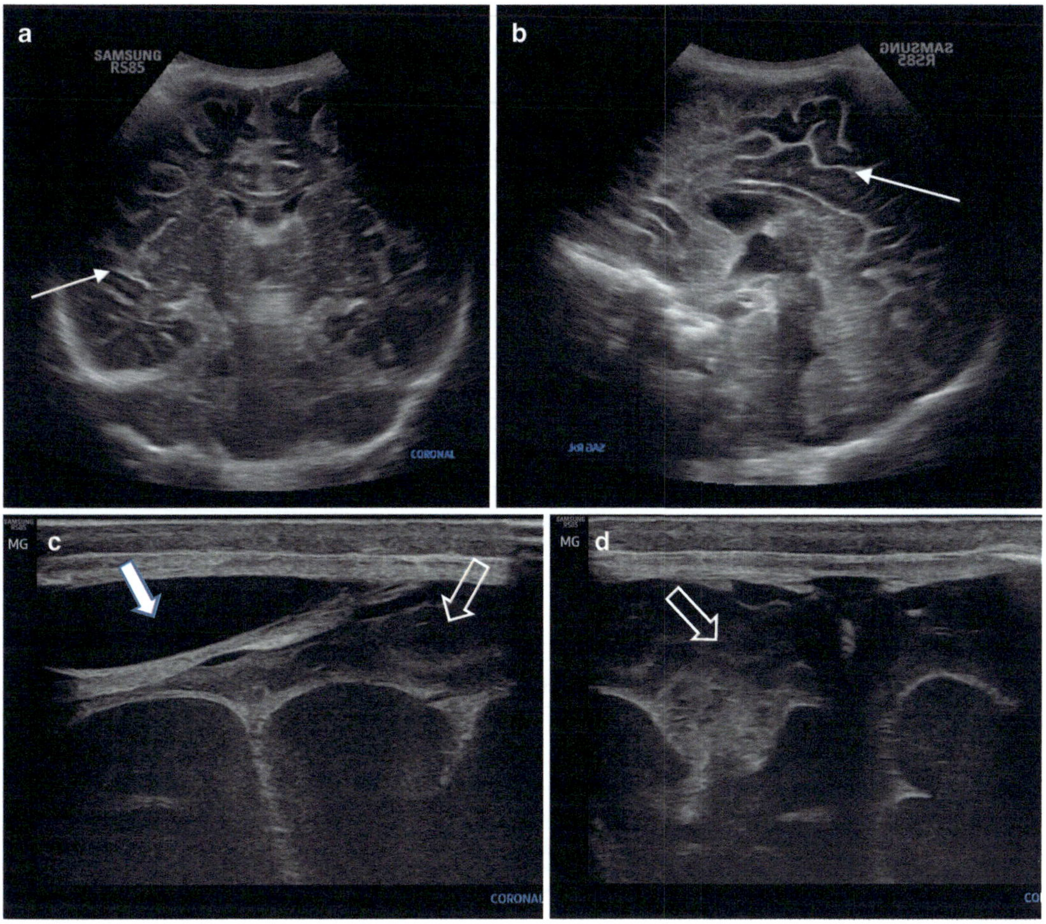

Fig. 2.14 (**a**–**d**) Meningitis in a neonate. Coronal (**a**) and mid-sagittal (**b**) US images show increased sulcal echogenicity (thin arrow). High resolution coronal ultrasound (**c**, **d**) showing subdural effusion (block arrow) and subarachnoid collection with thick debris (open arrows)

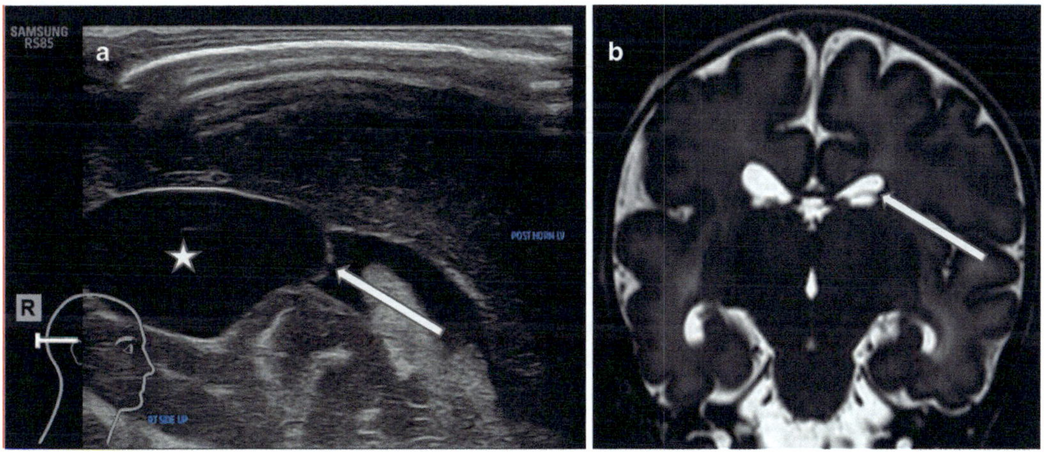

Fig. 2.15 (**a**, **b**) Intraventricular synechiae formation after meningitis. Axial US image through mastoid fontanelle (**a**) shows a synechia (arrow) and a trapped ventricular horn (asterisk). Coronal heavily T2W MR image (**b**) shows intraventricular synechia (arrow)

2.9 Congenital Malformations

While MRI is the imaging modality of choice in congenital brain malformations, CUS can act as a good initial screening modality [5]. In experienced hands, it is a very sensitive modality for screening of congenital anomalies.

- *Agenesis of the corpus callosum.*
- *Dandy-Walker spectrum.*
- *Arnold Chiari II malformation.*
- *Holoprosencephaly spectrum.*
- *Schizencephaly.*
- *Arachnoid cyst.*
- *Vein of Galen malformation.*
- *Disorders of neuronal migration/polymicrogyria.*

2.9.1 Corpus Callosal Agenesis

Congenital absence of the corpus callosum is manifested as an absence of the corpus callosum and radial arrangement of the mesial gyri in sagittal sections (Figs. 2.16 and 2.17). On the coronal images, the medial wall of the frontal horn of lateral ventricles appears to have indentations caused by the Probst bundles, giving rise to the "viking helmet" or "racing car" sign. Interhemispheric cyst or lipoma may be associated with it.

2.9.2 Dandy-Walker Phenotype

Dandy-Walker phenotype manifests as an enlarged posterior fossa, posterior fossa cyst communicating with the fourth ventricle, and vermian hypoplasia. In the absence of cerebellar hypoplasia, mega cisterna magna may present with a retrocerebellar cystic structure. However, the posterior fossa is not enlarged in mega cisterna magna. It can be associated with other congenital intracranial anomalies.

2.9.3 Arnold Chiari II Malformation

Arnold Chiari II malformation has a high association with lumbosacral myelomeningocele. The posterior fossa is small, and there is crowding of cerebellar tonsil around the brainstem at the level of foramen magnum. Tectal beaking can be appreciated on mid-sagittal images. The demonstration of cervicomedullary kink in the cervical spine can be challenging, due to difficult probe positioning at the neck and poor acoustic window. However,

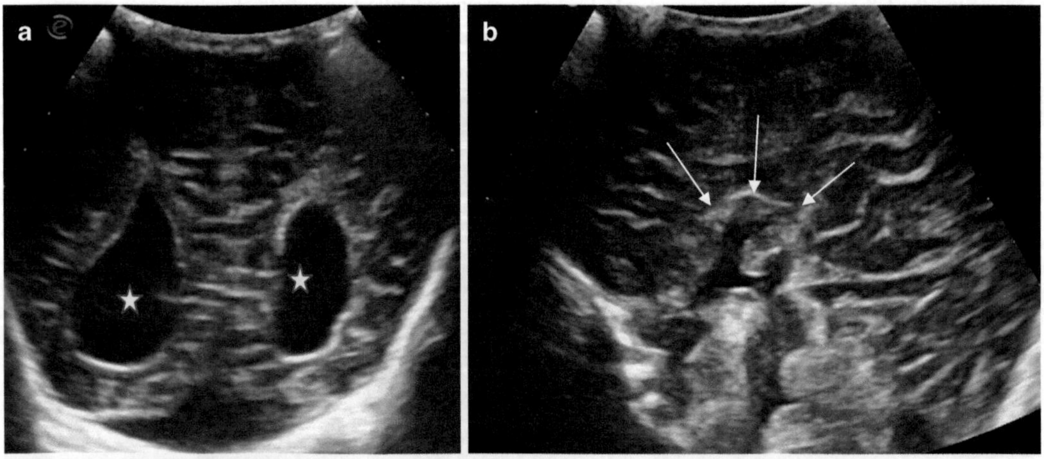

Fig. 2.16 (**a**, **b**) Agenesis of corpus callosum. (**a**) Coronal ultrasound image showing parallel orientation of the lateral ventricles (asterisk) with colpocephaly. (**b**) Mid-sagittal image showing absence of the corpus callosum with radially arranged gyri (arrows)

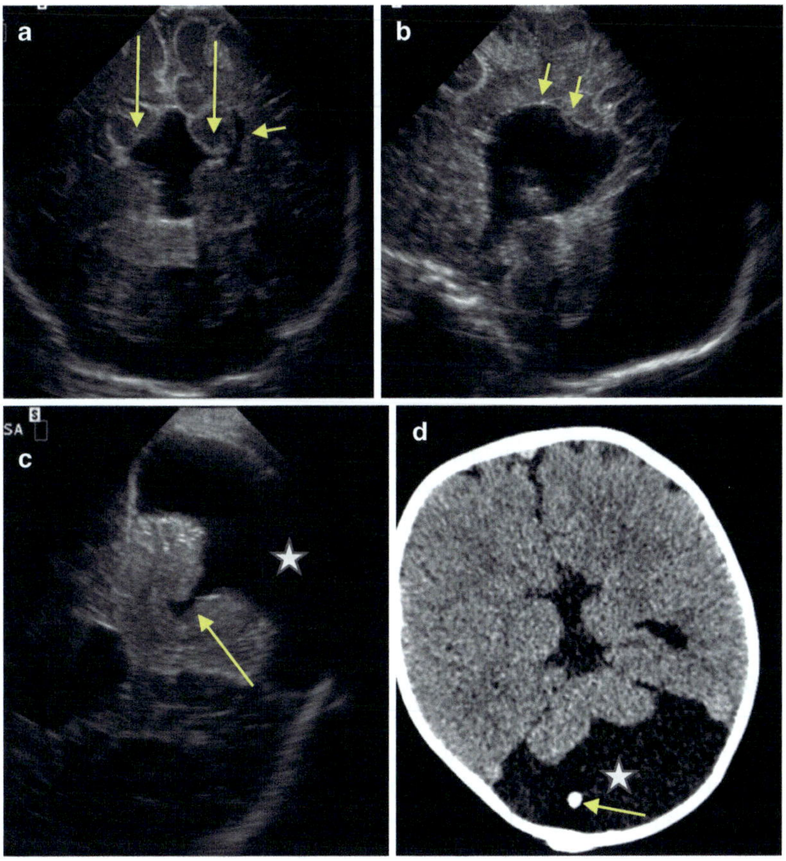

Fig. 2.17 (**a**–**d**) Corpus callosal agenesis with Dandy Walker phenotype. Coronal US image (**a**) showing 'viking helmet' appearance of the frontal horn (short arrow) of lateral ventricles and Probst bundles (long arrow). Parasagittal US image (**b**) showing radial orientation of the mesial gyri (arrows) in agenesis of corpus callosum. Axial US image through mastoid fontanelle (**c**) and axial NCCT brain (**d**) of the same patient showing a large posterior fossa cyst (asterisk) communicating with the 4th ventricle (arrow in **c**). Note the tip of the cysto-peritoneal shunt (arrow in **d**)

on occasions, insonation through the nuchal ligament with the neonate in the prone position is helpful in demonstrating vermian herniation.

2.9.4 Holoprosencephaly Spectrum

The three subtypes of holoprosencephaly (lobar, semilobar, alobar) present with variable fusion of the ventricles, deep gray matter, and the cerebellar hemispheres. In all the three subtypes, septum pellucidum is absent. Alobar holoprosencephaly shows fusion of the lateral ventricles and the basal ganglia and thalami along with absence of falx and interhemispheric fissure. The lobar variant may present with mild changes such as fusion of the frontal horn of the lateral ventricles and absent septum pellucidum.

2.9.5 Lissencephaly

While type I lissencephaly can be easily detected on cranial ultrasound, milder forms of type II lissencephaly and other forms of neuronal migration disorders are difficult to diagnose on cranial ultrasound and require MRI. In lissencephaly, the sulcal depth is reduced, along with a reduced number of gyri.

2.9.6 Schizencephaly

Schizencephaly refers to a gray mattered lined tract communicating with an extra-axial cystic lesion. Detection of open lip schizencephaly is easier on ultrasound than closed lip ones; as the ventricular communication is evident in the open lip variant. However, MRI is superior for detection of the cortical malformations associated with it.

2.9.7 Arachnoid Cyst

These are extra-axial fluid-containing lesions in various intracranial locations, having a variable mass effect on the adjacent brain parenchyma. On ultrasound, they are seen as anechoic lesions with no color flow on Doppler imaging.

2.9.8 Vein of Galen Malformation

This is seen as a tubular/rounded anechoic lesion inferior to the splenium of the corpus callosum on a mid-sagittal image. Use of Doppler imaging is of paramount importance so as not to misdiagnose it as a cystic lesion. Ultrasound can be used for follow-up imaging in these neonates.

MR remains the imaging investigation of choice.

2.10 Role of Contrast-Enhanced Ultrasound (CEUS)

CEUS performed after intravenous administration of ultrasound contrast agent (most commonly used sulfur hexafluoride microbubble, Sonovue/Lumason) is a unique investigation targeted at evaluation of the microvasculature of an organ. While it has been approved by the US-FDA for the evaluation of pediatric focal liver lesions, applications for other indications in children are still off-label use. CEUS in transcranial ultrasound is not used routinely, however, it has been reported to be of use in several conditions, namely, hypoxic ischemic encephalopathy, intracranial hemorrhage, intracranial infections, and tumors [23].

2.11 Conclusion

Cranial ultrasound can be a useful diagnostic modality in experienced hands, especially in neonatal hypoxic ischemic injury and germinal matrix hemorrhage. It can be a good screening tool for suspected congenital anomalies and cerebral venous sinus thrombosis.

References

1. Dudink J, Jeanne Steggerda S, Horsch S, Agut T, Alarcon A, Arena R, et al. State-of-the-art neonatal cerebral ultrasound: technique and reporting. Pediatric Res. 2020;87(Suppl. 1):3–12.
2. Anon. AIUM practice parameter for the performance of Neurosonography in neonates and infants. J Ultrasound Med. 2020;39(5):E57–61.
3. Dorner RA, Burton VJ, Allen MC, Robinson S, Soares BP. Preterm neuroimaging and neurodevelopmental outcome: a focus on intraventricular hemorrhage, post-hemorrhagic hydrocephalus, and associated brain injury. J Perinatol. 2018;38(11):1431–43.
4. Caro-Domínguez P, Lecacheux C, Hernandez-Herrera C, Llorens-Salvador R. Cranial ultrasound for beginners. Transl Pediatr. 2021;10(4):1117–37.
5. Yoon HK, Cho SW. Neonatal head ultrasound: systematic approach to congenital central nervous system anomalies. A pictorial essay. Med Ultrason. 2016;18(3):386–93.
6. Maller VV, Cohen HL. Neurosonography: assessing the premature infant. Pediatr Radiol. 2017;47(9):1031–45.
7. Hand IL, Shellhaas RA, Milla SS. Routine neuroimaging of the preterm brain. Pediatrics. 2020;146(5):e2020029082.
8. Papile LA, Burstein J, Burstein R, Koffler H. Incidence and evolution of subependymal and intraventricular hemorrhage: a study of infants with birth weights less than 1500 g. J Pediatr. 1978;92(4):529–34.
9. Parodi A, Govaert P, Horsch S, Bravo MC, Ramenghi LA, Agut T, et al. Cranial ultrasound findings in preterm germinal matrix haemorrhage, sequelae and outcome. Pediatr Res. 2020;87(Suppl. 1):13–24.
10. Roze E, Benders MJ, Kersbergen KJ, Van Der Aa NE, Groenendaal F, Van Haastert IC, et al. Neonatal DTI early after birth predicts motor outcome in preterm infants with periventricular hemorrhagic infarction. Pediatr Res. 2015;78(3):298–303.

11. Agut T, Alarcon A, Cabañas F, Bartocci M, Martinez-Biarge M, Horsch S, et al. Preterm white matter injury: ultrasound diagnosis and classification. Pediatr Res. 2020;87(Suppl. 1):37–49.
12. Steggerda SJ, de Vries LS. Neonatal stroke in premature neonates. Semin Perinatol. 2021;45(7):151471.
13. Hwang M. Gray-scale ultrasound findings of hypoxic-ischemic injury in term infants. Pediatr Radiol. 2021;51(9):1738–47.
14. Lally PJ, Montaldo P, Oliveira V, Soe A, Swamy R, Bassett P, et al. Magnetic resonance spectroscopy assessment of brain injury after moderate hypothermia in neonatal encephalopathy: a prospective multicentre cohort study. Lancet Neurol. 2019;18(1):35–45.
15. Naidich TP, Gusnard DA, Yousefzadeh DK. Sonography of the internal capsule and basal ganglia in infants: 1. Coronal sections. AJNR Am J Neuroradiol. 1985;6(6):909–17.
16. Leijser LM, de Vries LS, Cowan FM. Using cerebral ultrasound effectively in the newborn infant. Early Hum Dev. 2006;82(12):827–35.
17. Daneman A, Epelman M, Blaser S, Jarrin JR. Imaging of the brain in full-term neonates: does sonography still play a role? Pediatr Radiol. 2006;36(7):636–46.
18. Gonçalves FG, Hwang M. Superficial anatomy of the neonatal cerebrum—an ultrasonographic roadmap. Pediatr Radiol. 2021;51(3):353–70.
19. Chacko A, Andronikou S, Mian A, Gonçalves FG, Vedajallam S, Thai NJ. Cortical ischaemic patterns in term partial-prolonged hypoxic-ischaemic injury—the inter-arterial watershed demonstrated through atrophy, ulegyria and signal change on delayed MRI scans in children with cerebral palsy. Insights Imaging. 2020;11(1):53.
20. Raets MMA, Sol JJ, Govaert P, Lequin MH, Reiss IKM, Kroon AA, et al. Serial cranial US for detection of cerebral sinovenous thrombosis in preterm infants. Radiology. 2013;269(3):879–86.
21. Teele RL, Hernanz-Schulman M, Sotrel A. Echogenic vasculature in the basal ganglia of neonates: a sonographic sign of vasculopathy. Radiology. 1988;169(2):423–7. https://doi.org/10.1148/radiology.169.2.2845473.
22. Gupta P, Sodhi KS, Saxena AK, Khandelwal N, Singhi P. Neonatal cranial sonography: a concise review for clinicians. J Pediatr Neurosci. 2016;11(1):7–13.
23. Plut D, Prutki M, Slak P. The use of contrast-enhanced ultrasound (CEUS) in the evaluation of the neonatal brain. Children (Basel). 2023;10(8):1303.

3 Neonatal Ultrasound: Orbits, Face, and Neck

Youck Jen Siu Navarro, Austin Moats,
Abhay Srinivasan, Tamara Feygin,
and Karuna Shekdar

3.1 Introduction

The technique of B scan ultrasound (US) has been in use since 1950s. With technical progress in specifically designed probes, there has been significant improvement in the resolution of two-dimensional US and Doppler acquisition of various parts of the human body including the orbits, face, and neck [1, 2].

The easy availability, noninvasive nature, and wide spectrum of clinical applications make US an extremely useful modality in children including neonates. The utility of US imaging in the multimodality evaluation of various neonatal orbit, face, and neck pathologies will be emphasized in this chapter.

3.2 Biosafety

The eye and orbit are potentially sensitive to the thermal and mechanical effects of ultrasound. For ocular ultrasound, the maximum recommended values for thermal index (TI) and mechanical index (MI) are significantly lower than rest of the body tissues. So, it is recommended to use dedicated ocular settings. Limiting the acoustic output to Food and Drug Administration (FDA) recommended maximum levels is strongly advised [3]. This is also applicable for US of face and neck in the neonates.

The acoustic output in spectral (pulsed) and color Doppler modes is higher than gray scale US. Hence, adjusting settings to decrease acoustic output and limiting the time of the examination should be done when performing a Doppler examination [3, 4].

3.2.1 Orbit Ultrasound in Neonates

The location and cystic composition of the eye renders it suitable for US examination [4]. The advent of high-frequency transducers has remarkably improved the quality of information US evaluation of orbits can provide [4, 5]. Detailed cross-sectional anatomy of the entire globe and surrounding orbital structures can be visualized using conventional ultrasound transducers [6, 7]. Some of the seemingly incidental orbital lesions may be a first sign of an underlying systemic disorder [8].

US exams can often be compromised in neonates due to patient motion and movement of the eyes. Whenever feasible in neonates, US should be planned when baby is sleeping or when appli-

Y. J. S. Navarro · A. Moats · A. Srinivasan
T. Feygin · K. Shekdar (✉)
Department of Radiology, Perelman School of Medicine @ University of Pennsylvania,
The Children's Hospital of Philadelphia,
Philadelphia, PA, USA
e-mail: siunavarry@chop.edu; moatsa@chop.edu; srinivasaa@chop.edu; feygin@chop.edu; shekdar@chop.edu

K. S. Sodhi (ed.), *Neonatal Ultrasound*, https://doi.org/10.1007/978-981-97-8576-6_3

cable under the same sedation or anesthesia being done for another concurrent study or procedure.

3.2.2 Technique

Patient is placed in the supine position, and probe placed on the closed eyelids following gel application. Generous amount of gel will help to improve probe contact and prevent air gap. Sometimes a small and thin tape/tegaderm can help to keep the eyelids closed. A paper or drapery isolation field around the orbit may further prevent gel slippage. Additionally, the probe should rest lightly on top of the gel, decreasing the pressure on the eye. If there is too much pressure the anterior eye segment can collapse or get flattened, subsequently not visualized. For this reason, US is contraindicated in traumatic eye injuries and suspected eye rupture [6].

3.2.3 Equipment

High-frequency linear probes (7.5–15 MHz) are used to evaluate the internal structures of the globe. Smaller high-frequency linear probe, "hockey-stick" probe, with small footprint is ideally suited for ocular US evaluation in neonates [7, 8].

3.2.4 Protocol

US assessment should include both orbits. The orbit should be assessed in both transverse and sagittal planes. With the probe in the transverse plane, the sonographer should scan the globe from top to bottom. In the sagittal plane, the globe should be scanned from temporal to nasal side.

Color Doppler can be used for assessing vessels or a vascular lesion. Doppler parameters need to be adjusted for low flow. With the help of power or color Doppler, the presence of blood flow and depiction of even small vessels such as the central retinal ones is possible.

3.2.5 Orbit US Anatomy

Knowledge of the US technique and normal anatomy is essential for accurate and prompt diagnosis. The orbital cavity represents a large bony socket, containing the optic globe, with extra ocular muscles, nerves, blood vessels, and fat. The optic globe is anatomically divided into anterior and posterior segments.

The structures of the eye can be identified on US with echogenic lines and anechoic areas (Fig. 3.1). The cornea appears as a thin convex line that sometimes may be unseen. The anterior chamber, between the cornea and lens, is filled

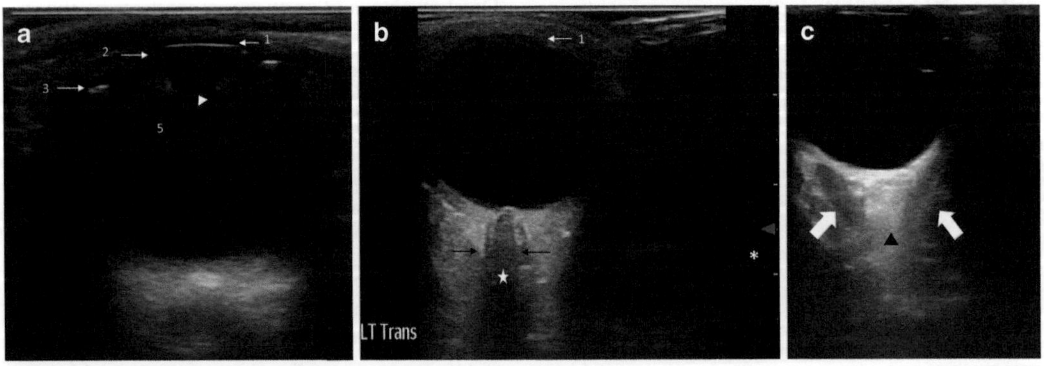

Fig. 3.1 Ocular ultrasound anatomy. Grayscale ultrasound of the optic globe in transverse plane. (**a**) Anterior segment anatomy: cornea (1), anterior chamber (2), iris/ciliary body (3), lens (white arrowhead). (**b**) Optic nerve (star) and optic sheath (black arrows) are well depicted. Imaging resolution improves when the focus is adjusted at the area of interest (asterisk). (**c**) Extraocular muscles (thick white arrows) and intraconal fat as echogenic area (black arrowhead)

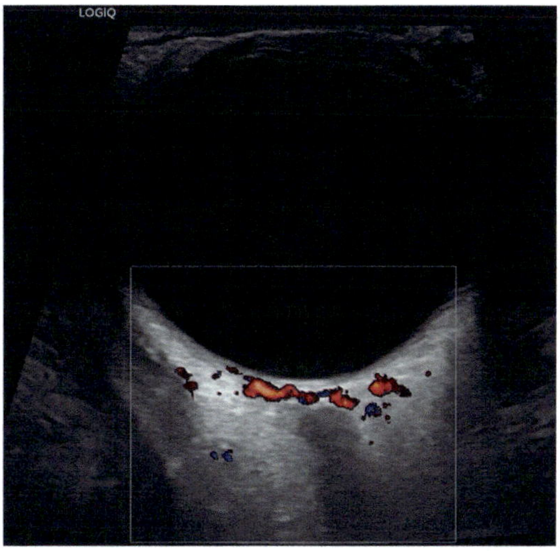

Fig. 3.2 Ocular color Doppler normal US. Normal color flow, depicting the tiny posterior ciliary arteries

with anechoic fluid, representing the aqueous humor. The ciliary bodies are seen on either side of the lens, appearing as hypoechoic structures. The posterior segment, which is larger and containing the vitreous body, is the anechoic area posterior to the lens. Posterior to the eye globe, the orbital fat appears hyperechoic, and extraocular muscles appear hypoechoic. The optic nerve is visible as a hypoechoic band posterior to the optic disc and extending posteriorly and medially [8]. The central retinal artery and short posterior tiny ciliary arteries are seen at color Doppler US [7] (Fig. 3.2).

3.2.6 Transient Phenomenon of the Newborn Eye

There are physiological changes which are transient, that occur in the eyes of neonates during the first month of life, particularly in the preterm neonates. Certain characteristics on B-mode ocular ultrasound should be considered normal in neonates which would be considered pathological in adults. These findings include visualization of the Tenon's capsule, sonolucent extraocular muscles, prominent superior ophthalmic vein, and vitreous opacities. Additional imaging may be warranted only if these findings persist beyond the perinatal period.

3.3 Common Indications for Ocular Ultrasound Evaluation in Neonates

3.3.1 Persistent Fetal Vasculature/Persistent Hyperplastic Primary Vitreous

Persistent fetal vasculature (PFV), also known as persistent hyperplastic primary vitreous (PHPV) is a congenital ocular abnormality in which the embryonic vasculature fails to regress partially or completely [9, 10]. PFV accounts for 5% of childhood blindness in western countries. The clinical presentation is of leukocoria with poor vision and small globe. PFV can be isolated posterior form (15–25%), isolated anterior form (5–25%), or mixed anterior and posterior form (50–80%). Majority of cases are unilateral, with less than 10% being bilateral. Bilateral PFV lesions are associated with syndromic conditions, like Norrie, Walker-Warburg, trisomy 13, congenital CMV and Rubella, metabolic disease like G6PD (glucose 6 phosphate dehydrogenase deficiency), and maternal cocaine use during pregnancy.

On imaging, there is a triangular retrolental soft tissue with a linear stalk of the hyaloid artery extending from retrolental region to the optic nerve head resulting in the classic "Martini glass" shape of the soft tissue. On US, hyperechoic retrolental tissue stalk is seen with the thickened hyaloid, seen as double line at pars plana (Fig. 3.3). On Color Doppler imaging, blood flow can be detected in the retrolental fibrovascular membrane tethering the lens into the vitreous [6] (Fig. 3.3).

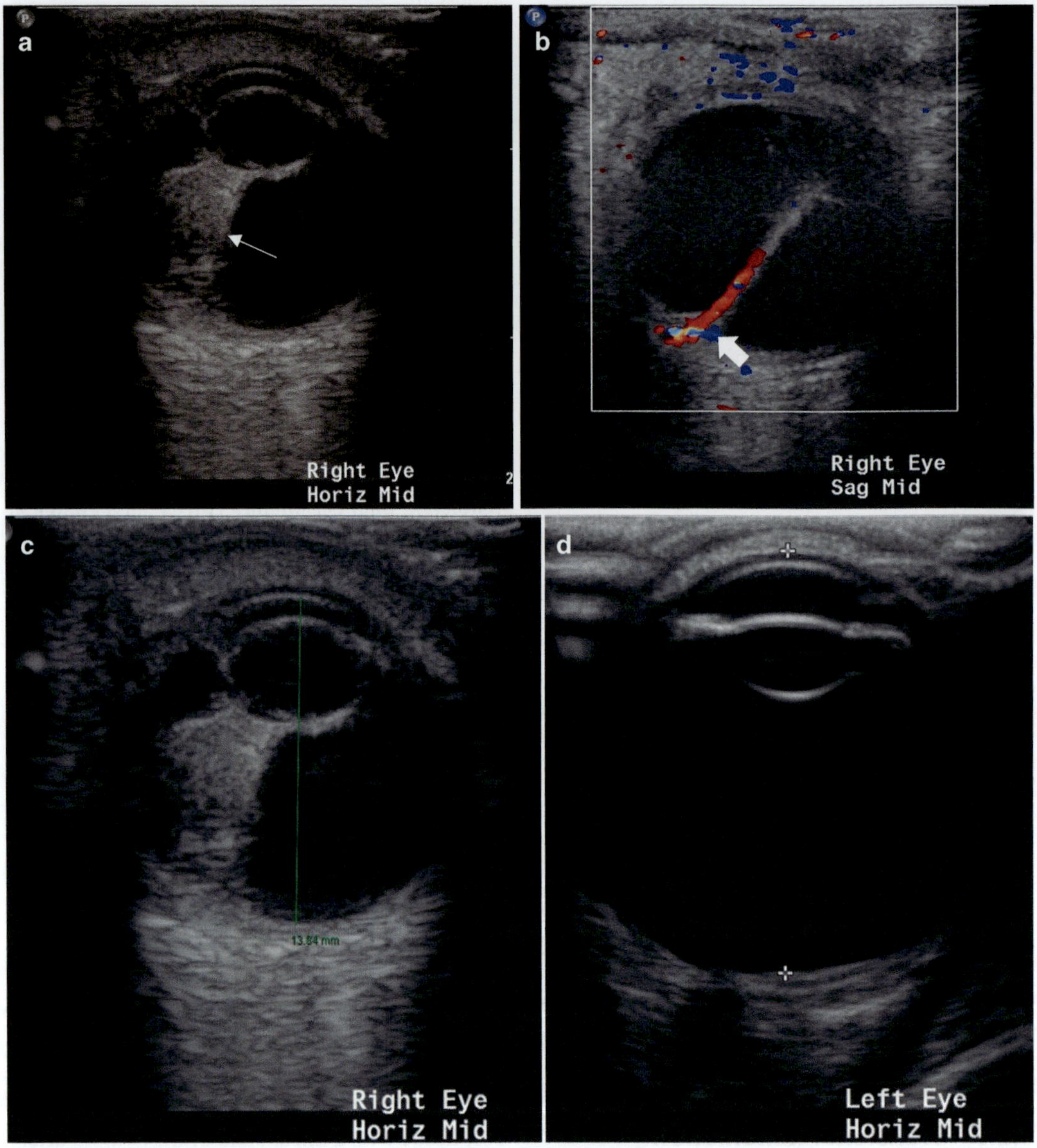

Fig. 3.3 PFV. Gray-scale image in a 4 weeks old with right eye leukocoria demonstrates (**a**) an echogenic band (thin white arrow) extending across the vitreous. (**b**) Color doppler demonstrates flow within the persistent hyaloid artery (thick white arrow). Side-by side comparison of small right globe with PFV (**c**), and normal left optic globe (**d**). Images courtesy: Dr. Ajay Taranath (Women's and Children's Hospital, Adelaide, SA, Australia)

3.3.2 Cataracts

A cataract results from clouding of the lens of one or both eyes. Neonates with cataracts are mostly congenital. Majority of the congenital cataracts are detected on antenatal US. On fetal and neonatal US, the normal lens appears as a hyperechoic ring with a hypoechoic center. Cataracts can be detected on ultrasound as echogenic area in the expected position of the lens and loss of the normal hypoechoic center of the lens. The edges of the lens may appear thickened and irregular (Fig. 3.4).

Intrauterine infections TORCH—toxoplasmosis, rubella, cytomegalovirus, herpes simplex virus, varicella and syphilis are common causes

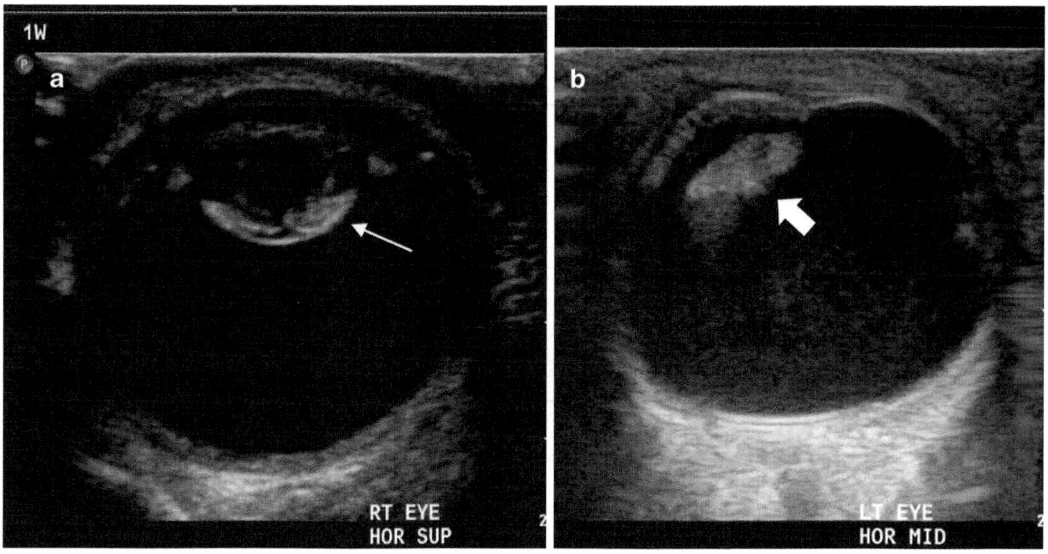

Fig. 3.4 Congenital cataract. Ocular Ultrasound images in two different neonates with cataract (**a**) Thick rim of increased echogenicity involving the right lens (**b**) Entire left lens is echogenic with somewhat irregular margin. Images courtesy: Dr. Ajay Taranath (Women's and Children's Hospital, Adelaide, SA, Australia)

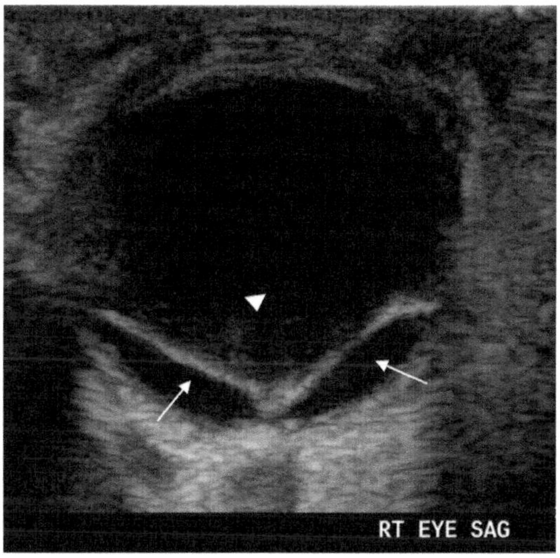

Fig. 3.5 Retinopathy of Prematurity (ROP). 28 weeks preterm infant with ROP. Ultrasound depicts retinal detachment (arrows) and subretinal exudate (arrowhead). Image courtesy: Dr. Ajay Taranath (Women's and Children's Hospital, Adelaide, SA, Australia)

of congenital cataracts. Chromosomal abnormalities (trisomy 13, 18, and 21) and metabolic diseases such as galactosemia, hypoparathyroidism, and maternal diabetes are other causes of congenital cataracts.

3.3.3 Retinopathy of Prematurity

Retinopathy of prematurity (ROP) referred to in older literature as "retrolental fibroplasia," is a vasoproliferative retinal disorder that occurs in premature infants born with immature retinal vasculature. Premature birth interrupts with the normal process of vasculogenesis, which results in incomplete vascularization of retina and hypoxia and causes abnormal neovascularization [9–11]. The common high risk factors for ROP include female gender, low birth weight, and low gestational age. US findings in ROP are usually bilateral but can be asymmetric with regards to amount of echogenic material in the vitreous chamber, and with extent of ocular detachments (Fig. 3.5). In advanced stages, the globe can become small and calcified-phthisis bulbi. US evaluation is useful in the documentation of the progression of ROP, especially in aggressive cases, and can demonstrate sequelae of ROP.

3.3.4 Dacryocystocele

A dacryocystocele (DC) is one of the most common abnormalities [12–14] of infant lacrimal

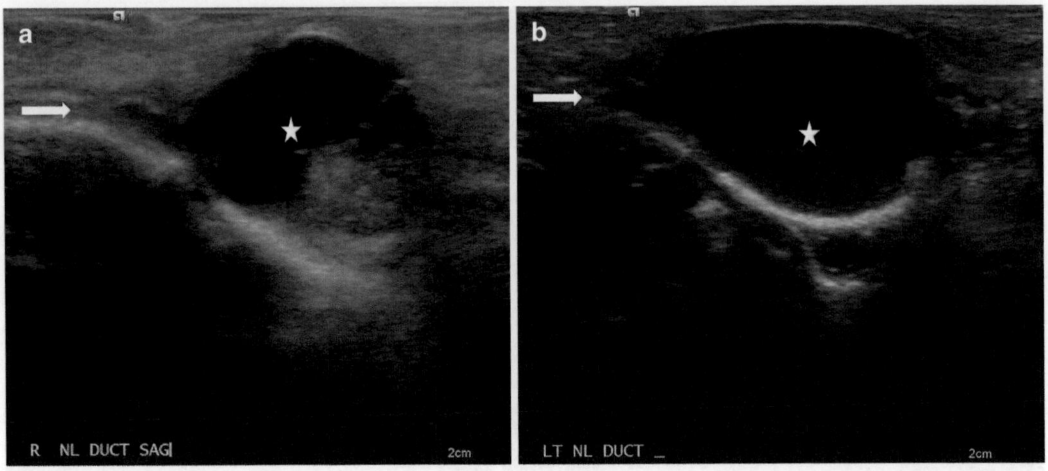

Fig. 3.6 Bilateral dacryocystocele. US images in sagittal planes of bilateral orbits, (**a**) right, (**b**) left, show fusiform dilation of both nasolacrimal ducts, containing mobile debris, right greater than left (star). Connection of dacryocystocele with tubular nasolacrimal duct is seen (arrow), consistent with bilateral dacryocystocele

apparatus. Congenital DC results from congenital nasolacrimal duct obstruction [14]. DC usually presents as a focal cystic swelling below or at the medial canthus [14, 15]. DC can be diagnosed by physical examination typically on the first day of life, with a mean age at presentation at 7 days. DC can be unilateral or bilateral [12]. On postnatal US, a DC appears as anechoic or hypoechoic round lesion with thin wall and increased through transmission at medial canthus. Connection with tubular nasolacrimal duct can be demonstrated in some cases (Fig. 3.6). DCs have no blood flow in or around them on color Doppler evaluation. It is important to differentiate DCs from other causes of periorbital cystic lesions. The differential diagnosis for dacryocystocele includes encephalocele, hemangioma, and dermoid cysts [13–15].

3.3.5 Congenital Orbit Malformations Spectrum

Coloboma is a defect in the posterior globe which results from failure of the embryonic choroidal fissure to close properly with vitreous fluid herniation via the defect. Small colobomas are better seen with MR than ultrasound.

Congenital cystic eye (CCE) is a rare abnormality which results from arrest of the globe formation at the vesicle stage due to incomplete or absent invagination of the optic vesicle [16, 17]. The optic globe is replaced by a cystic cavity lined by neuroglial tissue. CCE should be differentiated from microphthalmia with cyst and from severe posterior colobomas.

Congenital simple microphthalmia (MO) is characterized by a small globe containing normal anatomic structures and is typically unilateral [18, 19]. Congenital complex MO is usually bilateral and associated with other orbit anomalies like colobomas and brain anomalies [18, 19].

Anophthalmia (AO) is a congenital absence of one or both globes. It can be primary, due to failure of optic vesicle development or as part of general abnormality of forebrain development or degenerative AO, which is characterized by initial formation of the optic vesicle with subsequent degeneration [18, 19].

3.3.6 Neonatal Tumors of the Orbit

3.3.6.1 Dermoid and Epidermoid

Dermoid and epidermoid cysts are congenital inclusion cysts (ICs) resulting in choristomatous collection [20, 21]. Dermoid includes dermal appendages while epidermoid does not contain any dermal adnexal structures [21]. Dermoid cyst (dermoid) is the most common orbital cystic lesion in children, accounting for over 40% of all orbital lesions of childhood and for 89% of all orbital cystic lesions of childhood that need biopsy or surgical removal [22]. The typical presentation of ICs is of a nontender subcutaneous nodule near orbital rim, commonly at lateral eyebrow, at the glabella and nasal tip.

US evaluation can be adequate for simple superficial ICs without posterior extension. On US, ICs are seen as well-circumscribed mass with high internal reflectivity and variable attenuation (Fig. 3.7). Internal debris may at times impair determination of cystic nature of the lesion [20, 21].

3.3.6.2 Teratoma

Orbital teratomas are rare congenital tumors that present in a neonate. Teratomas contain tissue derived from all three germ cell layers and discussed in further detail with teratomas of the face and neck.

The most common presentation of an orbital teratoma is extreme unilateral proptosis in an otherwise healthy full-term infant. Typically, the tumor is heterogeneous with mixed cystic-solid components, and usually the bony orbit is markedly expanded. US can clearly delineate components of the teratoma and differentiate from other congenital lesions, such as microphthalmos with cyst, dermoid cyst, congenital cystic eye, hemangioma, and meningoencephalocele.

Vascular lesions of the orbit and periorbital region including hemangiomas, lymphatic malformations are discussed in detail along with the vascular lesions of the extracranial head, face, and neck.

3.4 Face and Neck Ultrasound

3.4.1 Technique

The face and neck structures are located close to the skin surface and can be easily evaluated by US examination even in the neonates. High-frequency probes (10–15 MHz) are used for the ultrasound examination on the patient lying in supine decubitus and with their neck stretched out. The complete scan of the neck includes the evaluation of the thyroid and salivary glands and the vascular structures as well as the lymph node analysis.

Some of the common indications requested for neck and face evaluation by ultrasound in neonates are discussed below.

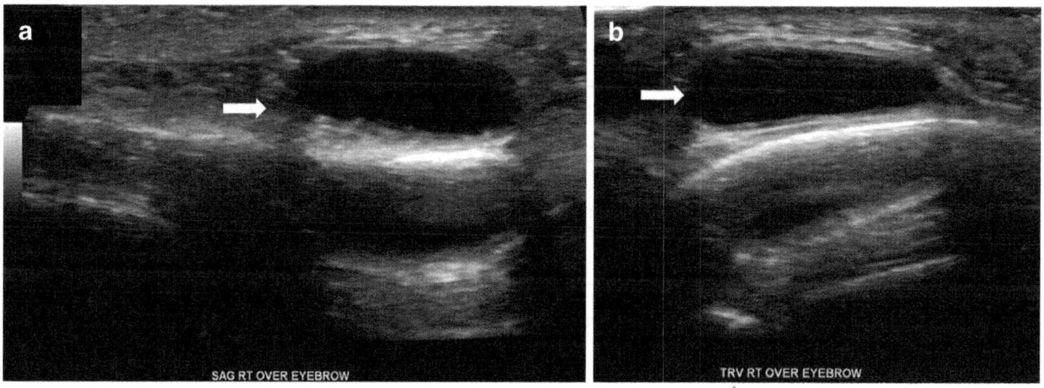

Fig. 3.7 Dermoid cyst. Ultrasound image in the sagittal plane (**a**) and transverse plane (**b**) demonstrate a subcutaneous, avascular, hypoechoic cystic lesion at the right eyebrow (arrow), representing a dermoid cyst. Underlying bony structure is intact

3.4.2 Fibromatosis Colli

Fibromatosis colli is a benign fusiform mass involving the sternocleidomastoid muscle in neonates. This entity is also known by the names of "sternocleidomastoid muscle (SCM) tumor of infancy" and "congenital muscular torticollis." This is a self-limited, painless benign mass of the SCM, thought to be due to a replacement of normal muscle fibers by fibrous tissue due to a "scar-like" reaction [22, 23]). The tumor typically does not extend beyond the muscle. Fibromatosis colli (FC) typically affects neonates with history of breech of neck mass or difficult obstetric history presenting with torticollis typically in the first 2–4 weeks of life. This has been reported to be common in first born neonates, and more common on the right side and rarely may be bilateral [2].

The affected portion of the SCM is enlarged and appears hyperechoic on US (Fig. 3.8) exam compared to the normal hypoechoic appearance of the muscle with thin echogenic lines of the muscle fascicles extending along the length of the muscle. Depending on the extent of SCM involvement, proportionate hyperechoic appearance is noted. The lower third of the SCM is found to be commonly involved in FC. With increasing severity, the middle third and the entire length of the SCM can be involved. Variable vascularity can be noted within and surrounding the lesion. There is usually no associated lymphadenopathy.

3.4.3 Vascular Lesions of Neonatal Orbit, Extracranial Head and Neck

Last revision of Mulliken and Glowacki classification of pediatric vascular pathology was accepted by the International Society for the Study of Vascular Anomalies in 2018 [24–26]. This classification divides vascular lesions in children as vascular tumors and non-tumoral congenital malformation, with further detailed subdivisions of each sections [26]. Vascular tumors are characterized as: (1) benign, (2) locally aggressive or borderline, and (3) malignant types. Congenital vascular malformations are categorized according to their flow pattern, as high or low-flow types; they are also described as (1) simple or combined (when several types of malformations co-exist in one lesion) and as (2) sporadic or with associated genetic mutation.

3.4.4 Lymphatic Malformations (LM)

LMs are the most common congenital non-neoplastic vascular lesions, consisting of a mixture of anomalous lymphatic and venous channels in different proportions. When there is an abundance of lymphatic tissue, the lesion is defined as "lymphatic malformation." Previous literature refers to them as "cystic hygromas" or "lymphan-

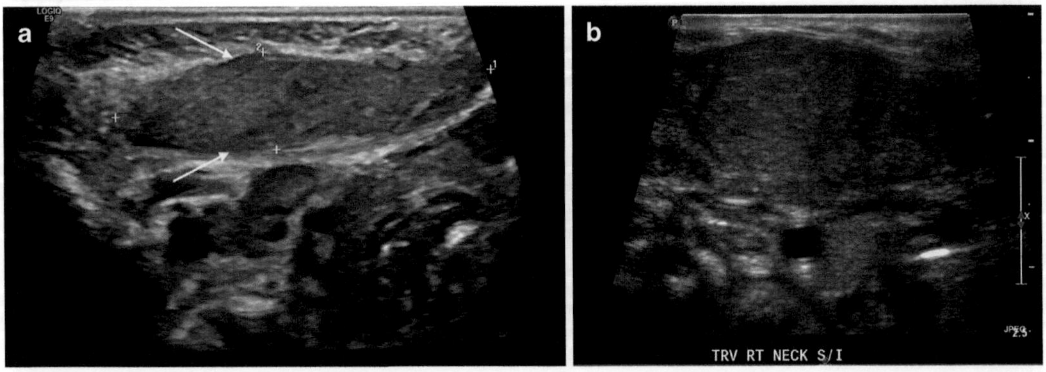

Fig. 3.8 Fibromatosis colli. Ultrasound image in the sagittal plane (**a**) demonstrates a slightly hypoechoic mass centered in the right sternocleidomastoid muscle with a fusiform shape consistent with fibromatosis colli. Similar findings are also seen within the right neck of another patient with fibromatosis colli (**b**)

giomas." LMs are thought to be derived from sequestration of primordial lymphatic sacs that fail to communicate with the peripheral draining channels. Malformations with predominant venous component usually manifest clinically later in life, and therefore rare to encounter in neonates. Extracranial head and neck are the most common locations for lymphatic malformations accounting for nearly 75% of all lymphatic malformations [27, 28].

LMs are easily recognized on US imaging as large multiloculated, trans-spatial, cystic masses with intervening septa and blood–fluid levels. US is especially helpful to reveal the macrocystic components of lymphatic malformations which appear as anechoic or hypoechoic cystic components. The micro-cystic components on US appear hyperechoic due to numerous wall interfaces. LMs typically do not show intrinsic increased vascularity or calcifications [29, 30]. LM typically have no or only minimal solid appearing portions; the resultant mass effect on surrounding tissue usually is mild, even for large lesions (Fig. 3.9). Colored Doppler provides helpful assessment of great neck vessels, providing vascular supply for the lesion. Lymphatic malformations may be quite different in volume, depending on size of their cysts, ranging from a few millimeters to a large cystic conglomerate, measuring several centimeters [28–30].

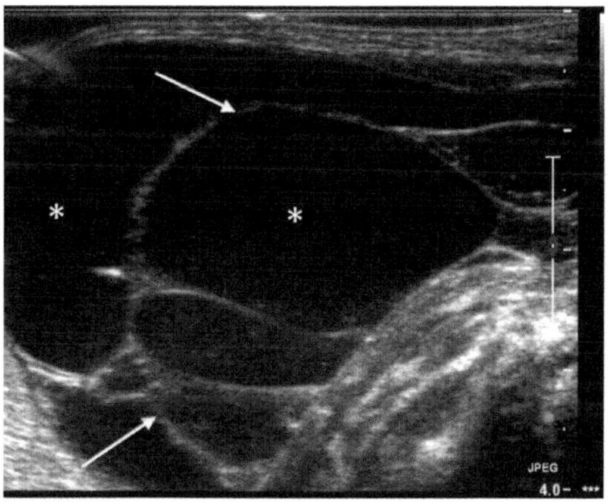

Fig. 3.9 Lymphatic malformation. Ultrasound image in the transverse plane demonstrates a large multiloculated-prdominantly anechoic cystic lesion with macro-cysts (white*) and thin septations (white arrows)

Many lymphatic malformations may be sufficiently assessed by sonography; however, some lesions may be challenging to distinguish from other cystic mass lesions of the neck because of its complex or atypical features [22].

Cystic teratoma is an important differential diagnosis.

LMs and teratomas have different prognosis and treatment options. The most helpful imaging sign to distinguish lymphatic malformation from teratoma is the infiltrative, trans-spatial pattern of LM, insinuating itself into the neighboring tissues. Teratoma usually demonstrates more sharp margins and tends to distort and exert mass effect on surrounding tissues. LM may invade sublingual space and tongue; it may affect the airway, but usually less severe than teratoma.

Venous malformations are low-flow vascular malformations composed of anomalous dilated venous channels with interspersed hamartomatous stroma [24, 25]. VMs are present at birth but may not become apparent until childhood or puberty when they can become more prominent.

3.4.5 Congenital Vascular Tumors

Updated ISSVA classification divides hemangioma into three types: the most common infantile type and rare congenital and intermediate types [26, 30].

3.4.6 Infantile Hemangioma

Infantile Hemangioma (IH) affects 2.5– 10% of young children and is the most common benign congenital vascular tumor of infancy. There is proliferation of endothelial cells and not a malformation [29–32]. There is widespread misuse of term "hemangioma" in literature. In IH, the GLUT1 immunohistochemical marker is positive in all phases of growth and regression which contrasts with GLUT1-negative congenital hemangioma [30, 32]. IH has a well-known clinical course with predictable phases of development and regression: proliferative phase (PP) in which there is rapid growth beginning few weeks after birth and continuing 6–24 months; involuting phase with gradual regression over next several years and involuted phase with a relatively small residual lesion.

Infantile hemangiomas are usually diagnosed by history and physical examination. On ultrasound, typically IHs are well-defined masses and with variable echogenicity, hypoechoic or hyperechoic masses, and few macroscopic vessels (Fig. 3.10). The echogenicity increases during involuting phase. A characteristic feature on color Doppler is markedly increased vascularity due to the presence of numerous smaller vessels. IHs have low resistance waveforms and high vessel density, typically greater than five vessels per square centimeter on color Doppler imaging. High peak arterial Doppler shift exceeding 2 kHz are noted [30, 32, 33] (Fig. 3.10). The lack of arterialized veins and non-elevated mean venous peak velocities are features helpful in distinguishing IHs from other masses including vascular malformations and other vascular tumors. Calcifications are usually not a feature of IHs.

Periorbital hemangioma may obscure the visual axis and cause deprivation amblyopia if not corrected early on.

There is known association between IH and PHACES syndrome (posterior fossa malformations, hemangiomas, arterial, cardiac anomalies, eye anomalies, sternal cleft syndrome).

3.4.7 Congenital Hemangioma

Congenital hemangioma is a clinical entity, distinct from the common infantile hemangioma. CHs are congenital vascular tumors, with some resemblance to infantile hemangiomas in appearance, but unlike IH, are fully developed at birth and do not undergo any further postnatal enlargement. They have been further divided into two categories: rapidly involuting congenital hemangioma (RICH) and non-involuting congenital hemangioma (NICH) [34, 35]. In the RICH lesions, the resolution starts almost immediately after birth and progresses faster than is seen with typical classic infantile hemangiomas, with the lesions often fully resolved by 1 year of age, sometimes with an area of resultant atrophy [35].

The sonographic features include uniform hypoechogenic lesion within the subcutaneous fat [36]. The periphery of the lesion is composed of small lobules of capillaries with plump endothelial cells. But the lobules are too small to be defined individually on US, so appear as a homogeneous mass. CHs are diffusely vascular, with multiple traversing vessels/centrilobular draining channels (Fig. 3.11). As CHs involute, the tortuous and compressible channels with a venous flow signal become the dominant feature [34, 35].

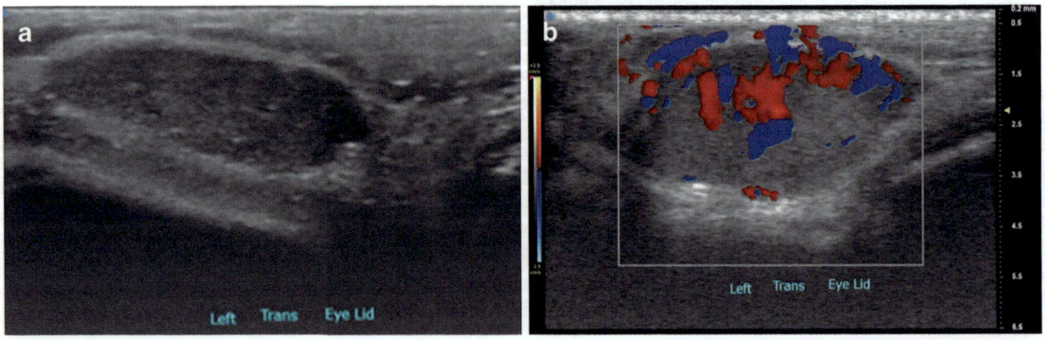

Fig. 3.10 Infantile hemangioma. (**a**) Ultrasound image in the sagittal plane shows a well-marginated hypoechoic lesion with through transmission in the superficial soft tissues. No calcification, necrosis or surrounding edema. On color doppler (**b**) demonstration of internal rich vascularity with both low resistant arterial and venous pattern, making this lesion to be most consistent with an infantile hemangioma

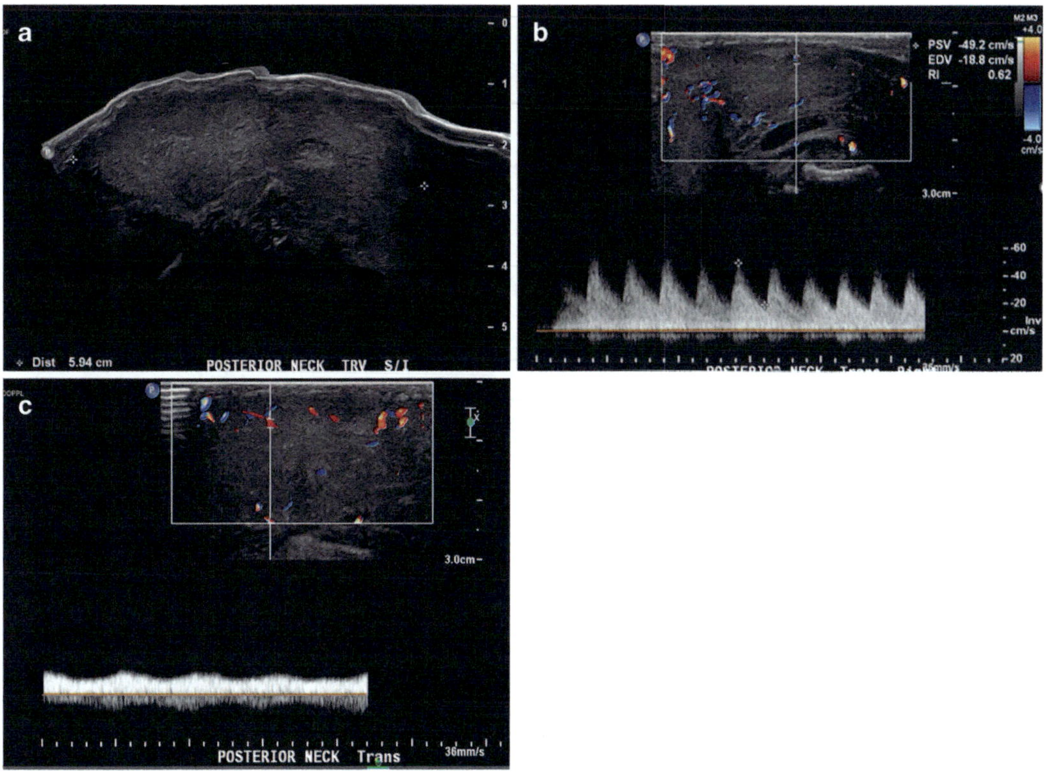

Fig. 3.11 Congenital Hemangioma. A panoramic gray-scale ultrasound image in the transverse plane (**a**) demonstrates a solid mass. Spectral doppler images confirm the presence of arterial waveforms (**b**) and venous waveforms (**c**) within the mass. This is consistent with a congenital hemangioma, which can be further classified by its course of involution as non-involuting congenital hemangioma (NICH), partially-involuting (PICH), or rapidly-involuting (RICH)

3.4.8 Kaposiform Hemangioendothelioma (KHE)

KHE is rare vascular tumor that can present in both the prenatal and neonatal period and is classified as a locally aggressive tumor, which results from abnormal angiogenesis and lymphangiogenesis, despite its mostly solid appearance [36–38]. KHE appears as an ill-defined solid vascular mass with subcutaneous fat stranding, intra-lesional calcification, and prominent feeding and draining vessels (Fig. 3.12). It tends to cause bony destruction. KHE can result in the development of Kasabach-Merritt phenomenon, a form of coagulopathy due to severe thrombocytopenia caused by platelet trapping within the vascular lesion, which may be observed in up to 70% of KHE [36, 38]. The diagnosis of KHE is challenging, the imaging and clinical features may be similar to that of infantile or congenital hemangioma or atypical Type IV veno-lymphatic malformation.

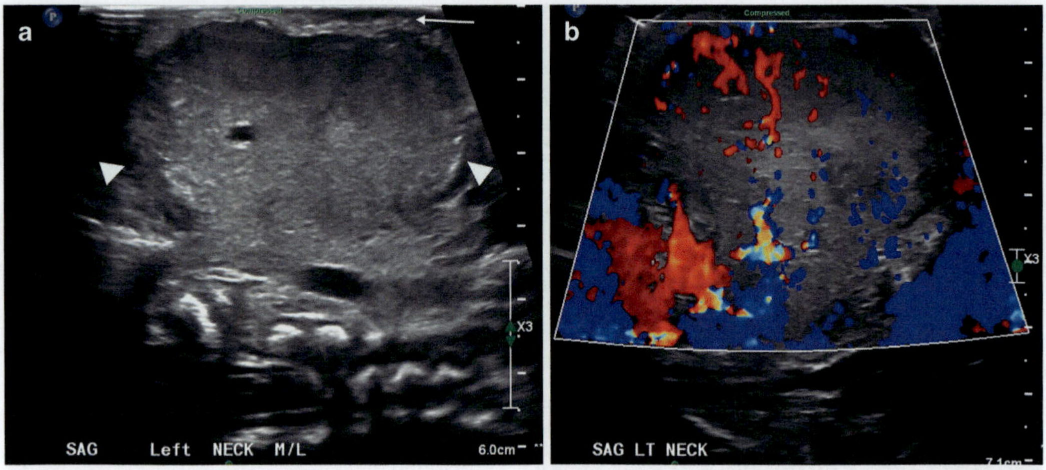

Fig. 3.12 Kaposiform hemangioendothelioma. Ultrasound image in the sagittal plane (**a**) demonstrates a solid mass (white arrowheads) with overlying skin thickening (white arrow) and areas with an ill-defined margin. Color Doppler shows hypervascularity characteristic of a fast-flow vascular tumor (**b**). This was biopsied and confirmed to be Kaposiform hemangioendothelioma (KHE)

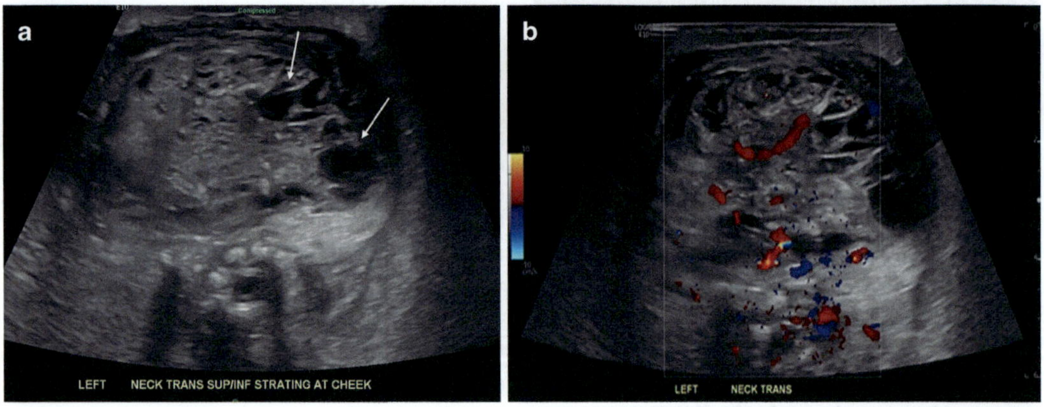

Fig. 3.13 Teratoma. Grayscale ultrasound image in the transverse plane (**a**) in the left neck demonstrates a heterogenous mass that is predominantly solid with cystic components (white arrows). Color Doppler confirms internal vascularity of the solid components (**b**). This was confirmed to be a teratoma

3.4.9 Teratoma (Neck)

Extracranial teratomas are the most common group of neonatal tumors [39–42]. Cervicofacial teratomas account for up to 15% of all teratomas [39]. Teratomas consist of tissues derived from all three germ cell layers—endoderm, mesoderm, and ectoderm. The lesions are generally well-circumscribed, heterogeneous, with cystic and solid components and calcifications and intra-lesion fat is near pathognomonic for teratoma, all these features are easily demonstrated by US (Fig. 3.13). Teratomas may cause high-output cardiac failure and hydrops which can be identified on US. Large palatal teratoma (epignathus) and cervical teratoma can result in impaired swallowing, resulting in polyhydramnios.

3.4.10 Fibrous Connective Tissue Tumors (Myofibroblastic Tumors)

Fibrous connective tissue tumors (myofibroblastic tumors) fall in the category of nonvascular soft tissue neoplasms in the neonates and infants [43, 44]. This group includes desmoid-type fibromatosis, infantile myofibromatosis, infantile fibrosarcoma, digital fibromatosis, and fibrous hamartoma of infancy. This group of tumors is second in incidence to teratomas in the newborn [44].

Myofibroma is a solitary, solid soft tissue mass in infants and neonates, which mostly occurs in the extremities, but in rare instances may be detected in the neonatal neck (Fig. 3.14). Myofibromas have variable appearance on US of amass with a purely anechoic center with a thick wall, a mass with a partially anechoic center, and a mass without anechoic components. In some cases, there can be multiple lesions of infantile myofibromatosis (IM), characterized by the development of nonmetastasizing tumors in the skin, muscle, bone, and viscera [2, 44]. Mutations in PDGFRB gene can cause autosomal-dominant infantile myofibromatosis [45].

Fibrosarcoma is the most common malignant soft tissue tumor in the fetus and infant [46].

A common presentation of infantile fibrosarcoma in a neonate is with a large soft tissue mass, often involving the extremities, and less frequently on the trunk, head, or neck [46]. The appearance on ultrasound examination is nonspecific, usually of a heterogeneous mass [46].

3.4.11 Lipoblastoma

Lipoblastoma is a rare benign neoplasm of embryonal fat tissue that occur almost exclusively in infants and children [47–49]. Two distinct types have been described—a localized and well-circumscribed lesion is termed "lipoblastoma" and the diffuse, multicentric lesion is termed "lipoblastomatosis." [49] The most common location of lipoblastoma is the soft tissue of the extremities but can be seen in the neck.

On ultrasound, lipoblastomas demonstrate variable appearance and can be hyperechoic, hypoechoic, or isoechoic and are usually heterogeneous (Fig. 3.15) [47, 48]. If there is a rapidly growing cervical mass of fatty tissue density in a neonate, a lipoblastoma should be considered. Evaluation with cross-sectional imaging modalities of computed tomography or magnetic resonance imaging confirms the fat density of the tumor (Fig. 3.15).

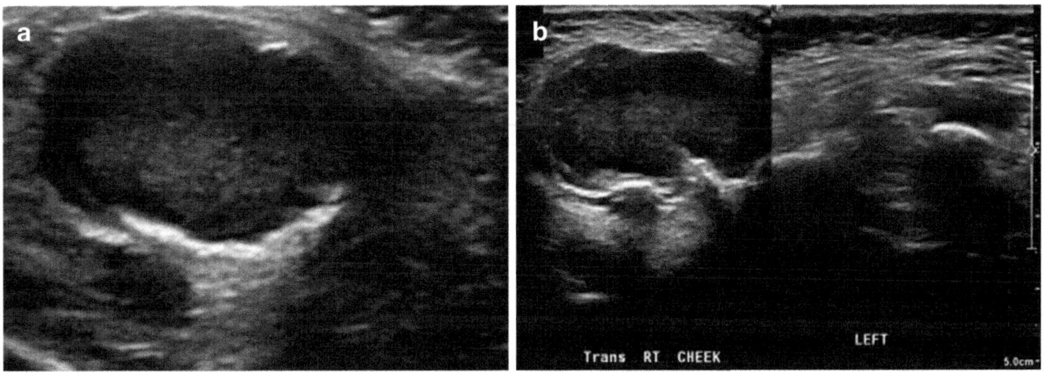

Fig. 3.14 Infantile myofibromatosis. Infantile myofibromatosis in a patient with family history of PDGFR mutation. Grayscale ultrasound image in the right cheek in the transverse plane (**a**) along with contralateral comparison (**b**) demonstrates a 2.1 cm subcutaneous oval solid mass. This lesion is hypoechoic compared to adjacent muscle

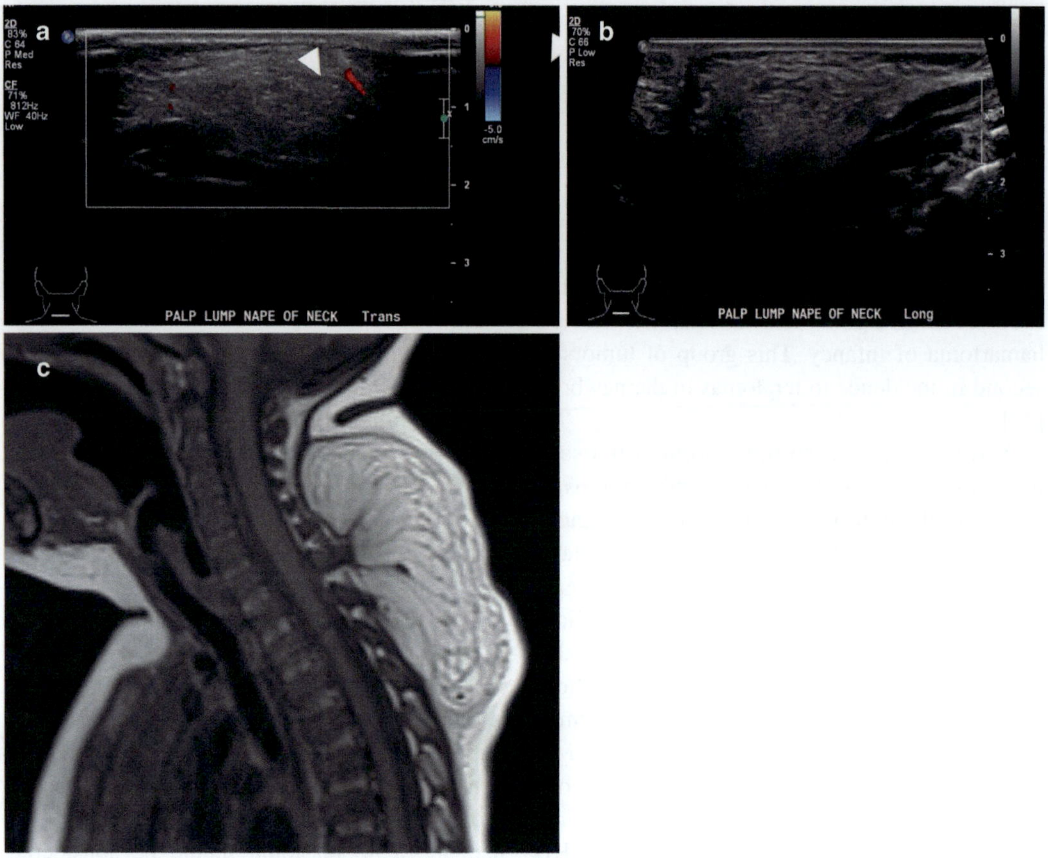

Fig. 3.15 Lipoblastoma. Color Doppler transverse (**a**) and grayscale longitudinal (**b**) images of the posterior neck demonstrate a mass (white arrowheads) that is ill-defined with similar echogenicity to the surrounding subcutaneous fat. Sagittal T1-weighted image from MRI study (**c**) shows T1 hyperintensity identical to fat with intervening septa and a lower signal region at the deep aspect. This was confirmed to be a lipoblastoma on histopathology

3.4.12 Branchial Cleft Cyst (BCC)

BCCs are anomalies/remnant of embryologic endodermal pouch, mesodermal arch, or ectodermal cleft. Although they commonly present in later childhood/adolescents, it can present as a mass/cyst, fistula, or sinus tract in the neck in neonates. US findings include thin-walled, hypoechoic cyst (Fig. 3.16). Mobile internal echoes may be present especially with infection or inflammation [50–52]. Communication to superficial draining sinus may be demonstrated on US in fluid-filled tracts. Differentiation of BCCs from other cystic lesions in the neck may require additional cross-sectional imaging with CT or MRI or tissue sampling. Different types of branchial cysts can be diagnosed based on their typical location.

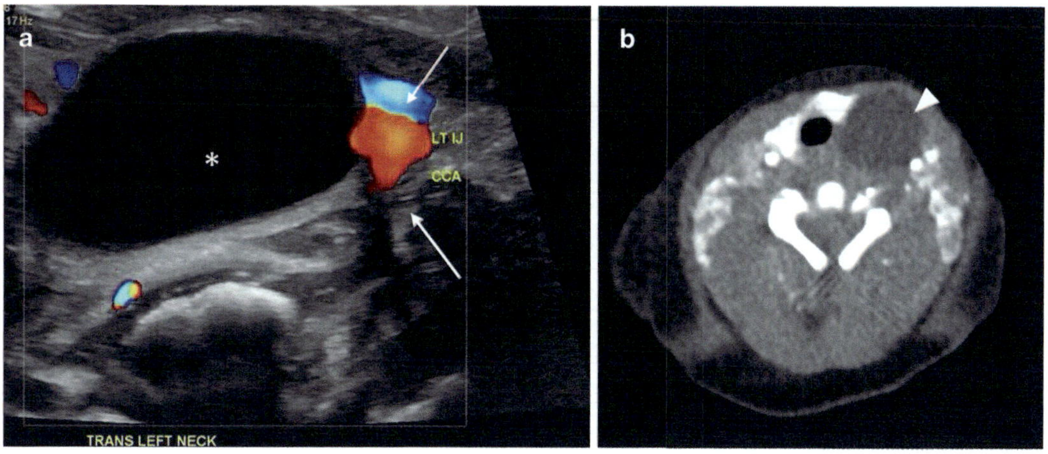

Fig. 3.16 Fourth branchial cleft cyst. Color Doppler ultrasound image in the transverse plane (**a**) demonstrates a simple appearing anechoic cyst without internal flow (*) within the left neck which has mass effect on the adjacent common carotid artery and internal jugular vein (white arrows). Axial contrast enhanced CT image (**b**) confirms a cyst (white arrowhead) with fluid attenuation and no enhancement displacing the left lobe of the thyroid, common carotid artery, and internal jugular vein. The relationship with the left thyroid is characteristic of a fourth branchial cleft cyst

3.4.13 Ectopic Thymus

Thymic tissue in an ectopic location in the neck can present as a soft tissue mass in the neonates and can be a diagnostic challenge. Ectopic cervical thymus can occur in various locations in the neck, typically in the expected path of the thymopharyngeal duct [2, 53]. The ultrasound appearance of thymic tissue is very characteristic, and the specific diagnosis of ectopic cervical thymus can be made based of ultrasound alone (Fig. 3.17) [53–56]. The ultrasound is distinct with hypo- and hyperechoic pattern with multiple linear and punctate echoes, "dot & dash" echoes, a fusiform shape, and well-demarcated contours [55, 56]. Additional imaging or biopsy may not be indicated when typical features can be identified on ultrasound.

3.4.14 Thyroid Abnormalities

Ultrasonography (US) is the imaging modality of choice for evaluating the neonatal thyroid gland. In newborns, one of the most common indications for thyroid ultrasound evaluation is congenital hypothyroidism which is typically detected on newborn screening of thyroid-stimulating hormone (TSH) levels.

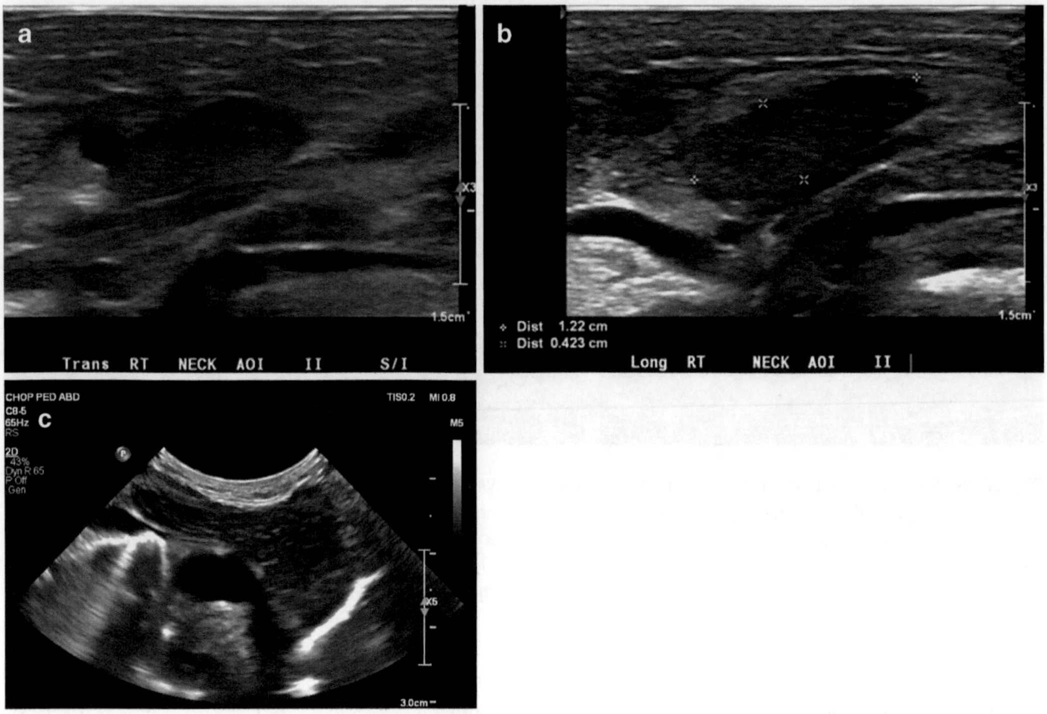

Fig. 3.17 Ectopic thymus. Grayscale ultrasound image in the transverse plane (**a**) and sagittal plane (**b**) in the right neck demonstrates a well-defined oblong hypoechoic mass. Coronal oblique plane of the upper chest (**c**) at the region of the aortic arch (*) shows that the thymus (white arrow) has the same echogenicity and echotexture as the mass suggesting that the mass is an ectopic thymus

US can be challenging in neonates due to short necks and excess fat. Care should be taken to support the neonatal neck during US evaluation of the thyroid gland. Every US thyroid scan should include evaluation of each lobe of the thyroid gland and isthmus in transverse and longitudinal planes (Fig. 3.18). The entire embryological path of the thyroid gland in the midline of the neck should be evaluated for thyroid tissue from the floor of the mouth to the thoracic inlet.

One of the most important roles of the ultrasound thyroid examination is to determine presence or absence of thyroid tissue in orthotopic location in the neck or ectopic locations on the embryological path of development [57–60].

Another important role of US after confirming presence of orthotopic thyroid gland is assessment of thyroid size; normal, hypoplastic, or enlarged as seen in congenital goiter. (Figs. 3.19 and 3.20) Measurements in orthogonal planes and volumes of the right and left lobes should be provided. There exist normative measurement data charts in term as well as preterm infants which can be referred to for evaluation [59, 60]. US should be complemented by scintigraphy and thyroid function tests [59, 60].

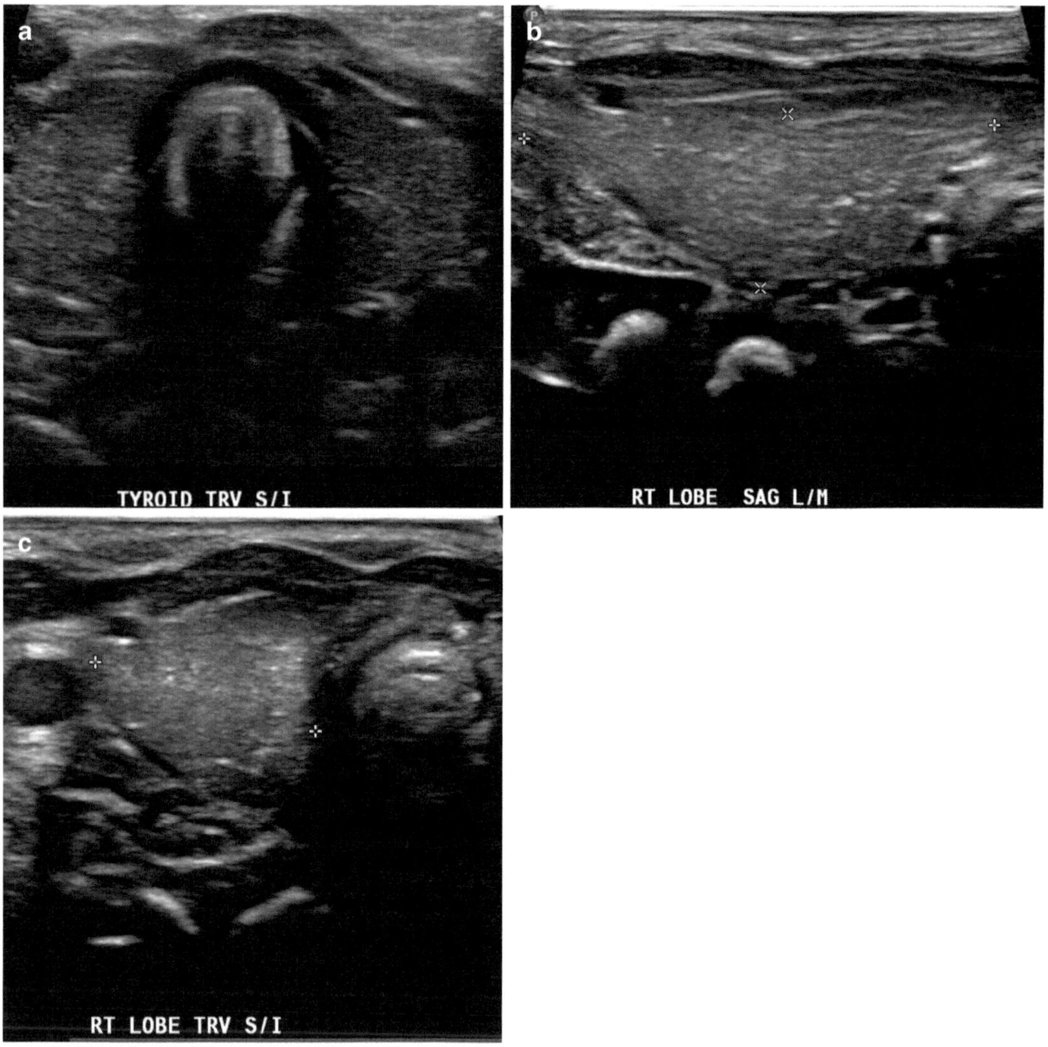

Fig. 3.18 Normal neonatal thyroid ultrasound. Six days old male presenting with increased thyroid stimulating hormone (TSH) on neonatal screening referred for evaluation of the thyroid gland. Grayscale ultrasound images shows thyroid gland in normal location in the neck. Image in the transverse plane through both thyroid lobes and isthmus (**a**), in the sagittal plane through right thyroid lobe (**b**), and in the transverse plane of the right lobe (**c**). Similar images through the left thyroid lobe were also obtained (not shown). Normal size/volume and echogenicity of the thyroid gland was noted without any focal lesions. Treatment with levothyroxine was initiated

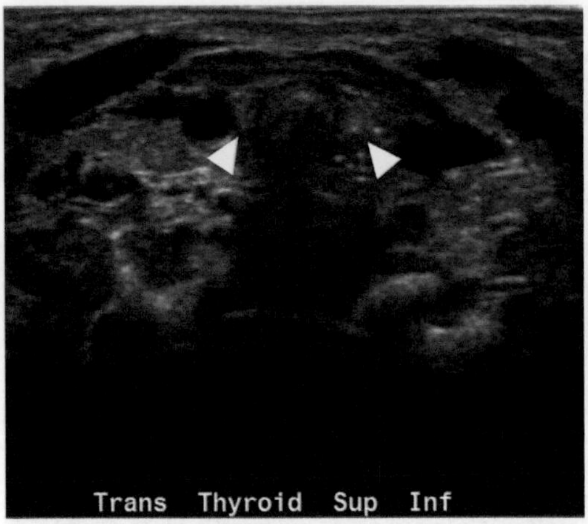

Fig. 3.19 Severely hypoplastic thyroid gland. Eight days old neonate had newborn screen with a low T4, high TSH. Grayscale ultrasound image in the region of the thyroid bed shows there is a small thyroid gland in orthotopic location. In the transverse plane, very small thyroid lobes are noted (white arrow heads) with size/volume consistent with a severely hypoplastic thyroid gland. There was no ultrasound evidence for midline cyst or base of tongue thyroid tissue

3.4.15 Cervical Lymphadenopathy

Suppurative lymphadenopathy in the neck is common in children between 4 and 8 years of age [61, 62]. Congenital malformations of the head and neck such as lymphatic malformations and branchial cleft cysts may present as a lump or swelling in the neonates that can be mistaken for lymph nodes, particularly if they become infected.

3.4.16 Neonatal Suppurative Submandibular Sialadenitis

Infection of the salivary glands is a rare clinical entity encountered in neonates and typically more commonly involves the parotid gland. However, isolated submandibular suppurative sialadenitis (ISSS) has been reported in neonates

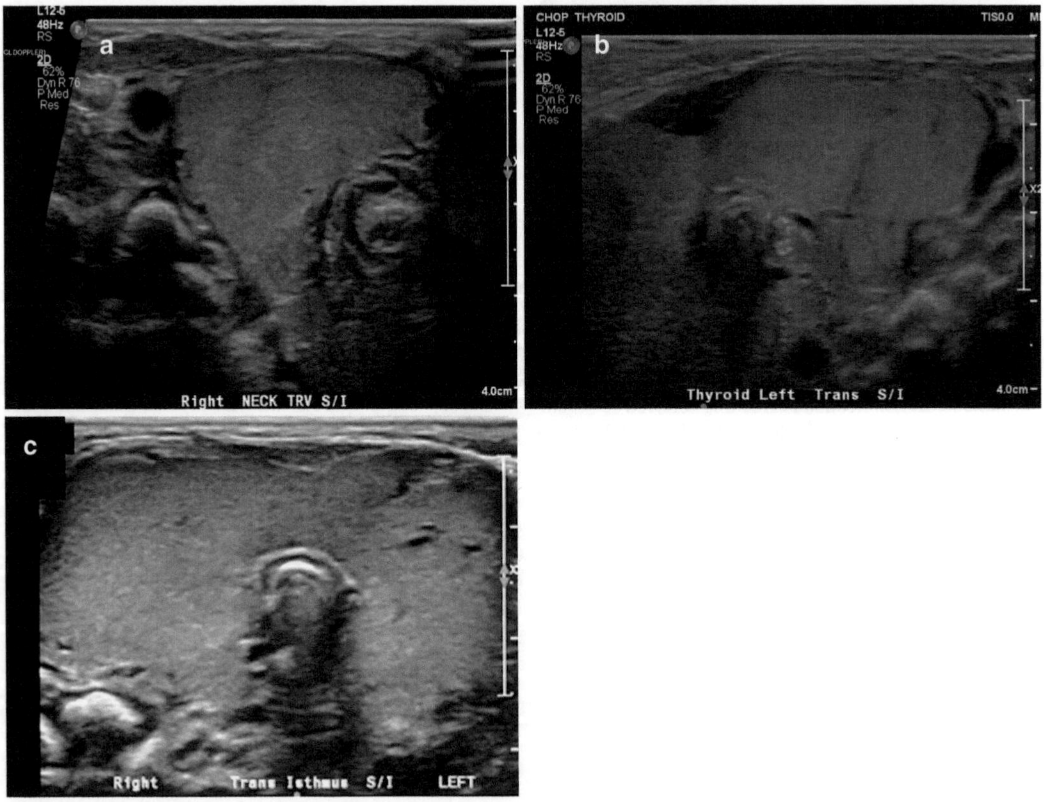

Fig. 3.20 Congenital goiter-hypothyroidism. Grayscale ultrasound images in the transverse plane of the right lobe (**a**), left lobe (**b**) and isthmus (**c**) demonstrate massive enlargement of the thyroid with normal echotexture and no focal lesion. The mother had a history of Hashimoto thyroiditis. The findings are consistent with a congenital goiter and hypothyroidism

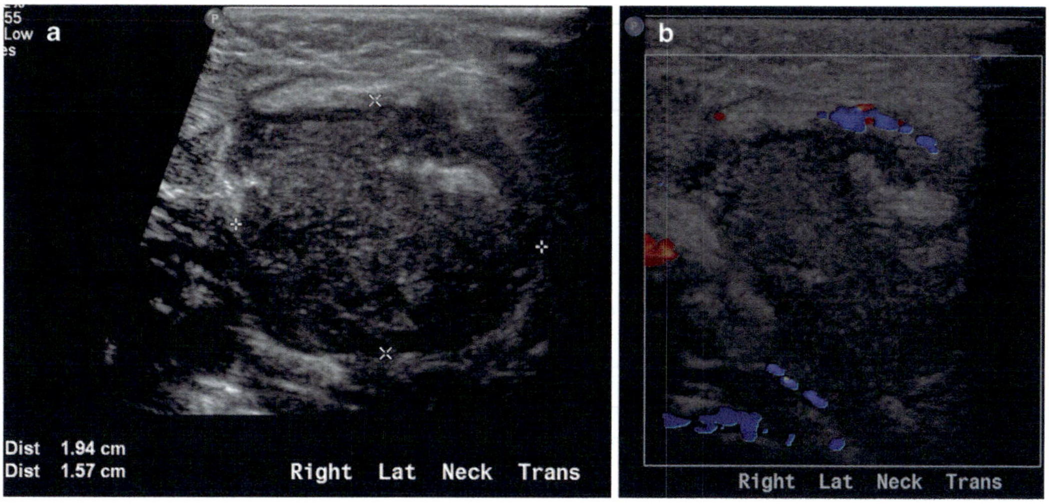

Fig. 3.21 Submandibular abscess. Ultrasound of right lateral neck in transverse plane (**a**) with color Doppler (**b**) in a 3-week-old former 29 weeks premature infant with submandibular swelling with a fluctuant collection involving the right lateral neck, subjacent to the sternocleidomastoid muscle, extending from the mandible to superior right thyroid lobe. Increased blood flow within the surrounding tissues on color Doppler (**b**), consistent with an abscess

especially in preterm infants [63, 64]. ISSS typically presents in neonates with an inflammatory swelling in the submandibular area and purulent material may be readily expressible from the Wharton's duct with gentle compression of the mass [64, 65]. Progression of ISSS to frank submandibular abscess has been seen in premature neonates [65] and can be identified on US evaluation demonstrates fluctuant collection containing internal debris, consistent with an abscess (Fig. 3.21).

3.5 Conclusion

The evaluation of disorders of the orbit, face, and neck requires multimodality imaging approach to balance the advantages and disadvantages of each method. Ultrasonography is a rapid and noninvasive test and, in some cases, may be the only imaging needed. In other cases, US may serve as a useful, noninvasive adjunct to clinical diagnosis. In addition, US is useful to guide diagnostic procedures such as biopsy or fine-needle aspiration and for therapeutic procedures like drainage and sclerotherapy.

References

1. Caprio MG, Di Serafino M, Pontillo G, Vezzali N, Rossi E, Esposito F, et al. Paediatric neck ultrasonography: a pictorial essay. J Ultrasound. 2019;22(2):215–26.
2. Bansal AG, Oudsema R, Masseaux JA, Rosenberg HK. US of pediatric superficial masses of the head and neck. Radiographics. 2018;38(4):1239–63.
3. Abramowicz JS, Adhikari S, Dickman E, Estroff JA, Harris GR, Nomura J, et al. Ocular ultrasound: review of bioeffects and safety, including fetal and point of care perspective: review of bioeffects and safety, including Fetal and point-of-care perspective. J Ultrasound Med. 2022;41(7):1609–22.
4. Gupta A, Arora SK, Seth R, Kumar R, Jana M. Paediatric orbital ultrasound: tips and tricks. Australas J Ultrasound Med. 2022;25(4):200–6.
5. Silva CT, Brockley CR, Crum A, Mandelstam SA. Pediatric ocular sonography. Semin Ultrasound CT MR. 2011;32(1):14–27.
6. Lorente-Ramos RM, Armán JA, Muñoz-Hernández A, Gómez JMG, Torre SBdl. US of the eye made easy: a comprehensive how-to review with Ophthalmoscopic correlation. Radiographics. 2012;32(5):E175–200.
7. Bates A, Goett HJ. Ocular ultrasound. In: StatPearls. Treasure Island (FL): StatPearls Publishing LLC; 2023.
8. Bedi DG, Gombos DS, Ng CS, Singh S. Sonography of the eye. AJR Am J Roentgenol. 2006;187(4):1061–72.
9. Chen C, Xiao H, Ding X. Persistent fetal vasculature. Asia Pac J Ophthalmol (Phila). 2019;8(1):86–95.

10. Chiaroni PM, Chapron T, Purcell Y, Zuber K, Savatovsky J, Caputo G, et al. Diagnostic accuracy of quantitative colour Doppler flow imaging in distinguishing persistent fetal vasculature from retinal detachment. Acta Ophthalmol. 2022;100(2):196–202.
11. Ludwig CA, Chen TA, Hernandez-Boussard T, Moshfeghi AA, Moshfeghi DM. The epidemiology of retinopathy of prematurity in the United States. Ophthalmic Surg Lasers Imaging Retina. 2017;48(7):553–62.
12. Cavazza S, Laffi GL, Lodi L, Tassinari G, Dall'Olio D. Congenital dacryocystocele: diagnosis and treatment. Acta Otorhinolaryngol Ital. 2008;28(6):298–301.
13. Ladeiras R, Nunes JS, Torres S, Duarte C, Pereira E, Rosmaninho A. An ultrasound diagnosis of a congenital periorbital rare condition. J Med Ultrasound. 2021;29(2):142–3.
14. Davies R, Watkins WJ, Kotecha S, Watts P. The presentation, clinical features, complications, and treatment of congenital dacryocystocele. Eye. 2018;32(3):522–6.
15. Miranda-Rivas A, Villegas VM, Nieves-Melendez JR, De La Vega A. Congenital dacryocystocele: sonographic evaluation of 11 cases. J AAPOS. 2018;22(5):390–2.
16. Bilaniuk LT, Farber M. Imaging of developmental anomalies of the eye and the orbit. AJNR Am J Neuroradiol. 1992;13(2):793–803.
17. Castillo M, Mukherji SK, Wagle NS. Imaging of the pediatric orbit. Neuroimaging Clin N Am. 2000;10(1):95–116. viii
18. Society for Maternal-Fetal M, Benacerraf BR, Bromley B, Jelin AC. Anophthalmia and Microphthalmia. Am J Obstet Gynecol. 2019;221(5):B20–B1.
19. Tortori-Donati P, Rossi A, Biancheri R, et al. Brain malformations. In: Tortori-Donati P, editor. Pediatric neuroradiology. Berlin: Springer Verlag; 2005.
20. Pushker N, Meel R, Kumar A, Kashyap S, Sen S, Bajaj MS. Orbital and periorbital dermoid/epidermoid cyst: a series of 280 cases and a brief review. Can J Ophthalmol. 2020;55(2):167–71.
21. Shields JA, Shields CL. Orbital cysts of childhood—classification, clinical features, and management. Surv Ophthalmol. 2004;49(3):281–99.
22. Tranvinh E, Yeom KW, Iv M. Imaging neck masses in the neonate and young infant. Semin Ultrasound CT MR. 2015;36(2):120–37. https://doi.org/10.1053/j.sult.2015.01.004.
23. Jecker P. Ultrasound anatomy of the head and the neck. In: Welkoborsky HJ, Jecker P, editors. Ultrasonography of the head and neck: an imaging atlas. Cham: Springer International Publishing; 2019. p. 15–39.
24. Mulliken JB, Glowacki J. Classification of pediatric vascular lesions. Plast Reconstr Surg. 1982;70(1):120–1.
25. Dasgupta R, Fishman SJ. ISSVA classification. Semin Pediatr Surg. 2014;23(4):158–61.
26. ISftSoV A. ISSVA Classification of Vascular Anomalies© 2018 International Society for the Study of Vascular Anomalies. Accessed March. 2022;14.
27. Shekdar K, Feygin T. Fetal neuroimaging. Neuroimaging Clin N Am. 2011;21(3):677–703. ix
28. Fordham LA, Chung CJ, Donnelly LF. Imaging of congenital vascular and lymphatic anomalies of the head and neck. Neuroimaging Clin N Am. 2000;10(1):117–36. viii
29. Restrepo R. Multimodality imaging of vascular anomalies. Pediatr Radiol. 2013;43(Suppl. 1):S141–54.
30. Gupta R, Bhandari A, Navarro OM. Pediatric vascular anomalies: a clinical and radiological perspective. Indian J Radiol Imaging. 2023;34(1):103–27.
31. North PE, Waner M, Mizeracki A, Mihm MC Jr. GLUT1: a newly discovered immunohistochemical marker for juvenile hemangiomas. Hum Pathol. 2000;31(1):11–22.
32. Dubois J, Alison M. Vascular anomalies: what a radiologist needs to know. Pediatr Radiol. 2010;40(6):895–905.
33. Habib AHI, El-Kaffas KH, Mustafa AS, Mashour SN. Role of ultrasound and colored Doppler examination in the diagnosis and the classification of the superficial soft tissue vascular anomalies. Egypt J Radiol Nucl Med. 2022;53(1):89.
34. HPW K. The pathology of rapidly involuting congenital hemangioma (RICH) and non-involuting congenital hemangioma (NICH). In: Vascular Anomalies 2001 meeting (18–19, 2001). New York, NY: New York University Medcial Center; 2001.
35. Enjolras O, Mulliken JB, Boon LM, Wassef M, Kozakewich HP, Burrows PE. Noninvoluting congenital hemangioma: a rare cutaneous vascular anomaly. Plast Reconstr Surg. 2001;107(7):1647–54.
36. Croteau SE, Liang MG, Kozakewich HP, Alomari AI, Fishman SJ, Mulliken JB, Trenor CC III. Kaposiform hemangioendothelioma: atypical features and risks of Kasabach-Merritt phenomenon in 107 referrals. J Pediatr. 2013;162(1):142–7.
37. Ji Y, Chen S, Yang K, Xia C, Li L. Kaposiform hemangioendothelioma: current knowledge and future perspectives. Orphanet J Rare Dis. 2020;15(1):39.
38. Sarkar M, Mulliken JB, Kozakewich HP, Robertson RL, Burrows PE. Thrombocytopenic coagulopathy (Kasabach-Merritt phenomenon) is associated with Kaposiform hemangioendothelioma and not with common infantile hemangioma. Plast Reconstr Surg. 1997;100(6):1377–86.
39. Brodsky JR, Irace AL, Didas A, Watters K, Estroff JA, Barnewolt CE, et al. Teratoma of the neonatal head and neck: a 41-year experience. Int J Pediatr Otorhinolaryngol. 2017;97:66–71.
40. Figueiredo G, Pinto PS, Graham EM, Huisman TA. Congenital giant cervical teratoma: pre-and post-natal imaging. Fetal Diagn Ther. 2010;27(4):231.
41. De Backer A, Madern GC, van De Ven CP, Tibboel D, Hazebroek FW. Strategy for management of newborns with cervical teratoma. J Perinat

Med. 2004;32(6):500–8. https://doi.org/10.1515/JPM.2004.122.
42. Laje P, Johnson MP, Howell LJ, Bebbington MW, Hedrick HL, Flake AW, et al. Ex utero intrapartum treatment in the management of giant cervical teratomas. J Pediatr Surg. 2012;47(6):1208–16.
43. Isaacs H. Soft tissue tumors. In: Tumors of the fetus and infant: An Atlas. Springer Science & Business Media; 2002. p. 37–111.
44. Hourani R, Taslakian B, Shabb NS, Nassar L, Hourani MH, Moukarbel R, et al. Fibroblastic and myofibroblastic tumors of the head and neck: comprehensive imaging-based review with pathologic correlation. Eur J Radiol. 2015;84(2):250–60.
45. Martignetti JA, Tian L, Li D, Ramirez MC, Camacho-Vanegas O, Camacho SC, et al. Mutations in PDGFRB cause autosomal-dominant infantile myofibromatosis. Am J Hum Genet. 2013;92(6):1001–7.
46. Hu Z, Chou PM, Jennings LJ, Arva NC. Infantile fibrosarcoma—a clinical and histologic mimicker of vascular malformations: case report and review of the literature. Pediatr Dev Pathol. 2013;16(5):357–63.
47. Pham NS, Poirier B, Fuller SC, Dublin AB, Tollefson TT. Pediatric lipoblastoma in the head and neck: a systematic review of 48 reported cases. Int J Pediatr Otorhinolaryngol. 2010;74(7):723–8.
48. Basaran UN, Inan M, Bilgi S, Pul M. Lipoblastoma: a rare cervical mass in childhood. Int J Pediatr Otorhinolaryngol. 2001;61(3):265–8.
49. Ratan SK, Gambhir A, Mullick S, Ratan J. Lipoblastoma of the neck. Indian J Pediatr. 2000;67:301–3.
50. Mukherji SK, Fatterpekar G, Castillo M, Stone JA, Chung CJ. Imaging of congenital anomalies of the branchial apparatus. Neuroimaging Clin N Am. 2000;10(1):75–93. viii
51. Thomas B, Shroff M, Forte V, Blaser S, James A. Revisiting imaging features and the embryologic basis of third and fourth branchial anomalies. AJNR Am J Neuroradiol. 2010;31(4):755–60.
52. Fanous A, Morcrette G, Fabre M, Couloigner V, Galmiche-Rolland L. Diagnostic approach to congenital cystic masses of the neck from a clinical and pathological perspective. Dermatopathology (Basel). 2021;8(3):342–58.
53. Han BK, Yoon HK, Suh YL. Thymic ultrasound. II. Diagnosis of aberrant cervical thymus. Pediatr Radiol. 2001;31(7):480–7.
54. Yildiz AE, Elhan AH, Fitoz S. Prevalence and sonographic features of ectopic thyroidal thymus in children: a retrospective analysis. J Clin Ultrasound. 2018;46(6):375–9.
55. Song I, Yoo SY, Kim JH, Hong E, Yoon HK. Aberrant cervical thymus: imaging and clinical findings in 13 children. Clin Radiol. 2011;66(1):38–42.
56. Andreozzi L, Sacchi C, Biagi C, Dondi A, Baldazzi M, Carfagnini F, et al. Abnormal locations of thymic tissue as an uncommon cause of neck masses in children: a practical approach. Life (Basel). 2023;13(3):685.
57. Perry RJ, Hollman AS, Wood AM, Donaldson MD. Ultrasound of the thyroid gland in the newborn: normative data. Arch Dis Child Fetal Neonatal Ed. 2002;87(3):F209–11.
58. Khan SS, Hong-McAtee I, Kriss VM, Stevens S, Crawford T, Hanna M, et al. Thyroid gland volumes in premature infants using serial ultrasounds. J Perinatol. 2018;38(10):1353–8.
59. Hashemipour M, Rostampour N, Nasry P, Hovsepian S, Basiratnia R, Hekmatnia A, et al. The role of ultrasonography in primary congenital hypothyroidism. J Res Med Sci. 2011;16(9):1122–8.
60. Tritou I, Vakaki M, Sfakiotaki R, Kalaitzaki K, Raissaki M. Pediatric thyroid ultrasound: a radiologist's checklist. Pediatr Radiol. 2020;50(4):563–74.
61. Leung AK, Davies HD. Cervical lymphadenitis: etiology, diagnosis, and management. Curr Infect Dis Rep. 2009;11:183–9.
62. Twist CJ, Link MP. Assessment of lymphadenopathy in children. Pediatr Clin N Am. 2002;49(5):1009–25.
63. Garavello W, Romagnoli M, Somigliana E, Zorloni C, Sordo L, Gaini RM. The intriguing association between prematurity and neonatal isolated submandibular suppurative sialadenitis. Int J Pediatr Otorhinolaryngol. 2002;62(1):41–4.
64. Banks WW, Handler SD, Glade GB, Turner HD. Neonatal submandibular sialadenitis. Am J Otolaryngol. 1980;1(3):261–3.
65. Bova R, Walker P. Neonatal submandibular sialadenitis progressing to submandibular gland abscess. Int J Pediatr Otorhinolaryngol. 2000;53(1):73–5.

4 Neonatal Chest Wall and Pleura

Santiago Martinez-Correa and Hansel J. Otero

Highlights

- Ultrasound is a valuable imaging modality for evaluating chest wall and pleural pathologies in newborns.
- Smaller patient size and acoustic windows provided by unossified cartilage allow for detailed real-time assessment with excellent detail and tissue characterization to help diagnose and follow-up most entities presenting in this age group.
- Neonatal chest ultrasound utilizes high-frequency linear transducers and various approaches, including intercostal, parasternal, subxiphoid, and posterior paraspinal acoustic windows. In addition to high-resolution grayscale images, color and spectral Doppler images are necessary to fully characterize chest wall and pleural lesions and their vascularity.
- Key applications include characterizing pleural effusions and pleural-based tumors as well as the diagnosis and full characterization of skin lesions, palpable and symptomatic breast lesions, as well as ribs and chest wall abnormalities. In addition to diagnosis and follow-up, ultrasound can be used for guiding interventions.

S. Martinez-Correa (✉)
Department of Radiology, Children's Hospital of Philadelphia, Philadelphia, PA, USA
e-mail: martinezcs@chop.edu; martinezcs.md@gmail.com

H. J. Otero
Department of Pediatric Radiology, Children's Hospital of Philadelphia, Philadelphia, PA, USA

Department of Radiology, Perelman School of Medicine, University of Pennsylvania, Philadelphia, PA, USA

4.1 Introduction

Ultrasound is an extremely valuable imaging modality for the evaluation of chest wall pathologies in the newborn [1, 2]. Increased availability and technological improvements, combined with concerns about cumulative ionizing radiation exposure in children, have expanded the role of ultrasound in evaluating common thoracic diseases from palpable superficial abnormalities to lung parenchymal pathology [3–5]. The smaller patient size and acoustic windows provided by unossified cartilage provide unique opportunities for real-time detailed assessment. Neonatal chest ultrasound involves various approaches utilizing high-frequency linear transducers for superficial structures, taking full advantage of intercostal, parasternal, subxiphoid, and posterior paraspinal acoustic windows [6]. Key applications include characterizing pleural effusions and skin, breast, chest wall, and pleural lesions as well as guiding interventions [7–11]. By understanding the expanding role of pediatric chest ultrasound techniques, clinicians can use this versatile modality to safely diagnose and manage various thoracic diseases in neonates.

K. S. Sodhi (ed.), *Neonatal Ultrasound*, https://doi.org/10.1007/978-981-97-8576-6_4

4.2 Indications and Technique

Like most ultrasound applications, there are several special technical considerations for performing neonatal chest ultrasound. First, it is crucial to tailor the exam to answer the specific clinical question and use the most direct approach to evaluate the anatomical structures of interest [2]. The target region is usually determined by physical exam or caretaker's concern over a palpable abnormality or skin discoloration. Abnormal or inconclusive findings from prenatal ultrasound or postnatal chest radiographs also necessitate ultrasound evaluation. Ultrasound is also beneficial for evaluating suspected rib fractures or costochondral injuries as well as for complete characterization of pleural effusions, which in children are most commonly parapneumonic and associated with infectious causes but, could also be hemo- or chylothoraces of various causes.

In general, the use of the highest frequency transducer that allows for penetration of the adjacent structure is recommended. Commonly available high-frequency linear transducers range between 9 and 17 MHz and provide excellent spatial resolution for visualizing superficial structures, like the chest wall and the pleura in neonates [4, 12]. The superficial nature of chest wall diseases paired with the small size and unossified thorax of the neonate allow for the full evaluation and characterization of most pathologies. A basic protocol for palpable abnormalities and areas of skin discoloration includes grayscale imaging of the area of concern in both sagittal and transverse planes, followed by color Doppler images (and spectral as needed) as well as comparison views of similar anatomy in the contralateral side or an unaffected area. An additional useful tool is the use of panoramic views for lesions incompletely visualized in a single image.

For deeper lesions within the thoracic cage, including pleural-based diseases, the suprasternal, supraclavicular, parasternal, and intercostal spaces permit imaging anteriorly, while the paraspinal and trans diaphragmatic approaches can be used to image posterior chest structures. The liver and spleen can also be used as acoustic windows to visualize the diaphragmatic and caudal pleural spaces.

4.3 Normal Chest Wall Anatomy

The skin appears as two parallel echogenic lines representing the epidermal entry echo and the underlying echogenic dermis. The subcutaneous tissues have a characteristic lobulated appearance with curvilinear hyperechoic lines from acoustic reflections of interdigitating fascia [7]. The musculature is slightly hypoechoic with a striated texture compared to fat, while the cartilaginous portions of the rib cage are hypoechoic as opposed to ossified ribs that are markedly hyperechoic with posterior acoustic shadowing. The normal neonatal chest wall structures are shown in Fig. 4.1.

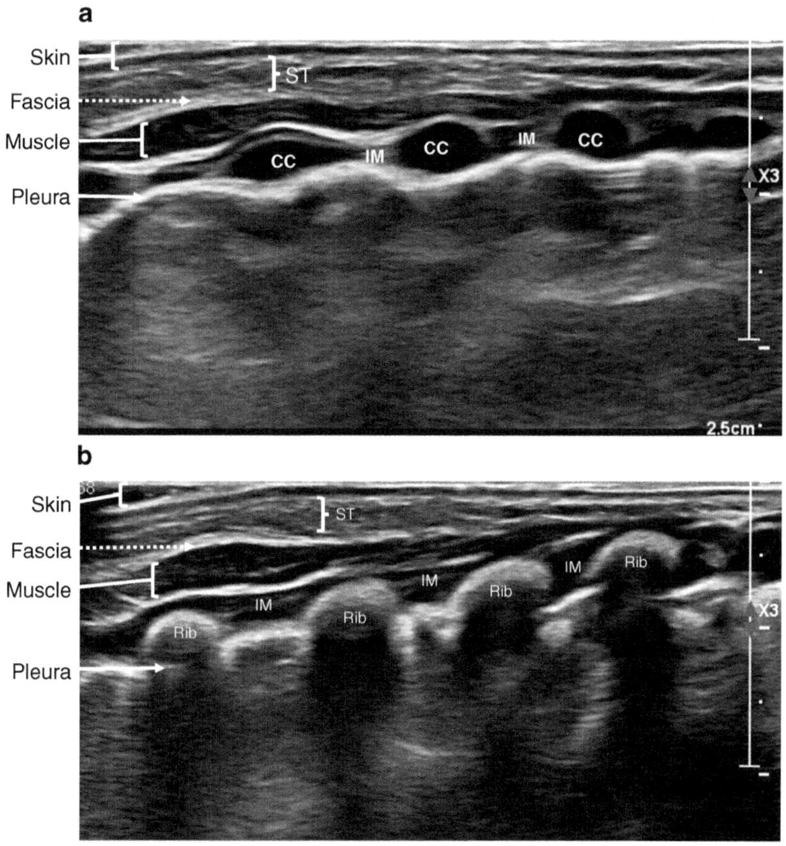

Fig. 4.1 Normal chest wall anatomy in an 11-day-old girl. (**a**, **b**) Sagittal ultrasound images showing chest wall layers from outer to inside. The skin appears as parallel echogenic lines, followed by subcutaneous tissues (ST), fascia (dashed arrow), and muscles with striated texture. Then, costal cartilages (CC), intercostal muscles (IM), and ribs are appreciated. The pleura appears deep as an hyperechogenic line (solid arrow)

Normal anatomic variants like asymmetric cartilage fusion or convex angulation of the ribs can be sources of concern and can be confused with pathology [12]. The pleura is a smooth echogenic line adjacent to the normally air-filled lung which produces fluttering reverberation artifacts. Vascular structures have an anechoic appearance with verification of flow on color and spectral Doppler imaging. The contralateral asymptomatic hemithorax serves as internal reference for symmetry to distinguish normal anatomy from potential abnormalities [4].

4.4 Breast and Soft Tissues

Although palpable breast masses in the pediatric population may be alarming, most are benign [13]. To our knowledge, no breast malignancies have been reported in neonates. The breast during the neonatal period is an immature organ with identical histology in both sexes. It consists of simple branched ducts supported by stromal connective tissue and is capable of responding to hormonal stimuli [14, 15]. Ultrasound serves as an essential tool to evaluate different breast conditions on the neonatal period due to its lack of ionizing radiation, portability, and wide availability.

4.4.1 Neonatal Breast Enlargement

Neonatal breast enlargement is a transient benign condition caused by an exaggerated response to maternal estrogens that enter the newborn's bloodstream through the placental circulation. It is seen in approximately 70% of neonates, usually presents bilaterally during the first week of life, is independent of the sex of the child, and has spontaneous resolution within 6 months of age [16]. Classically, ultrasound shows a hypoechoic retroareolar tissue or hypoechoic retroareolar nodule with central star-shaped or linear hypoechoic areas that represents primitive ducts with some degree of branching and supporting stroma (Fig. 4.2). Of note, no lobular parenchyma or fat is seen at this age, as the breast bud is composed of secretory ducts only [17].

4.4.2 Neonatal Mastitis and Abscess

Neonatal mastitis is an inflammatory process of the breast tissue that usually presents within the first 5 weeks of life, with peak incidence at 3 weeks of age. Neonatal mastitis is more common in full-term infants, usually presents unilaterally with no side predilection, and, after the second week of life, is more likely to be found in girls than boys [18]. Neonatal mastitis etiology is mainly due to *Staphylococcus aureus* in 83–88% of all cases, but other Gram-negative organisms have also been implicated [19]. Diagnosis can be made clinically when typical symptoms, such as erythema, swelling, tenderness, and induration of the area, are present. Ultrasound usually

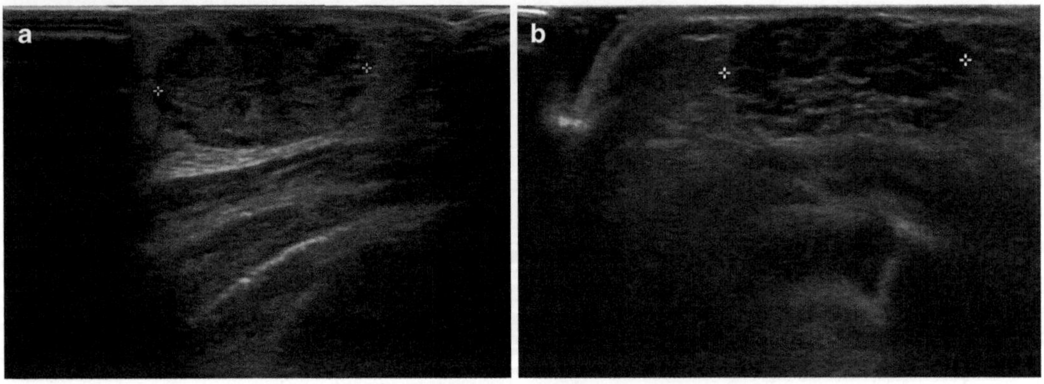

Fig. 4.2 Normal breast. A 20-day-old girl presenting with bilateral breast enlargement and concern for mastitis. Right (**a**) and left (**b**) transverse chest wall ultrasound images demonstrate bilateral breast bud enlargement, related to hormonal status. No signs of mastitis or abscess. Asterisks delimiting the breast tissue

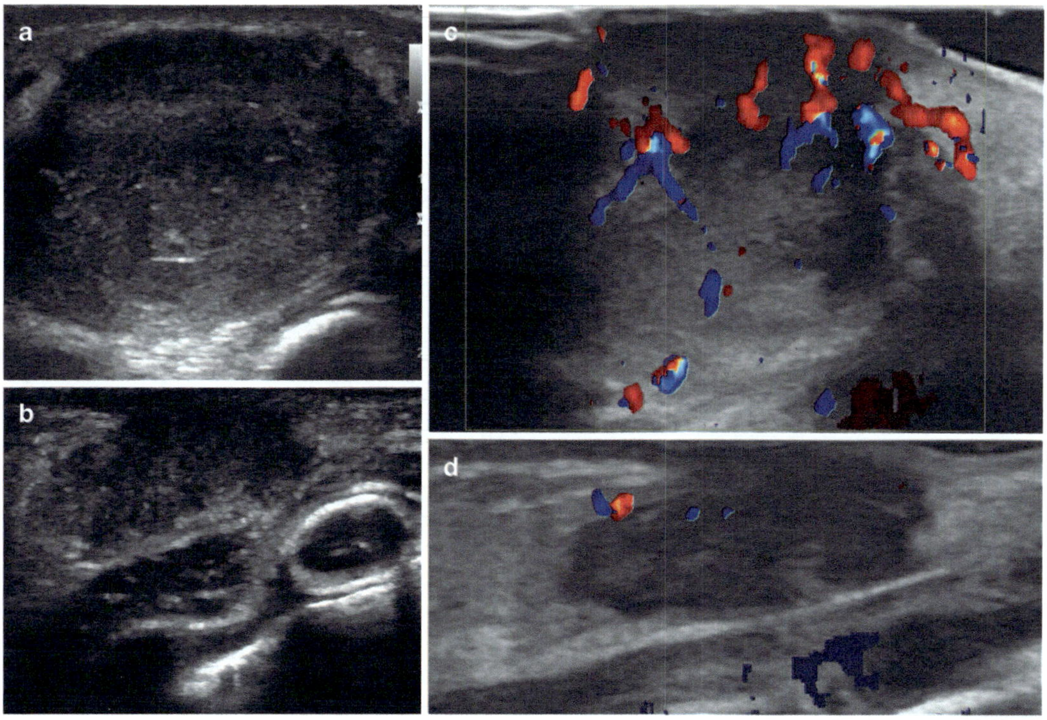

Fig. 4.3 Neonatal mastitis. A 20-day-old girl presenting with left breast enlargement. Sagittal left (**a**) chest ultrasound demonstrates increased thickening and echogenicity in the left breast with surrounding soft tissue edema. Sagittal right (**b**) chest ultrasound for comparison. Additionally, color Doppler demonstrates mild left breast hyperemia (**c**) compared to the contralateral side (**d**)

shows enlargement and indistinctness of the breast bud, with varying degrees of enhanced echogenicity and straining of the surrounding subcutaneous soft tissues, as well as hyperemia on color Doppler (Fig. 4.3) [14, 20]. Conversely, abscesses show avascular anechoic fluid collections with echogenic wall, debris, and peripheral hyperemia (Fig. 4.4). Ultrasound can also serve as guidance during needle aspiration of abscesses.

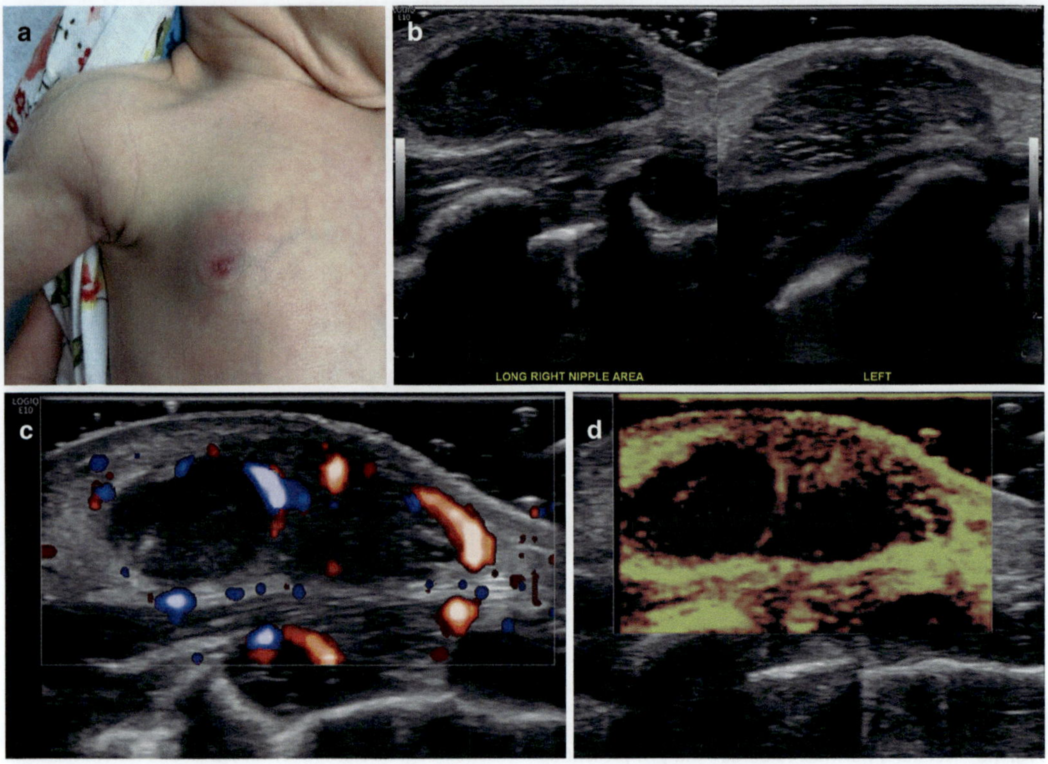

Fig. 4.4 Breast abscess. A 14-day-old girl presenting with swelling and inflammatory changes in the right nipple (**a**). (**b**) Transverse ultrasound image demonstrates a focal hypoechoic area in the right nipple (left side of the image). (**c**, **d**) Color Doppler and microvascular imaging images demonstrate absent internal flow. A comparison view between the right (affected) and left (normal) sides is also provided. Overall, findings are consistent with a right breast abscess

4.4.3 Accessory Breast Tissue

Accessory breast tissue consists of residual breast tissue that persists from normal embryologic development. Accessory breast tissue can be found anywhere along the "milk line" (supernumerary breast) or accessory fragments outside the periphery of the breast gland (aberrant breast) [21]. This condition is a relatively common finding in women and can be found in up to 6% of the general population [21]. This condition has been previously described in newborns in the literature [22]. Accessory breast tissue appears the same as normal breast tissue on ultrasound, irrespective of location.

4.4.4 Chest Wall Abscess

Primary abscesses of the thoracic wall are extremely rare condition [23]. More commonly, these lesions can be due to hematogenous dissemination [24]. Similar to abscesses in other body areas, ultrasound imaging reveals an anechoic or hypoechoic fluid collection with poorly defined borders, indicating the presence of purulent material within the affected tissue (Fig. 4.5).

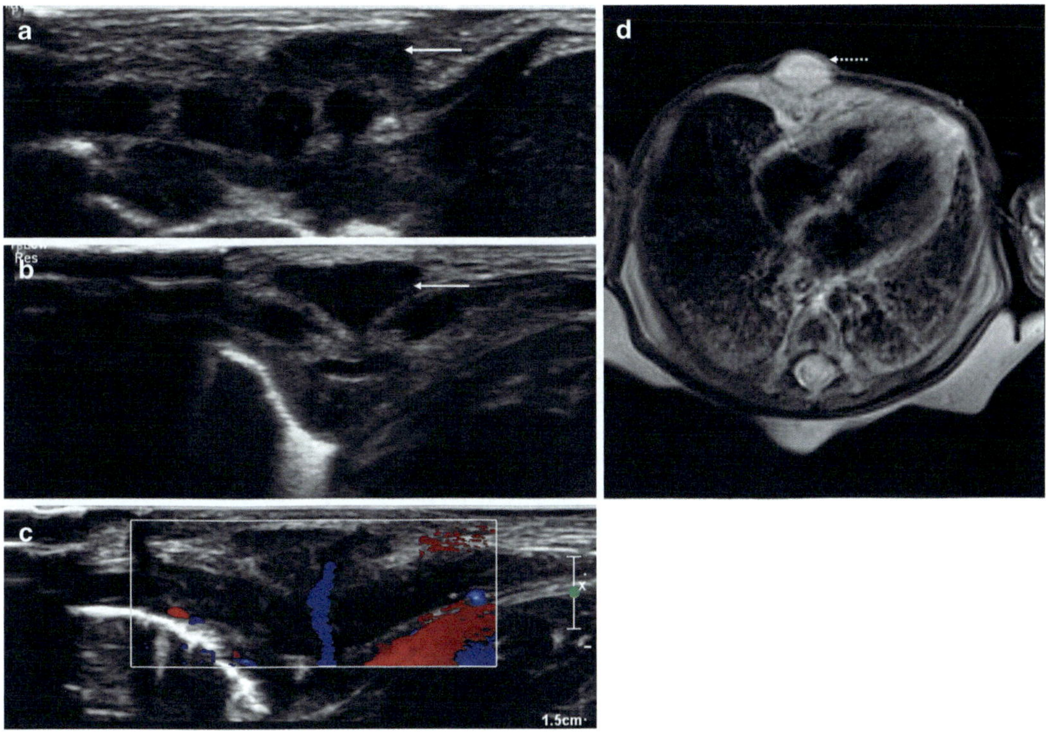

Fig. 4.5 Chest wall abscess. A 13-day-old boy born at 29 weeks of gestation and history of disseminated methicillin susceptible *Staphylococcus aureus* bacteriemia presenting with a subxiphoid lump. Sagittal (**a**) and transverse (**b**) chest ultrasound demonstrate a homogenous echogenic fluid collection extending from the xiphoid process (arrow). Color Doppler (**c**) image shows no internal vascularity. Subsequent T2 (**d**) MRI image shows a collection in the subxiphoid region (dashed arrow) with extension to the mediastinum

4.5 Rib Cage

Most non-tender palpable chest wall abnormalities in children represent developmental variants with no clinical significance and no required treatment; however, imaging may be necessary to rule out malignant processes. These abnormalities may result in palpable masses, especially in the setting of asymmetry. The sonographic appearance of chest wall structures may be confusing because many structures exist in proximity. Therefore, it is of utmost importance that radiologists are familiar with the appearance of normal variants to help improve diagnostic confidence and minimize the need for additional imaging and diagnostic procedures [7].

4.5.1 Congenital Costochondral Abnormalities

Variations in the anterior chest wall are common and present in almost one-third of children [7]. The most common variations include tilted sternum, prominent convexity of the anterior rib, prominent asymmetric costal cartilage, paracostal subcutaneous nodules, and pectus excavatum/carinatum. In addition, costochondral subluxation from either acute trauma or connective tissue diseases might also be present. Many of these findings are radiographically occult, while ultrasound offers additional insights on location, tissue characteristics, and perfusion in the area of interest (Fig. 4.6) [7, 25].

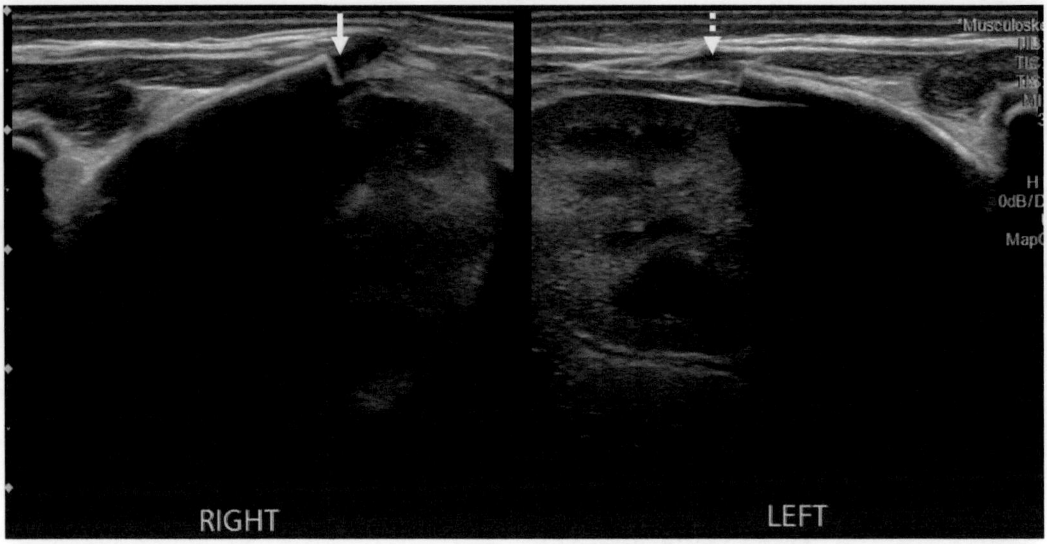

Fig. 4.6 Costochondral abnormality. A 26-day-old boy presented with a palpable mass in the right thoracolumbar junction. Ultrasound shows a protuberant 12th right rib protruding into the soft tissues of the back (arrow). Contralateral image demonstrates normal rib anatomy (dashed arrow). No associated mass or fluid collections are seen

4.5.2 Rib Fractures

Rib fractures in neonates are concerning for non-accidental injury (NAI), especially if the posterior ribs are involved. Some authors have preliminarily reported a positive predictive value as high as 95% for a rib fracture as an indicator of NAI [26]. To a lesser extent, rib fractures might result from delivery, but these cases are very rare [27]. Moreover, the traumatic separation of the costochondral cartilage has been associated with child abuse, which is readily visible on ultrasound but not on radiographs. Ultrasound can help detect slight fragment displacement that may be difficult to visualize on radiographs. Additionally, ultrasound can clearly show the disruption of the cortical surface of the rib, dislocation, and/or angulation of the broken end, adjacent hematomas, or callous formation, depending on the time of injury [5, 28].

4.6 Pleural Space

Several pleural conditions, particularly pleural effusions, can be easily evaluated using ultrasound. This modality allows direct visualization of the pleura and the adjacent lung parenchyma and helps distinguish between a large amount of fluid and a significant consolidation. Although ultrasound does not always allow definitive disease characterization, the classification of pleural fluid plays a significant role in clinical management [12, 29–31].

4.6.1 Pleural Effusions

Total lung volumes obtained post-mortem in neonates without respiratory pathology range between 39.3 and 47.3 ml/kg [32]. In adults, it has been demonstrated that pleural fluid less

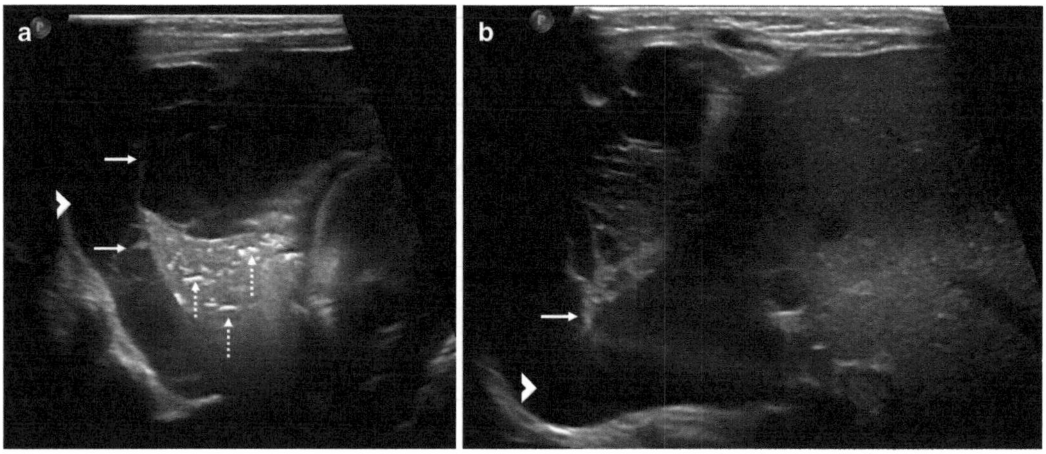

Fig. 4.7 Pleural effusion. A 20-day-old girl with history of trisomy 21 underwent a chest ultrasound. (**a**, **b**) Large complex pleural effusion (chevrons) with multiple septations (arrows) in the right hemithorax with air bronchogram (dashed lines) were seen

than 200 ml may not be visible in a lateral sulcus on a frontal chest radiograph, and a volume <50 ml may not be visible in the posterior sulcus on a lateral radiograph [33]. These limitations can affect the evaluation of small pleural effusions in newborns. Ultrasound plays a crucial role in evaluating and characterizing pleural effusions in this population due to its higher sensitivity, as it can detect effusions as small as 3–5 ml [4, 12]. Furthermore, ultrasound enables better characterization of the nature of pleural fluid (Fig. 4.7). For instance, depending on the sonographic features, it may help to differentiate between a transudate and an exudate. The presence of echoes within the fluid suggests an exudate or hemothorax. Simple, non-loculated collections can be seen to change shape with patients breathing or changing position. As collections progress, they can organize to form fibrinous strands that produce a honeycomb-like pleural space in which fluid no longer moves with changes in patient position or respiration [5]. The presence or absence of septations helps decide whether children require drainage, fibrinolytic therapy, or even video-assisted thoracoscopy [4, 31, 34]. Furthermore, given its lack of ionizing radiation and portability, ultrasound can serve as a follow-up modality for pleural effusions [12].

4.6.2 Pleural Tumors

Pleural tumors in neonates are extremely rare, but the most common type that can occur is congenital pleuropulmonary blastoma, with an incidence of 25–50 cases per year in the United States (Fig. 4.8) [35]. This condition is often mistaken for a congenital pulmonary airway malformation, as the two entities have similar appearances on imaging and pathology. Ultrasound can demonstrate a pleural-based multicystic lesion in a neonate with respiratory distress [36]. Metastatic pleural disease is rare in children compared to adults. However, it can occur after a Wilms tumor, neuroblastoma, or sarcoma. These growths are typically accompanied by large effusions with hemorrhage, which can be seen as echogenic debris-filled fluid during an ultrasound. If pleural masses are visible on ultrasound, they can be easily biopsied with ultrasound guidance, leading to a proper diagnosis [5].

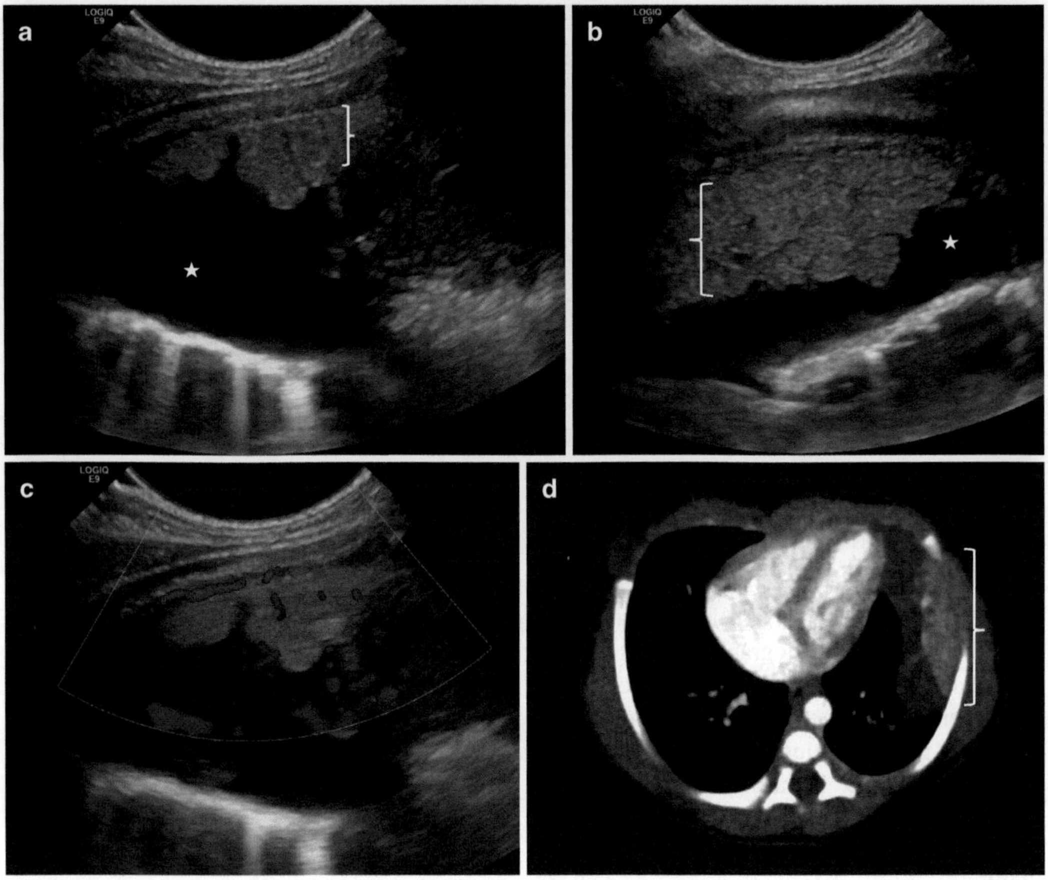

Fig. 4.8 Pleural tumor. A 1-day-old boy with a congenital left chest mass. (**a**–**c**) Ultrasound demonstrates a pleural base lobulated soft tissue mass (brackets) along the left lateral chest wall with large vessels and moderate reactive pleural effusion (stars). Axial (**d**) contrast-enhanced chest angiography shows a pleural-based lesion along the left lateral hemithorax with associated reactive pleural effusion, representing a pleuropulmonary blastoma

4.7 Infantile Hemangioma and Vascular Malformations of the Chest Wall

Most infantile hemangiomas and vascular malformations are congenital or present shortly after birth and progress over time. By using color Doppler, ultrasound allows proper characterization of these lesions and helps to distinguish from other soft tissue abnormalities.

4.7.1 Infantile Hemangioma

Infantile hemangiomas usually present shortly after birth and reach their maximal size between 3 and 5 months of age. Around 60% of cases are found in the head and neck, while 25% are found on the trunk and 15% on the extremities [37]. The physical examination may show the classic cherry-red or strawberry lesion appearance if present in the epidermis of superficial dermis. In

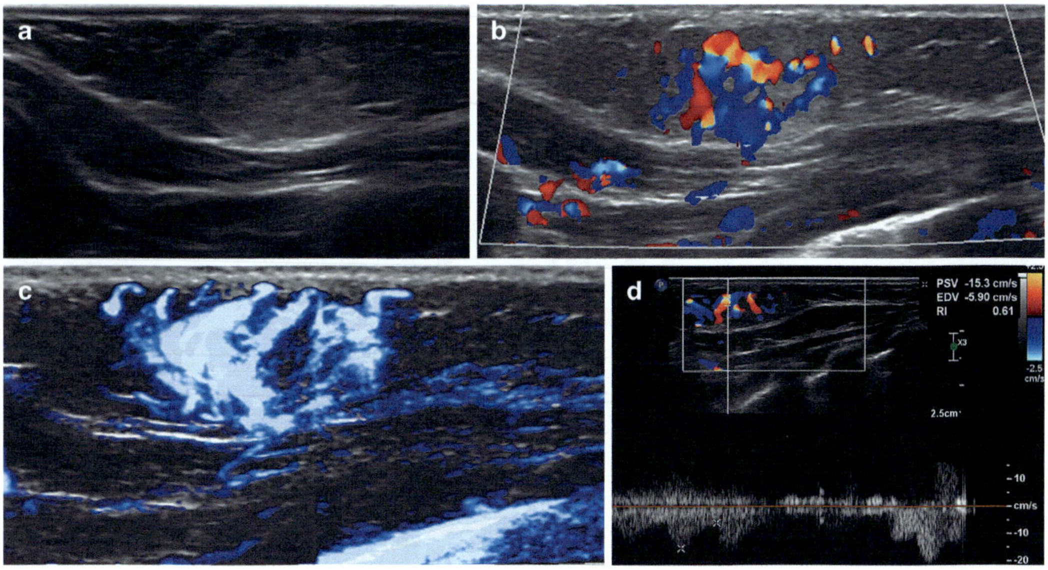

Fig. 4.9 Hemangioma. A 29-day-old girl presented with a blue tone nodule in the right upper chest. (**a**) Heterogeneously hyperechoic soft tissue lesion. (**b**, **c**) Color Doppler and microvascular imaging images demonstrate increased internal vascularity containing arterial spectral flows (**d**), suggestive of an infantile hemangioma

contrast, if located more deeply, the lesion could show a blue tone. Ultrasound demonstrates a well-circumscribed heterogeneous mass with variable echogenicity with marked internal vascularity in color Doppler (Fig. 4.9). Real-time spectral Doppler analysis can be used to differentiate infantile hemangiomas from other vascular tumors by evaluating vascularity density (≥5 vessels/cm^2), and high peak arterial Doppler shift (>2 kHz) [38]. Spectral Doppler has shown utility to predict response to treatment at 6 months [38].

4.7.2 Vascular Malformations

Vascular malformations are lesions present at birth that involve abnormalities of blood and lymph vessels. They can be categorized based on flow characteristics and vessel type. Ultrasound imaging plays a key role in evaluating vascular malformations by determining their features and guiding treatment decisions.

Venous malformations, the most common vascular malformation, appear variable on ultrasound but often show a tangled network of veins or a spongy structure with heterogeneous echogenicity [7, 39, 40]. Spectral Doppler reveals low velocity, monophasic venous waveforms within the malformation (Fig. 4.10). Clinically, these lesions are compressible and may increase in size with Valsalva maneuvers.

Lymphatic malformations are the second most common type and arise in the axilla in around 20% of cases [37, 41]. Based on lesion size, lymphatic malformations are classified as microcystic (<1 cm), macrocystic (≥1 cm), or mixed [42]. Ultrasound typically shows a lobulated cystic mass with thin internal septations. Color Doppler may demonstrate flow within the septations although this is variable (Fig. 4.11). Opposed to venous malformations, lymphatic malformations should not change in appearance with compression or repositioning [7].

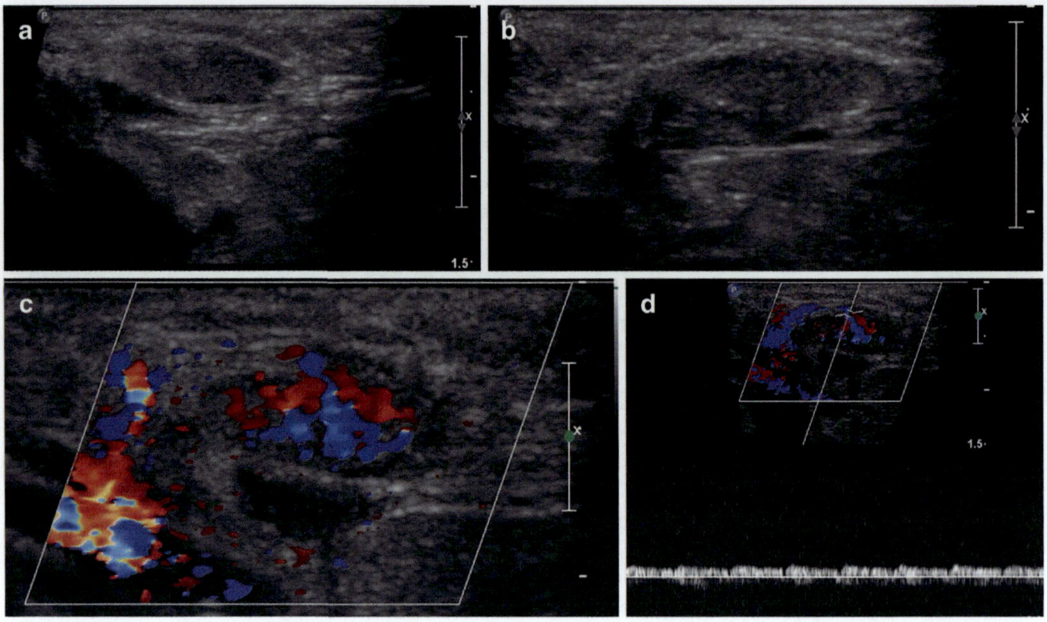

Fig. 4.10 Venous malformation. A 5-day-old girl with palpable chest lump. Sagittal (**a**) and transverse (**b**) grayscale ultrasound images show a lobular hypoechoic mass in the right axilla. Corresponding color Doppler image (**c**) shows internal vascularity and (**d**) spectral Doppler demonstrates venous waveforms, compatible with a venous malformation

Fig. 4.11 Lymphatic malformation. A 1-day-old boy was born with a right chest wall mass. (**a**) Grayscale ultrasound demonstrates large mixed microcystic and macrocystic masses involving the right chest (arrows). (**b**) No internal vascularity seen within the masses. (**c**) Coronal magnetic resonance imaging of the chest wall shows the extent of the large lymphatic malformation (bracket)

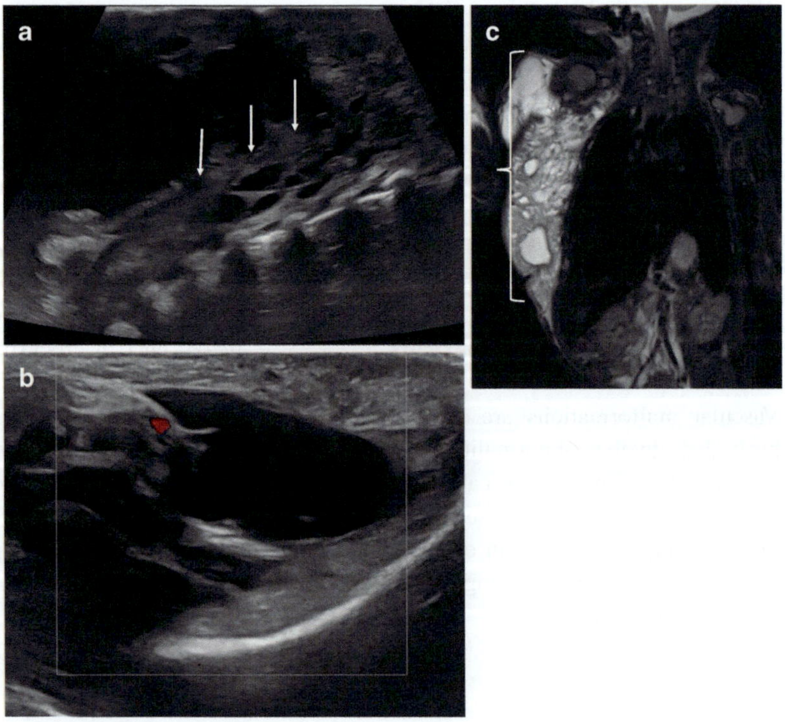

Acknowledgements We would like to thank Victoria Ramirez, PSM, medical science writer at the Children's Hospital of Philadelphia, for reviewing and editing this manuscript.

Declarations and Funding Statements The authors have no conflicts of interest to declare. No specific funding was received for the development of this project.

References

1. Joshi P, Vasishta A, Gupta M. Ultrasound of the pediatric chest. Br J Radiol. 2019;92:20190058. https://doi.org/10.1259/bjr.20190058.
2. Cox M, Soudack M, Podberesky DJ, Epelman M. Pediatric chest ultrasound: a practical approach. Pediatr Radiol. 2017;47:1058–68. https://doi.org/10.1007/s00247-017-3896-8.
3. Claudon M, Tranquart F, Evans DH, et al. Advances in ultrasound. Eur Radiol. 2002;12:7–18. https://doi.org/10.1007/s00330-001-1185-1.
4. Mong A, Epelman M, Darge K. Ultrasound of the pediatric chest. Pediatr Radiol. 2012;42:1287–97. https://doi.org/10.1007/s00247-012-2401-7.
5. Coley BD. Pediatric chest ultrasound. Radiol Clin North Am. 2005;43:405–18. https://doi.org/10.1016/j.rcl.2004.12.003.
6. Riccabona M. Ultrasound of the chest in children (mediastinum excluded). Eur Radiol. 2008;18:390–9. https://doi.org/10.1007/s00330-007-0754-3.
7. Colucci PG, Cohen SA, Baad M, et al. Pediatric chest wall masses: spectrum of benign findings on ultrasound. Pediatr Radiol. 2022;52:429–44. https://doi.org/10.1007/s00247-021-05196-4.
8. Lichtenstein DA, Mauriat P. Lung ultrasound in the critically ill neonate. Curr Pediatr Rev. 2012;8:217–23. https://doi.org/10.2174/157339612802139389.
9. Nasseri F, Eftekhari F. Clinical and radiologic review of the normal and abnormal thymus: pearls and pitfalls. Radiographics. 2010;30:413–28. https://doi.org/10.1148/rg.302095131.
10. Feola GP, Shaw LCA, Coburn L. Management of complicated parapneumonic effusions in children. Tech Vasc Interv Radiol. 2003;6:197–04. https://doi.org/10.1053/j.tvir.2003.10.004.
11. Kim OH, Kim WS, Kim MJ, et al. US in the diagnosis of pediatric chest diseases. Radiographics. 2000;20:653–71. https://doi.org/10.1148/radiographics.20.3.g00ma05653.
12. Goh Y, Kapur J. Sonography of the pediatric chest. J Ultrasound Med. 2016;35:1067–80. https://doi.org/10.7863/ultra.15.06006.
13. Valeur NS, Rahbar H, Chapman T. Ultrasound of pediatric breast masses: what to do with lumps and bumps. Pediatr Radiol. 2015;45:1584–99; quiz 1581. https://doi.org/10.1007/s00247-015-3402-0.
14. Restrepo R, Cervantes LF, Swirsky AM, Diaz A. Breast development in pediatric patients from birth to puberty: physiology, pathology and imaging correlation. Pediatr Radiol. 2021;51:1959–69. https://doi.org/10.1007/s00247-021-05099-4.
15. Howard BA, Gusterson BA. Human breast development. J Mammary Gland Biol Neoplasia. 2000;5:119–37. https://doi.org/10.1023/a:1026487120779.
16. Amer A, Fischer H. Images in clinical medicine. Neonatal breast enlargement. N Engl J Med. 2009;360:1445. https://doi.org/10.1056/NEJMicm0707832.
17. Jawahar A, Vade A. Sonographic features of physiologic neonatal breast enlargement. J Clin Neonatol. 2014;3:106–8. https://doi.org/10.4103/2249-4847.134701.
18. D'Auria D, Ferrara D, Aragione N, et al. Role of ultrasound in diagnosis of neonatal breast enlargement: a newborn case report. Radiol Case Rep. 2021;16:2692–6. https://doi.org/10.1016/j.radcr.2021.06.057.
19. Masoodi T, Mufti GN, Bhat JI, et al. Neonatal mastitis: a clinico-microbiological study. J Neonatal Surg. 2014;3:2.
20. Borders H, Mychaliska G, Gebarski KS. Sonographic features of neonatal mastitis and breast abscess. Pediatr Radiol. 2009;39:955–8. https://doi.org/10.1007/s00247-009-1310-x.
21. DeFilippis EM, Arleo EK. The ABCs of accessory breast tissue: basic information every radiologist should know. AJR Am J Roentgenol. 2014;202:1157–62. https://doi.org/10.2214/AJR.13.10930.
22. Calle-Toro JS, Kelly A, Ford EJ, et al. Incidental findings during ultrasound of thyroid, breast, testis, uterus and ovary in healthy term neonates. J Ultrasound. 2019;22:395–400. https://doi.org/10.1007/s40477-019-00365-6.
23. Correia RS, Fonseca JP, Delgado M. Primary chest wall abscess caused by pseudomonas aeruginosa and staphylococcus epidermidis. Cureus. 2023;15:e48544. https://doi.org/10.7759/cureus.48544.
24. Yamaoka Y, Yamamura J, Masuda N, et al. Primary chest wall abscess mimicking a breast tumor that occurred after blunt chest trauma: a case report. Case Report Med. 2014;2014:620876. https://doi.org/10.1155/2014/620876.
25. Supakul N, Karmazyn B. Ultrasound evaluation of costochondral abnormalities in children presenting with anterior chest wall mass. AJR Am J Roentgenol. 2013;201:W336–41. https://doi.org/10.2214/AJR.12.9792.
26. Barsness KA, Cha E-S, Bensard DD, et al. The positive predictive value of rib fractures as an indicator of nonaccidental trauma in children. J Trauma. 2003;54:1107–10. https://doi.org/10.1097/01.TA.0000068992.01030.A8.
27. van Rijn RR, Bilo RAC, Robben SGF. Birth-related mid-posterior rib fractures in neonates: a report of three cases (and a possible fourth case) and a review

of the literature. Pediatr Radiol. 2009;39:30–4. https://doi.org/10.1007/s00247-008-1035-2.
28. Liu J. Using ultrasound to diagnose neonatal clavicle and rib fracture. Chest. 2021;160:A1950. https://doi.org/10.1016/j.chest.2021.07.1729.
29. Chiu C-Y, Wong K-S, Huang Y-C, et al. Echo-guided management of complicated parapneumonic effusion in children. Pediatr Pulmonol. 2006;41:1226–32. https://doi.org/10.1002/ppul.20528.
30. Ekingen G, Güvenç BH, Sözübir S, et al. Fibrinolytic treatment of complicated pediatric thoracic empyemas with intrapleural streptokinase. Eur J Cardiothorac Surg. 2004;26:503–7. https://doi.org/10.1016/j.ejcts.2004.05.032.
31. Gates RL, Hogan M, Weinstein S, Arca MJ. Drainage, fibrinolytics, or surgery: a comparison of treatment options in pediatric empyema. J Pediatr Surg. 2004;39:1638–42. https://doi.org/10.1016/j.jpedsurg.2004.07.015.
32. Dassios T. Critical functional lung volumes in neonatal intensive care: evidence and clinical applications. Pediatr Res. 2023;94:82–8. https://doi.org/10.1038/s41390-022-02450-9.
33. Brogi E, Gargani L, Bignami E, et al. Thoracic ultrasound for pleural effusion in the intensive care unit: a narrative review from diagnosis to treatment. Crit Care. 2017;21:325. https://doi.org/10.1186/s13054-017-1897-5.
34. Kalfa N, Allal H, Lopez M, et al. Thoracoscopy in pediatric pleural empyema: a prospective study of prognostic factors. J Pediatr Surg. 2006;41:1732–7. https://doi.org/10.1016/j.jpedsurg.2006.05.066.
35. Priest JR, Andic D, Arbuckle S, et al. Great vessel/cardiac extension and tumor embolism in pleuropulmonary blastoma: a report from the International Pleuropulmonary Blastoma Registry. Pediatr Blood Cancer. 2011;56:604–9. https://doi.org/10.1002/pbc.22583.
36. Lyle ANJ, Ohlsen TJD, Miller DE, et al. Congenital pleuropulmonary blastoma in a newborn with a variant of uncertain significance in DICER1 evaluated by RNA-sequencing. Matern Health Neonatol Perinatol. 2023;9:4. https://doi.org/10.1186/s40748-023-00148-2.
37. Mulligan PR, Prajapati HJS, Martin LG, Patel TH. Vascular anomalies: classification, imaging characteristics and implications for interventional radiology treatment approaches. Br J Radiol. 2014;87:20130392. https://doi.org/10.1259/bjr.20130392.
38. He L, Huang G. Spectral Doppler ultrasound for predicting long-term response to topical timolol in children with infantile hemangioma. J Clin Ultrasound. 2017;45:480–7. https://doi.org/10.1002/jcu.22471.
39. Flors L, Leiva-Salinas C, Maged IM, et al. MR imaging of soft-tissue vascular malformations: diagnosis, classification, and therapy follow-up. Radiographics. 2011;31:1321–40.; discussion 1340. https://doi.org/10.1148/rg.315105213.
40. Olivieri B, White CL, Restrepo R, et al. Low-flow vascular malformation pitfalls: from clinical examination to practical imaging evaluation—Part 2, venous malformation mimickers. AJR Am J Roentgenol. 2016;206:952–62. https://doi.org/10.2214/AJR.15.15794.
41. Puig S, Casati B, Staudenherz A, Paya K. Vascular low-flow malformations in children: current concepts for classification, diagnosis and therapy. Eur J Radiol. 2005;53:35–45. https://doi.org/10.1016/j.ejrad.2004.07.023.
42. Merrow AC, Gupta A, Patel MN, Adams DM. 2014 revised classification of vascular lesions from the International Society for the Study of Vascular Anomalies: radiologic-pathologic update. Radiographics. 2016;36:1494–516. https://doi.org/10.1148/rg.2016150197.

5 Neonatal Lungs and Mediastinum

Priscilla Joshi, Shriyash Pinglikar, and Vandana Jahanvi

Highlights
- Introduction
- Procedure and Protocols
- Indications for Neonatal Lung Ultrasound
- Appearances of Normal and Abnormal Lung on Ultrasound
- Ultrasound of the Mediastinum

5.1 Introduction

Air in the lungs was earlier looked upon as a deterrent for evaluation of the lungs. However, in the recent past, the same artefacts produced by air in the lungs are being used for the diagnosis of various lung conditions.

Neonatal respiratory distress, which is responsible for a high proportion of mortality occurs due to various causes [1], of these, prematurity with resultant surfactant deficiency is one of the commoner causes. Ultrasound has been found to be superior to conventional radiography in the diagnosis and follow-up of this condition [2]. Lung ultrasound (LUS) is less expensive, available at the bedside, quicker and does not expose patients to ionizing radiation and hence reduces the risks of radiation [3].

Ultrasound also provides real-time imaging, hence allowing evaluation of dynamic changes in lung tissue during breathing. It also allows the evaluation of pleural effusions, pneumothorax and diaphragmatic movements.

5.2 Procedure and Protocols

5.2.1 Scanning Protocol for Common Neonatal Lung Conditions

5.2.1.1 Equipment and Probe Selection

Linear high frequency transducers with a frequency of 5–12 and 12–18 MHz are used for lung and mediastinal ultrasound [4]. The smaller the footprint, the greater is the ease of scanning the patients. Lower frequency transducers can be used for evaluating deeper structures or evaluating neonates with an increased birth weight.

Each lung is divided by the anterior and posterior axillary lines which divide them into three areas vertically and further by a horizontal line midway through each lung further dividing each lung into six areas (Fig. 5.1) [5].

P. Joshi (✉) · S. Pinglikar
Department of Radiodiagnosis, Bharati Vidyapeeth (DU) Medical College and Hospital, Pune, Maharashtra, India

V. Jahanvi
Department of Radiodiagnosis, Paras Hospitals, Gurgaon, Haryana, India

K. S. Sodhi (ed.), *Neonatal Ultrasound*, https://doi.org/10.1007/978-981-97-8576-6_5

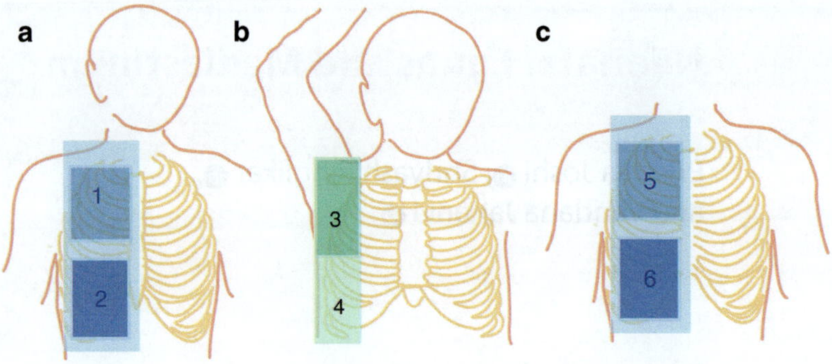

Fig. 5.1 Frontal view: Line diagram showing the six areas of the pediatric chest. Each lung is divided by the anterior and posterior axillary lines into three areas vertically and by a horizontal line midway through each lung further dividing each lung into six areas. (**a**) Frontal view showing 1 and 2 the anterior superior and inferior areas, (**b**) showing 3 and 4 the lateral superior and inferior areas, and (**c**) posterior aspect of chest showing 5 and 6 the postero superior and inferior areas

5.3 Acoustic Windows for Scanning

In neonates and infants, lack of costal cartilage ossification and low bone mineral content improve trans-osseous trans-sternal and trans-costal visualization.

The windows which can be used for scanning are the:

1. Intercostal spaces.
2. Parasternal region.
3. Suprasternal notch.
4. Transdiaphragmatic approach—subcostal and subxiphoid.

5.3.1 Scanning Techniques and Positions

The neonate is scanned in the supine, lateral decubitus and prone positions for evaluation of each lung [5].

While evaluating each lung the transducers are placed in the vertical plane perpendicular to the horizontally oriented ribs.

Scanning is also done in the transverse plane parallel to the ribs.

Inclined transverse and inclined longitudinal scans may also be performed by tilting the transducer.

In case the scan is for evaluation of an opacity seen on a chest radiograph, the neonate is also scanned on the presumed location of the lesion based on the radiographic findings.

Subcostal scans are done with the transducer placed horizontally and obliquely, below the rib cage in the subcostal position, to evaluate the right lung base and look for the presence of the mirror image artefact of the liver in the lung which is seen in case the lung base is normally aerated. It is prudent to also evaluate the diaphragm and diaphragmatic movements as well as the liver in each patient to complete the study.

B mode, M mode ultrasound and colour Doppler are used.

5.3.2 B Mode

B mode ultrasound or brightness mode ultrasound produces two-dimensional, real-time images of internal structures based on the echoes of sound waves. This is used for lung pathologies like consolidation, RDS (respiratory distress syndrome), MAS (Meconium aspiration syndrome),

TTN (Transient tachypnoea of the newborn) and for pleural pathologies like effusion and pneumothorax [6].

5.3.3 M Mode

M mode ultrasound (motion mode) is a type of ultrasound imaging that displays motion over time. In the chest, it is used to confirm normal lung and to evaluate pathologies like pneumothorax, lung sliding and diaphragmatic motion.

Colour Doppler is used for the visualization of the normal vascular anatomy. It is also used for evaluating the vascularity of mediastinal masses. Colour Doppler helps demonstrate abnormal vessel. It is also used to differentiate between, CPAM and sequestration [7].

5.4 Indications for Neonatal Lung Ultrasound

The following are the indications for a neonatal chest ultrasound:

1. Evaluation of a case of respiratory distress in the newborn for the underlying cause which includes [6]:
   (a) Respiratory Distress Syndrome or Surfactant Deficiency Disorder.
   (b) Transient tachyponea of the newborn (TTN).
   (c) Meconium aspiration syndrome (MAS).
   (d) Pneumonia.
2. Evaluating an opacity detected on a chest radiograph.
3. Detection of a pneumothorax.
4. Congenital lung abnormalities.

5.4.1 Normal Lung Appearance on Ultrasound

On a longitudinal scan of the chest, the most superficial structures seen are the skin, below which lies the subcutaneous tissue. The intercostal muscles lie deep to the subcutaneous tissues, between the ribs. The ribs are seen as echogenic structures at regular intervals and show distal shadowing (Fig. 5.2).

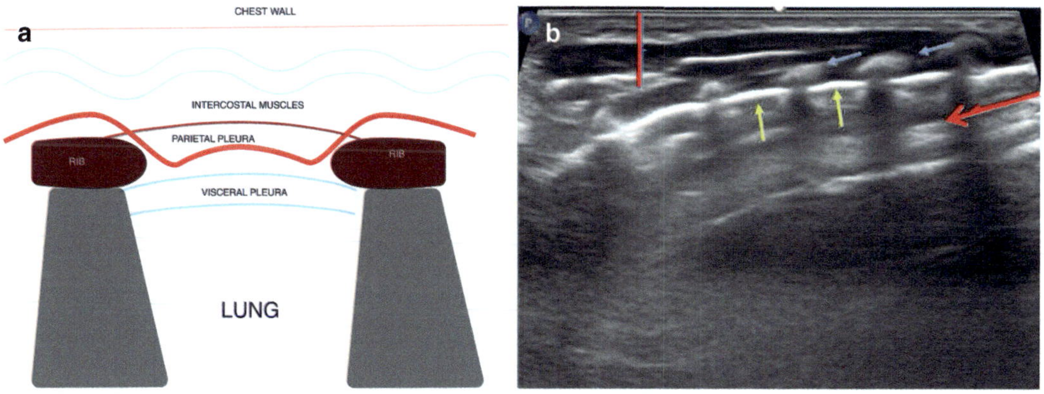

Fig. 5.2 (**a**) Schematic diagram of normal lung showing the ribs (brown) with the intervening intercostal muscles. Overlying skin and subcutaneous tissue is seen. The parietal and visceral pleura are seen in blue below or posterior to the intercostal muscles."Bats wing" appearance (a red line is seen) formed by the adjoining ribs and the pleural line—the wings are formed by the ribs. (**b**) Longitudinal B scan ultrasound image using a linear transducer showing the echogenic pleura (yellow arrow), horizontal echogenic A lines (red arrow). Ribs appear hyperechoic with distal shadowing (blue arrow) with intercostal muscles in between. Overlying subcutaneous tissue and skin appearing hypoechoic (vertical red line)

The parietal and visceral layers of pleura lie below the ribs and intercostal muscles and appose each other. Together they appear as a bright hyperechoic line less than a millimetre in thickness (Fig. 5.4b). The movement of the parietal pleura against the visceral pleura and the underlying lung during inspiration and expiration is called as "lung sliding" [8]. Presence of "lung sliding" indicates the underlying lung and pleura are disease free.

"**Seashore Sign**": The image obtained in the M mode with the cursor on the pleura shows as a linear pattern in the tissues superficial to the pleural line (referred to as the "sea") and as a grainy or "sandy" look deeper to the pleural line (referred to as the "shore"), forming the "seashore sign" (Fig. 5.3a, b) [9].

"**Bat Sign**": The bat's wings are depicted on B mode imaging by two neighbouring ribs with posterior shadowing, while the echogenic pleural line represents the body (Fig. 5.2) [9].

"**A**" **Lines**: The air in the normally aerated lungs produces reverberation artefacts which are horizontally placed bright lines, parallel to the ribs and pleura called as the "A" lines [9]. These are equidistant from each other (Fig. 5.2). Absence of these "A" lines indicates a possible abnormality in the underlying lung.

"**B**" **Lines**: These are lines perpendicular to the chest wall, reaching up to the end of the screen, not moving with respiration. These are hyperechoic with the overlying pleura appearing thick and irregular. They indicate presence of fluid within the interstitium (Fig. 5.4).

In children and adults, B lines signal the presence of pathology; however, in term neonates few B lines may be seen in the first 48 h after birth. These may be seen for longer in pre-term neonates.

"**Comet Tail**" **Artefacts**: The "B lines" should be differentiated from "Comet tail" artefacts which are shorter [10]. The comet tail artefacts do not erase/mask the A lines and do not reach up to the edge of the screen. The overlying pleura appears normal (Fig. 5.4c).

"**Mirror Image**" **Artefact**: On a subcostal scan, if the lung base is normal, i.e. the lung is aerated, the image of the liver is mirrored in the lung base (Fig. 5.5). Absence of "mirror image" artefact occurs if the lung base is abnormal.

Lung Pulse Sign [10]: Cardiac pulsations may be conducted to the adjoining atelectatic lung in contact with the heart.

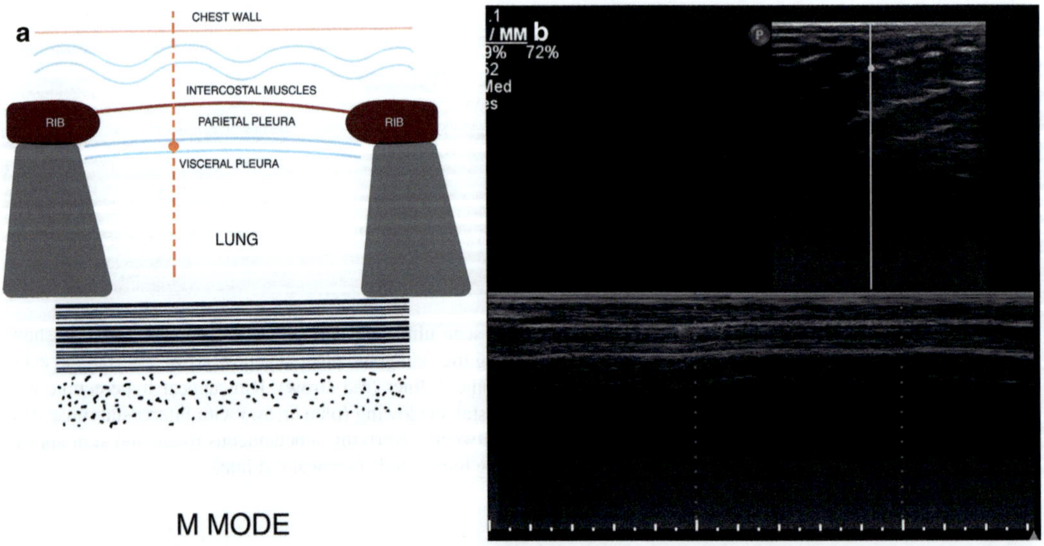

Fig. 5.3 (**a**) Diagrammatic representation showing seashore sign. (**b**) M Mode (static) ultrasound images of normal lung showing seashore sign

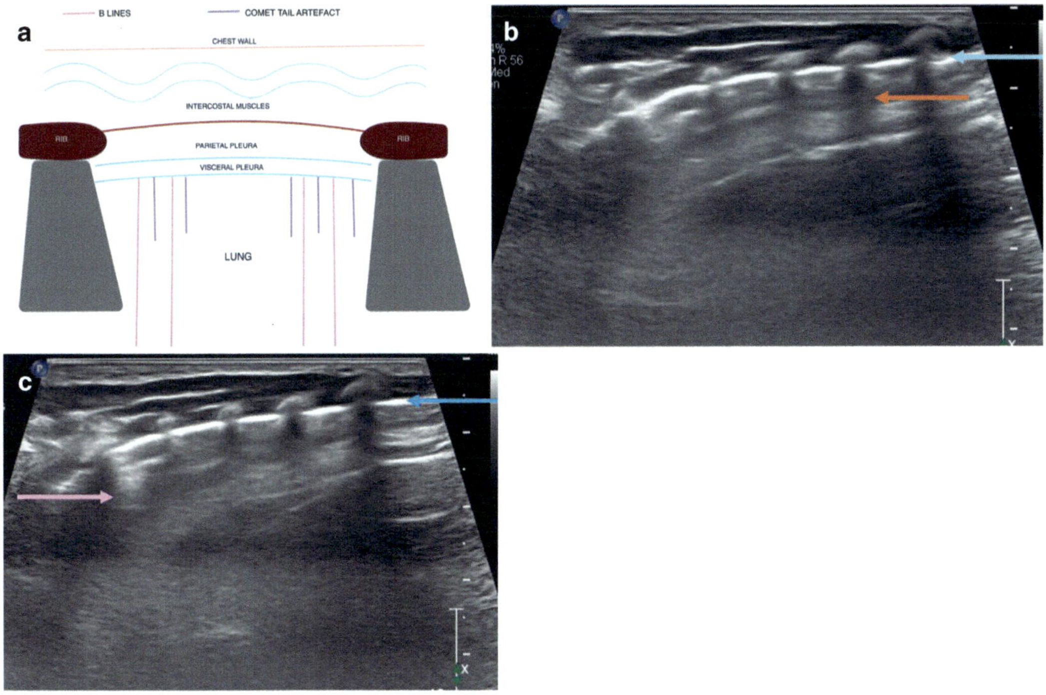

Fig. 5.4 Ultrasound images of lung showing comet tail artefact. (**a**) Schematic diagram. The short vertical purple lines are comet tail artefacts. These do not reach upto the border (periphery) of the screen. The pink vertical lines reach upto the border (periphery) of the screen are B lines. The horizontally oriented blue lines are the visceral and parietal pleura. (**b**) Longitudinal ultrasound image using a linear transducer blue arrow shows pleural line formed by apposed visceral and parietal layers of pleura. Orange arrow shows shadowing from ribs (**c**) Comet tail artefact, short echogenic lines perpendicular to the chest wall not reaching upto the border (periphery) of the screen not erasing A lines (pink arrow). Overlying normal echogenic line is the pleural line (blue arrow)

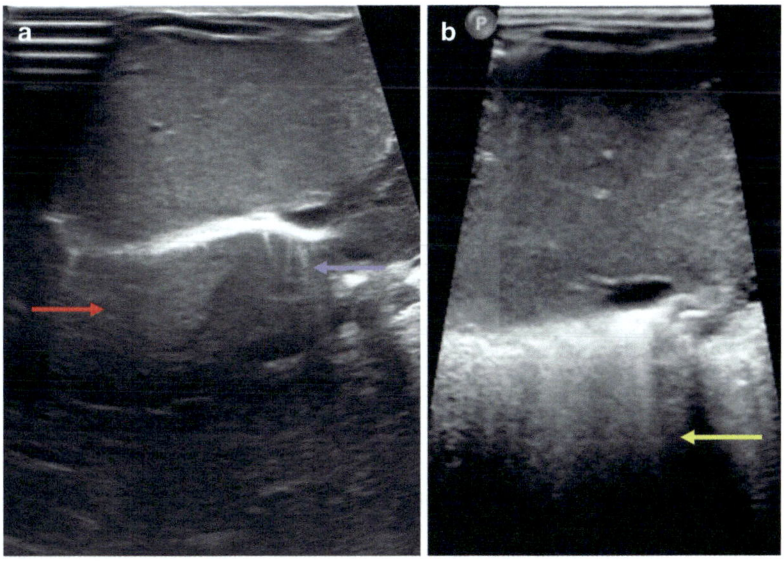

Fig. 5.5 Mirror image artefact: (**a**) Showing a normal mirror image artefact of the liver in the lung base (red arrow). This is seen if the lung base is normal Note the comet tail artefacts in (**a**) (purple arrow). (**b**) Subcostal scan of right lung base showing the normal mirror image artefact is replaced by condensed B lines which are fairly densely packed in a pre term neonate with RDS (yellow arrow)

A lines	B lines	Comet tail artefact
Horizontal lines, equidistant occur parallel to the chest wall	Vertical lines perpendicular to the chest wall erase the A lines reach up to the end of the screen	Short vertical lines. Perpendicular to the chest wall do not reach up to the end of the screen do not erase A lines
Seen in normal lung	In the early post-natal period, few B lines maybe normal. Condensed B lines are abnormal	
	Overlying pleura may be thick and irregular	Overlying pleura is normal

5.4.2 Abnormal Findings in Various Lung Pathologies

Lung ultrasound has in the recent past shown its utility in the diagnosis of respiratory distress syndrome and also in replacing conventional radiographs in the follow-up of neonates with respiratory distress syndrome. It can also differentiate TTN from RDS, thus improving the outcome in these patients. It is helpful in the evaluation and follow-up of neonates with consolidation especially where there is a delayed resolution.

5.4.3 Surfactant Deficiency Disorder/Respiratory Distress Syndrome (RDS)

The overlying pleural line is thick and irregular. Small areas of consolidation may also be seen [11, 12](Fig. 5.6).

Ultrasound is useful in the diagnosis of this condition, as well as in the follow-up in these neonates [13, 14].

Several lung ultrasound scores are available. The decision to administer surfactant depends on these scores [15]. The scores are also helpful in the follow-up of these neonates.

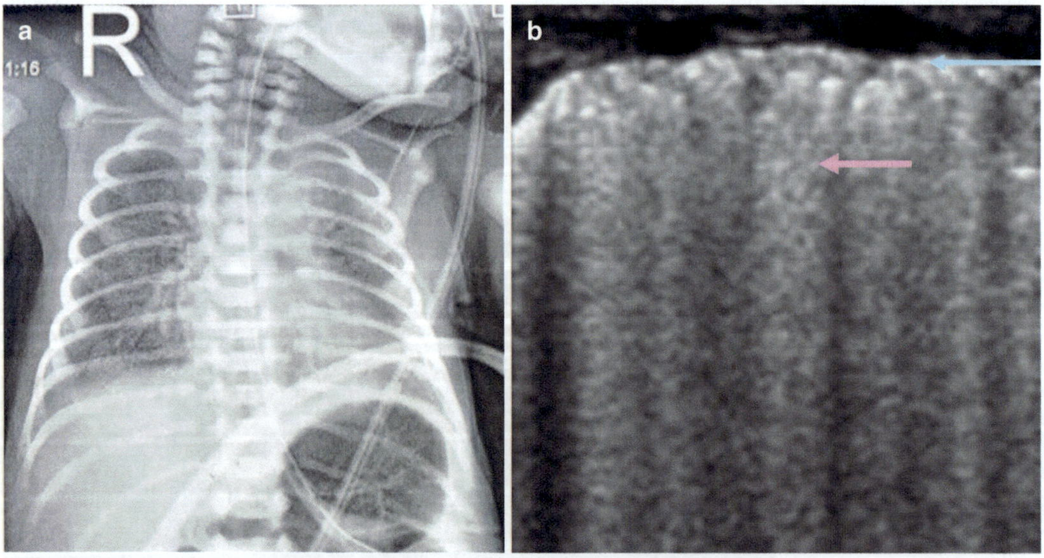

Fig. 5.6 Thirty-two week preterm neonate with tachpnoea. Respiratory distress syndrome. (**a**) Frontal chest radiograph shows subtle granular opacities in both lungs. Ultrasound was performed as RDS was suspected. The findings served as a base line for follow up. (**b**) Longitudinal B mode ultrasound of lung showing condensed B lines (pink arrow). The overlying pleural line is shaggy and irregular (blue arrow). Lung sliding seen on real time imaging was reduced

Lung ultrasound score:

There are several scoring systems used to assess lung ultrasound findings in neonates, especially in the context of respiratory distress syndrome (RDS) [16]. These scores help clinicians evaluate the severity of lung disease, monitor response to treatment [17] and guide clinical decision-making [14, 18]. Here are two commonly used lung ultrasound scores for RDS:

LUS:

Components: The LUS is often based on the evaluation of multiple lung zones, typically divided into anterior, lateral and posterior regions on each side of the chest [19].

Scoring Criteria: Each lung zone is scored based on specific ultrasound findings, such as the presence of A lines (normal aeration), B lines (indicating interstitial syndrome), consolidation or other abnormalities. The severity of each finding is assigned a numerical score [20].

Interpretation: The total LUS is the sum of scores from all examined zones, providing an overall assessment of lung aeration. Higher scores indicate more severe lung pathology.

Brat et al. also devised a score where a 0 to 3 point score was given [16]:

Scoring Criteria [20]

- 0: where only A lines were present.

1: with three or more well-spaced B lines.

2: with the presence of crowded and coalescent B lines with or without consolidations limited to the subpleural space.

3: with extensive consolidations.

Interpretation

- Higher BRAT scores suggest decreased lung aeration and increased severity of respiratory distress.

5.4.3.1 Transient Tachypnoea of the Newborn (TTN)

This happens as a result of the fluid in the lungs clearing more slowly. Normal labour involves the vaginal squeezing of the chest to eliminate the fluid that is present in the lungs prior to birth. There is delayed fluid drainage in the first 3 h after birth [21], as a result of the fluid in the lungs clearing more slowly; therefore, the disease is more common in newborns delivered by Caesarean section (Fig. 5.7).

A chest radiograph has been considered the gold standard for the diagnosis; however in the recent past, ultrasound has been increasingly used in the diagnosis [22, 23].

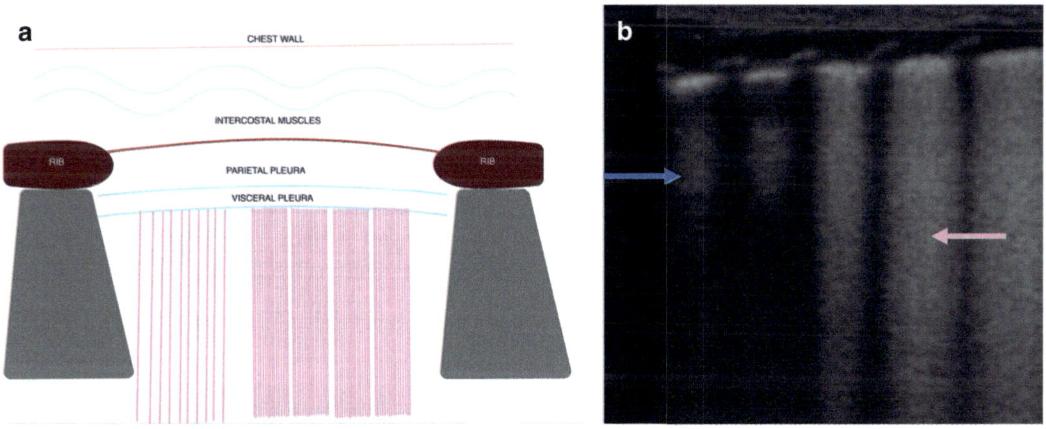

Fig. 5.7 Term neonate LSCS delivery. Respiratory distress after birth. (**a**) Diagrammatic representation showing densely packed B lines (vertical pink lines) caudally with less densely packed B lines cranially (vertically oriented pink lines). (**b**) Longitudinal B scan ultrasound image revealing densely packed B lines caudally (pink arrow) with less densely packed B lines cranially (blue arrow) suggestive of a double lung point diagnostic of transient tachypnoea of new born

Findings

TTN is characterized by the presence of a "double lung" point. This means that the B lines are condensed at the lung base and are relatively less condensed above [24].

Double lung point therefore helps differentiate surfactant deficiency disorder from TTN. In contrast to respiratory distress syndrome surfactant deficiency disorder the overlying pleural line is normal [25].

Surfactant Deficiency Disorder (SDD)	Transient Tachypnoea of the Newborn (TTN)
Condensed B lines	Double lung point-condensed B lines caudally without condensed lines cranially
Overlying pleural line is thick and "shaggy"	Normal thin echogenic pleural line

5.4.3.2 Meconium Aspiration Syndrome

Antepartum or puerperal inhalation of meconium or amniotic fluid stained with meconium can result in respiratory distress [26]. This can occur in term or post-term neonates. Birth asphyxia and neonates born via a caesarean section are more commonly affected. Subpleural areas of consolidation are seen on lung ultrasound with air bronchogram. Other findings seen are presence of B lines, absence of A lines, irregular/thick pleura.

Complications include pneumothorax in 15–30% of cases. The condition results in mortality in <12% patients [27].

5.4.3.3 Pneumonia

Both viral and bacterial pneumonias which are life threatening present with respiratory distress [6].

Lung infection may occur intrapartum, during delivery or post-partum. The foetus can acquire the infection from maternal cervical secretions or contaminated amniotic fluid. Intrapartum infection can be transmitted through the blood circulating the placenta and amniotic membranes secondary to premature rupture of membranes [28].

Infection primarily occurs through the respiratory tract but can also be blood borne or iatrogenic. *E. coli* and *Staphylococcus aureus* are the common bacteria responsible. Viruses include herpes simplex, cytomegalovirus, rubella, chicken pox and Coxsackie. Other organisms include Klebsiella, Listeria, Chlamydia and Mycoplasma.

On ultrasound, lung consolidation is seen. Other findings seen are irregularity and thickening of the pleura, absence of lung sliding, presence of pleural effusion [29].

Consolidation appears as "lung hepatization". The lung appears hypoechoic, akin to the liver with the air in the bronchi appearing "hyperechoic" and showing a branching pattern. This is termed as the ultrasound "air bronchogram" [30] (Fig. 5.8a).

The air bronchogram in consolidation is a "dynamic air bronchogram", i.e. the air within the bronchi shows a centrifugal movement.

In atelectasis or where there is a bronchial occlusion a "static" air bronchogram is seen (Fig. 5.8b).

Ultrasound is able to detect areas of "necrosis" and pneumatocoele formation in a consolidation, much earlier than plain radiographs and hence is important in the follow-up of patients with pneumonia, especially in necrotising pneumonias and neonates not responding to antibiotic therapy (Fig. 5.9).

5.4.4 Pulmonary Haemorrhage of the Newborn

This has an incidence 1–12 per 1000 live births [31] with risk factors including RDS, severe intrauterine infection and severe birth asphyxia. Other causes include prematurity, intrauterine growth retardation (IUGR), patent ductus arteriosus (PDA), disseminated intravascular coagulation (DIC), meconium aspiration syndrome (MAS) and sepsis.

In three fourths of the patients, this occurs in the first 24 h of life with around 80% developing pulmonary haemorrhage within 3 days and 90% within a week of birth. Condensed B lines are seen, which appear more hyperechoic than those seen in RDS. It has a high mortality rate [31, 32].

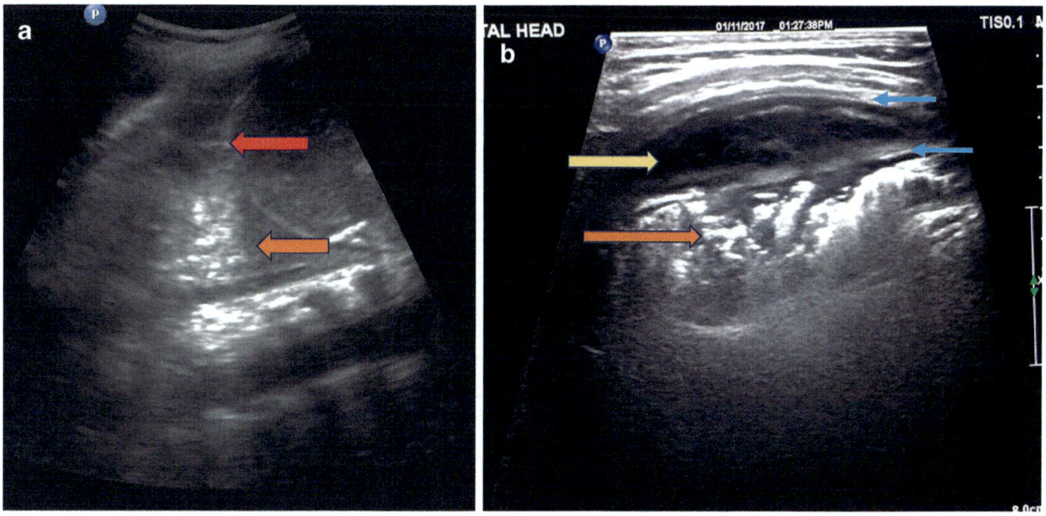

Fig. 5.8 (**a**) Consolidation – Note the air bronchogram and lung hepatization, seen i.e. the appearance of the lung akin to the liver in consolidation (orange arrow, red arrow). (**b**) Atelectasis –where crowding of lung markings is seen. There is overlying loculated pleural effusion (yellow arrow, orange arrow) with thickening of the parietal and visceral pleura (blue arrows)

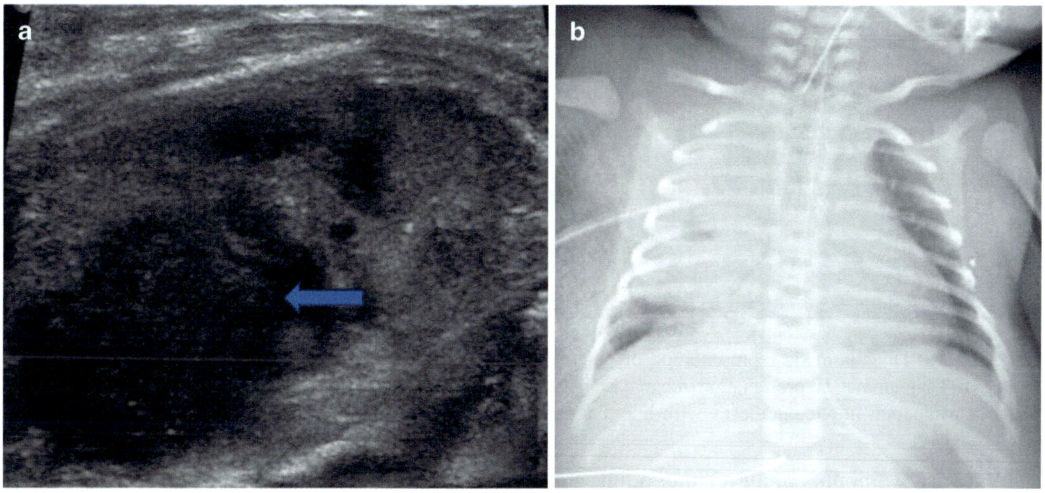

Fig. 5.9 Early detection of areas of breakdown—necrotizing pneumonia on ultrasound. (**a**) Ultrasound images showing hypo to anechoic areas in the areas of consolidation. (**b**) Frontal chest radiograph showing large homogenous opacity right upper and mid zones suggestive of consolidation. No apparent findings suggestive of breakdown are seen

5.4.5 Air Leak Syndromes

Inappropriate mechanical ventilation in lungs, which are fragile and immature, results in air leak syndromes, which manifest as pneumothorax, pneumomediastinum and pulmonary interstitial emphysema.

Pulmonary air leak occurs more frequently in the newborn period than at any other time of life and spontaneous pneumothorax may be seen in 1–2% of neonates [33].

In pneumothorax, the A lines and pleural sliding are no longer seen. A "lung point" may be seen due to separation of the parietal and visceral pleura by the air. This is seen better with smaller amounts of air separating the two reflections of pleura (Fig. 5.10).

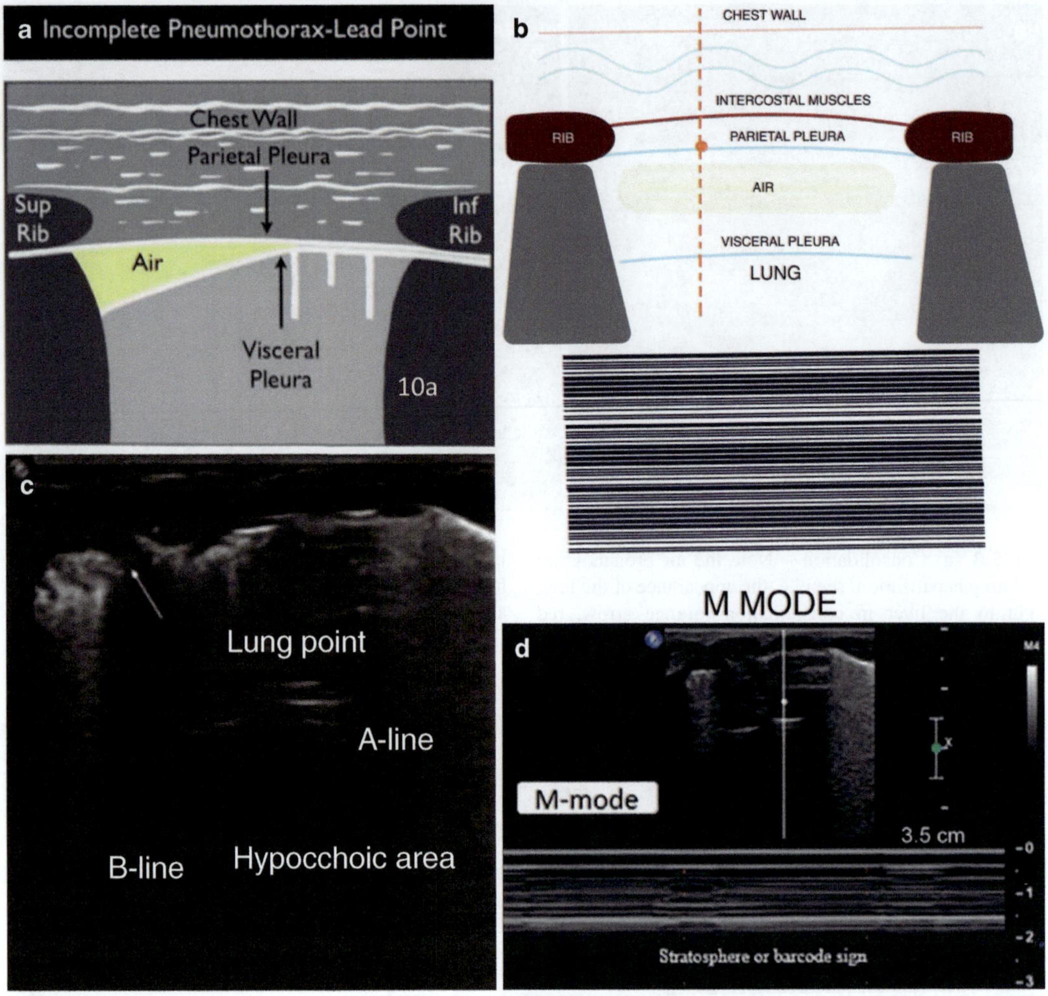

Fig. 5.10 (**a**) Diagrammatic representation of pneumothorax. (**b**) Diagrammatic representation of barcode sign on M mode evaluation in pneumothorax with line diagram. (**c**) Lung point in a neonate with pneumothorax on ultrasound. (**d**) M mode ultrasound depicting the barcode sign. (**c**, **d**: Image courtesy Dr. Pradeep Suryavanshi)

With larger amounts of air a "lung point" may not be discernible.

5.4.6 Pneumothorax

Pneumothorax is more common in neonates on mechanical ventilation. Tension pneumothorax can occur either due to mechanical ventilation or due to the original disease [34, 35].

Normal lung on B mode imaging reveals presence of A lines with normal lung sliding and presence of a seashore sign on M mode imaging.

Separation of the parietal and visceral layers of the pleura by a small amount of air causes absence of "lung sliding" and formation of a "Lung point" (Fig. 5.10 a–c). The reported sensitivity and specificity of ultrasound for detecting pneumothorax is up to 96.7% and 100%, respectively [36].

With larger amounts of air a "lung point" may not be seen [9].

On M mode ultrasound, when the cursor is placed on the pleura, the chest wall which is not moving will show multiple parallel horizontal lines as will the absence of normal lung movement in the lungs, hence producing the "stratosphere" or barcode sign [37] (Fig. 5.10d).

It should be remembered that both A and B lines will not be seen in pneumothorax. Presence of B lines has a 100% negative predictive value for pneumothorax [38].

5.4.7 Atelectasis

Collapse of a part of the lung is known as atelectasis [39]. This causes an impairment of gas exchange. Atelectasis can result from airway obstruction, lung compression either by an extra-pulmonary or a pulmonary lesion. Thick mucus or meconium causing airway obstruction is one of the commoner causes. In intubated and mechanically ventilated neonates, right upper lobe collapse can occur due to traumatic injury to the right bronchi's mucosa. This area of consolidation with disruption of A lines is visible on ultrasonography. Lung hepatization and lung sliding will be present or absent, depending on the degree and severity of the condition.

Severe atelectasis may cause a lung pulse sign, in which the collapsed lung is pulsating with each heartbeat.

The air bronchogram observed in atelectasis is static [40] and must be differentiated from dynamic air bronchogram seen in consolidation. Ultrasound helps differentiate atelectasis from small pleural effusion, both of which may be seen as linear opacities on a chest radiograph (Fig. 5.8b).

Ultrasound has shown has a higher sensitivity in the diagnosis in contrast to chest radiographs which have been reported to have a sensitivity of 75% [41]. Bronchoalveolar lavage under ultrasound monitoring has been found to be effective in the treatment of these patients.

5.4.8 Differentiating Between Atelectasis, Consolidation

In consolidation and atelectasis, there is lung hepatization. However, in atelectasis there is crowding of the air containing bronchi due to volume loss. The dynamic air bronchogram sign may also not be seen. In contradistinction, in consolidation, the air bronchogram which is seen shows normal disposition of the bronchi.

Consolidation	Atelectasis
Lung hepatization	Lung hepatization seen in larger atelectasis
[b]Dynamic air bronchogram	[a]Static air bronchogram
Lung pulsation not seen	Lung pulsation may be present
Normal disposition of bronchi	Crowding of bronchi
On colour Doppler normal branching and disposition of vessels	On colour Doppler crowding of vessels
Overlying pleural line is thick and irregular	

[a] Static air bronchogram seen in resorptive atelectasis, there is no movement within the air bronchogram because of bronchial occlusion

[b] Dynamic air bronchogram seen in consolidation, there is "movement" within the air bronchogram during inspiration and expiration

5.4.9 Bronchopulmonary Dysplasia (BPD)

This is a common complication of RDS and is seen in one third of extremely low birth neonates.

This occurs due to injury to the immature lung causing an imbalance with the repair which occurs. Lung ultrasound allows early prediction of BPD [42, 43].

On ultrasound, unequally distributed B lines are seen with thickening of the pleural line and small subsegmental subpleural consolidations.

5.4.10 Evaluation of an Opacity Seen on a Chest Radiograph

Ultrasound can be very useful in evaluation of an opacity seen on an initial chest radiograph. The opacity can be a mass, loculated effusion, consolidation or subsegmental atelectasis. The incidence of masses, for example, pleuropulmonary blastomas and other neoplastic lesions detected at birth is very low [44]. Air bronchogram and normal branching of vessels will not be seen in a mass.

5.4.11 Congenital Lung Abnormalities

Congenital lung anomalies which may have been detected antenatally and may require post-natal evaluation include :

1. Pulmonary sequestration.
2. Congenital pulmonary airway malformation.
3. Hybrid lesions.
4. Congenital diaphragmatic hernia.
5. Diaphragmatic eventration.
6. Bronchogenic cysts.

Antenatally detected lung abnormalities require post-natal follow-up.

It is important to know the antenatal findings and review foetal MRs if any, prior to performing the lung ultrasound.

5.4.11.1 Pulmonary Sequestration

Pulmonary sequestration is a condition where non-functional dysplastic lung tissue exists with no communication with the rest of the tracheobronchial tree. A segment or lobe is involved. The sequestrated lung receives an anomalous systemic vascular supply, from the aorta separate from the rest of the lung.

Sequestration can be further divided into

(a) Intralobar: Intralobar sequestration is present within the visceral pleura of the functioning lung. It is commoner in the left lower lobe commoner in the posterior basal segment (75%). Scimitar syndrome (partial anomalous pulmonary venous connection) is associated with right-sided lesions.
(b) Extralobar: A separate visceral pleura and venous drainage is seen into the systemic veins, frequently the lower lobe vein, azygos vein or hemiazygos vein. Drainage into the subclavian and portal vein have also been reported.

Arterial supply is commonly from the descending thoracic aorta, celiac axis. The other arteries which may supply the sequestrated segment include the pericardiophrenic, right coronary artery, subclavian and internal thoracic arteries.

Sequestrated segment may be seen between the diaphragm and the lower lobes and rarely may be infra-diaphragmatic.

On lung ultrasound, it is seen at the lung bases and shows an appearance similar to consolidation (Fig. 5.11a). If searched for carefully on colour Doppler examination, a vessel from the aorta will be seen going directly into this lesion (Fig. 5.11b) suggesting this is an extrapulmonary sequestration. The vascular supply and the venous drainage may be further confirmed on a CT angiography.

5.4.11.2 Congenital Pulmonary Airway Malformation (CPAM)

This was formerly known as congenital cystic adenomatoid malformation (CCAM). It is an abnormality which occurs during embryogenesis leading to anomalous bronchial morphology. It is frequently antenatally diagnosed and followed up in the neonatal period. The neonates may be asymptomatic or present with respiratory distress.

CPAM is of five major subtypes as per the Stocker classification [45] depending on the site of origin from the bronchial tree, morphology and size of the cysts.

Antenatally, the cysts are filled with fluid and are detected on ultrasound and foetal MRI.

In case there is a prenatal diagnosis of CPAM, a chest radiograph should be done after birth (Fig. 5.12a). Post-natally, if the cysts are small and air filled or not in contact with the chest wall, they may not be detected on ultrasound. However, they are in contact with the chest wall they will

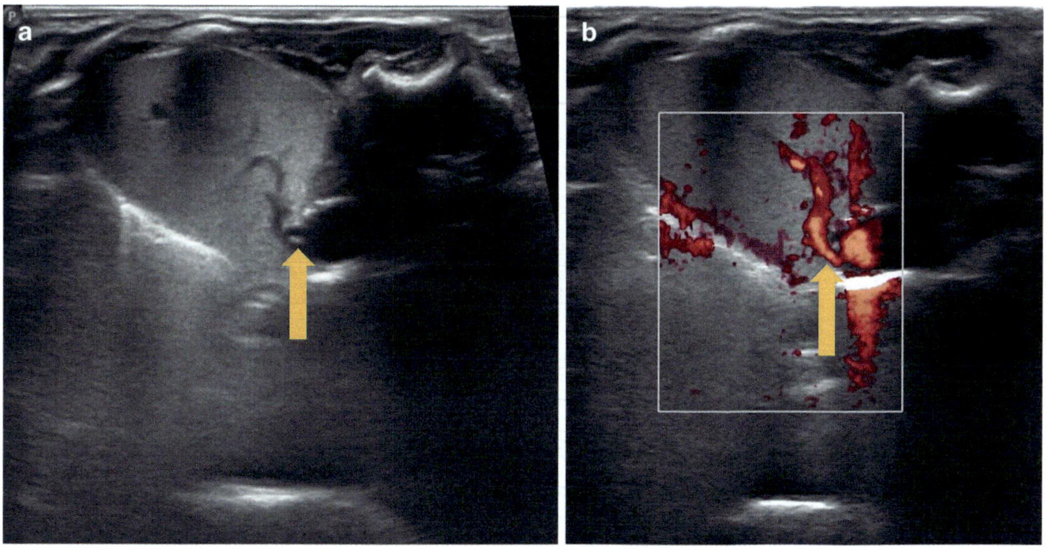

Fig. 5.11 Term neonate with antenatally detected lung lesion. (**a**) Subcostal B mode ultrasound image showing a solid hypoechoic lesion in the right lung base. A vessel from the aorta is seen going into this lesion (arrow). (**b**) Color Doppler evaluation confirming the feeding vessel going towards the solid lesion arrow). Diagnosis: Extrapulmonary sequestration

be seen as anechoic structures, with or without septations (Fig. 5.12 b and c). A differential diagnosis would include a bronchogenic cyst, especially if the lesion is mediastinal in location. CT may be unable to differentiate between the two conditions [46, 47].

Bronchogenic cysts have smooth borders with variable shapes, such as round or oval, depending on their location and growth pattern. While the cystic portion is typically anechoic, some bronchogenic cysts may show internal echoes, debris or septations within the cystic fluid. The presence of internal echoes may help differentiate bronchogenic cysts from other mediastinal cystic lesions. Bronchogenic cysts are typically avascular.

CPAM may undergo spontaneous regression. However, the lungs should be carefully evaluated post-natally as the incidence of malignancy is higher in these patients. In case these are not abutting the chest wall, they may not be appreciable on ultrasound and may require an MRI/CT scan for further evaluation.

CPAM can be associated with bronchopulmonary sequestration (i.e. Hybrid lesion) [48]. An anomalous systemic artery from the systemic circulation can confirm the diagnosis of associated sequestration.

5.4.11.3 Congenital Diaphragmatic Hernia

Congenital diaphragmatic hernia is a defect of the diaphragm which is developmental. There is herniation of abdominal viscera/bowel loops into the abdomen. This is usually detected antenatally [49]. The earlier the abnormality is picked up the worse the prognosis. Diaphragmatic hernia results in lung hypoplasia which results in a poor prognosis. On ultrasound examination, there is interruption of the diaphragm. Herniation of the bowel

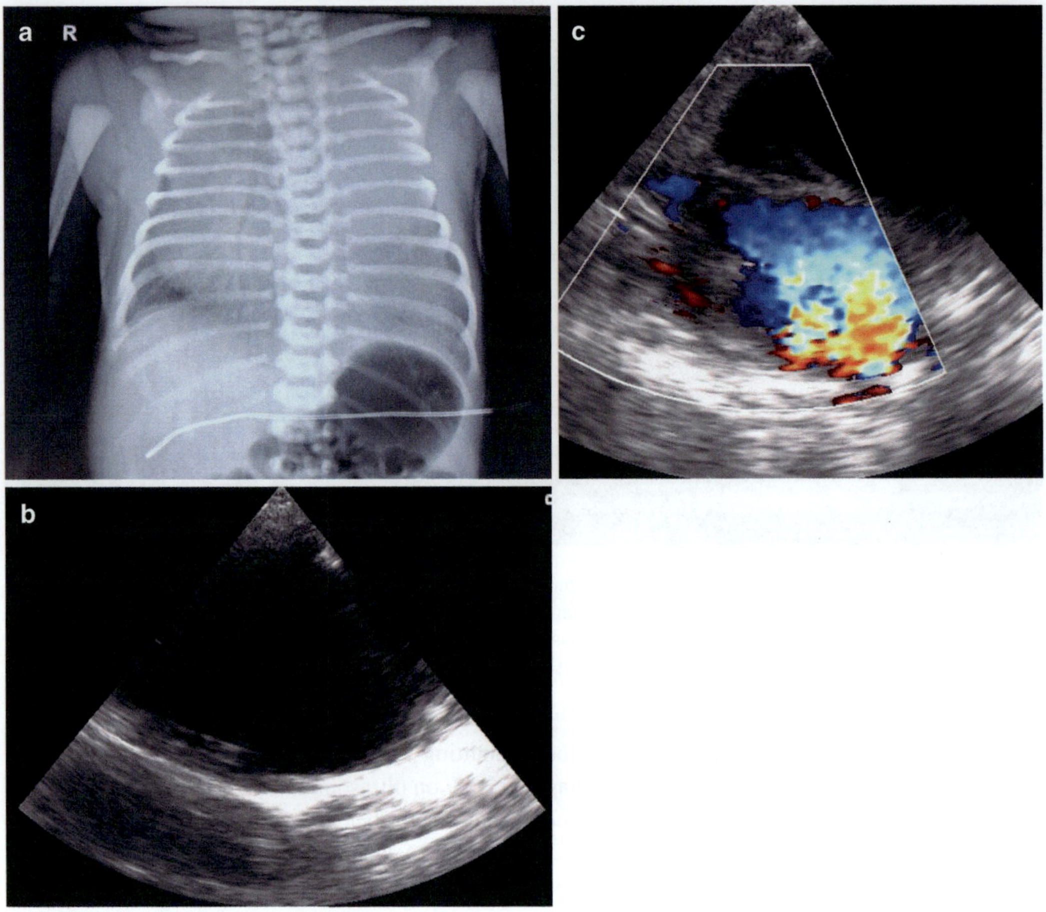

Fig. 5.12 Term neonate. Antenatally detected Congenital Pulmonary Airway Malformation. (**a**) Frontal chest radiograph showing a homogenous opacity occupying the entire left lung causing contralateral mediastinal shift. (**b**) B mode ultrasound image showing an anechoic lesion with posterior acoustic enhancement suggestive of a cyst. (**c**) Color Doppler image showing no colour uptake by this lesion

loops into the abdomen is seen. The bowel loops are air and fluid containing and appear echogenic. The bowel loops are seen at the same level as the heart and show peristalsis within, helping confirm their presence as contents of the hernia (Fig. 5.13).

In right-sided hernias, herniation of liver can also occur which worsens the prognosis.

5.4.11.4 Diaphragmatic Eventration

Diaphragmatic hernia needs to be differentiated from diaphragmatic eventration where a part of the diaphragm is elevated as compared to a diaphragmatic palsy, where the entire diaphragm is elevated and shows paradoxical movements on ultrasound. There is no defect in the diaphragm in eventration [50].

While doing a lung ultrasound, it is imperative to look below the diaphragm, at the liver and other structures. This may give a clue to abdominal pathologies, causing respiratory distress and tachycardia, for example, collections, masses and anomalous pulmonary venous return (Fig. 5.14).

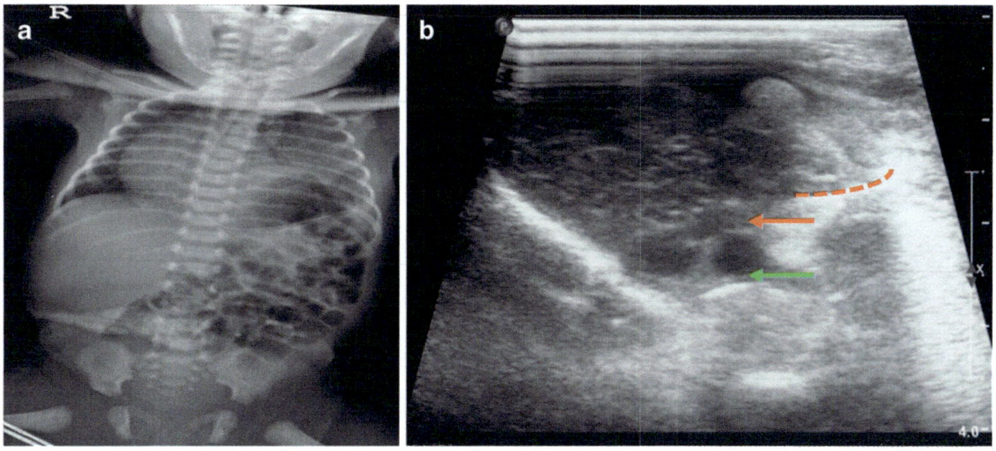

Fig. 5.13 Diaphragmatic hernia. (**a**) Chest radiograph showing indistinct outline of the left hemidiaphragm with diaphragmatic discontinuity. Multiple lucencies are seen in the left hemithorax. (**b**) Ultrasound with a linear high frequency transducer reveals multiple anechoic areas within the left hemithorax. These showed peristalsis on real time imaging confirming they were bowel loops. Note the defect in the diaphragm delineated by arrows (orange arrow, green arrow)

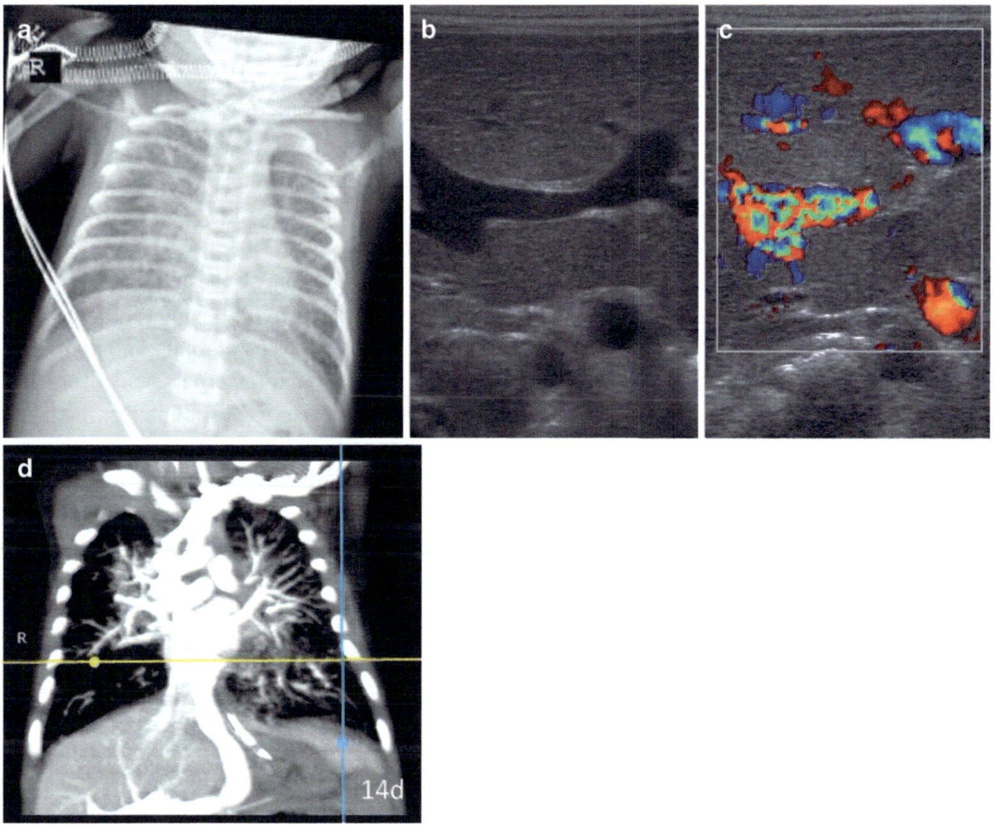

Fig. 5.14 Twenty-three day old neonate with Respiratory distress. Functional echocardiography revealed pulmonary hypertension. (**a**) Chest radiograph showing haziness in both lungs, indicative of pulmonary edema. (**b**) B mode ultrasound image showing a dilated portal vein. (**c**) Colour Doppler image. (**d**) Coronal contrast enhanced CT images show right and left superior and inferior pulmonary veins draining into a vertically oriented vessel seen posterior to the left atrium showing an "inverted fir tree" like appearance consistent with Total Anomalous Pulmonary Venous Connection. This example stresses the importance of infra-diaphragmatic scanning

5.4.12 Limitations

Limitations of lung ultrasound are that it is operator dependant with a learning curve and the structures not in contact with the chest wall will not be delineated.

5.4.13 Mediastinum

Neonatal mediastinal ultrasound is a crucial non-invasive imaging method used to diagnose and manage a wide range of congenital and acquired mediastinal abnormalities.

As the neonatal skeleton is immature, visualization of the anterior mediastinal structures is possible trans-sternally and para-sternally as well as through intercostal spaces. Anterior mediastinal lesions will be easy to image.

Ultrasonographic evaluation of the posterior and middle mediastinum may be relatively difficult. Several factors like air in the bronchi and alveoli limit ultrasound examination of the middle and posterior mediastinum. Reverberation artefacts lead to difficulty in diagnosis, as they can be mistaken for normal morphology of the lung. Movements due to respiration reduce the diagnostic accuracy.

5.4.14 Role of Doppler

Colour Doppler allows visualization of major vessels such as the ascending, descending thoracic aorta, the aortic arch and its branches, i.e. the right brachiocephalic trunk, left common carotid artery and the left subclavian artery (Figs. 5.15 and 5.16). The superior vena cava pulmonary trunk, right and left main pulmonary arteries (Fig. 5.17) are also well visualized and can be assessed. While assessing the mediastinum on USG, it is imperative to evaluate these vessels.

5.4.14.1 Techniques

Neonatal ultrasound requires high frequency linear transducer. Frequency modulation, harmonic imaging are useful tools to visualize the area of interest [51].

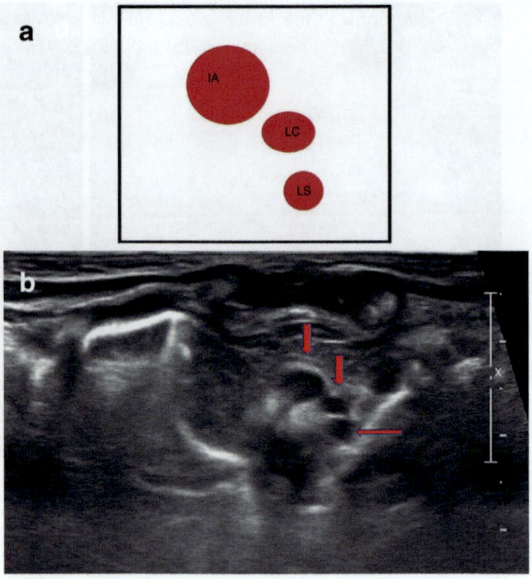

Fig. 5.15 (**a**) Line diagram and (**b**) ultrasound image showing the three great vessels—right brachiocephalic artery, left common carotid artery and left subclavian artery taking off from the aortic arch

The use of Doppler and real-time imaging allow evaluation of mediastinal vessels and to look for vascular lesions. Mediastinal ultrasound examination is generally preferred in supine position.

The examination of the mediastinum is performed in longitudinal, axial and oblique planes. In addition to trans-sternal and parasternal approach, the suprasternal and subxiphoid approaches are also used for anterior mediastinal evaluation [51, 52].

The procedure involves placing the transducer on the chest of the newborn, using gel to facilitate sound wave transmission. The sonographer or radiologist then captures images of the mediastinum in various planes to obtain a comprehensive view.

5.4.14.2 Normal Anatomy

Thymic and superior mediastinal evaluation is mainly performed through suprasternal approach. Thymus in one of the main mediastinal organs assessed on ultrasonography. On USG, thymus has a typical stippled appearance or "starry-sky" appearance [53]. It appears hypoechoic with echogenic specks. However, in few neonates, it may appear homogeneously hypoechoic. The

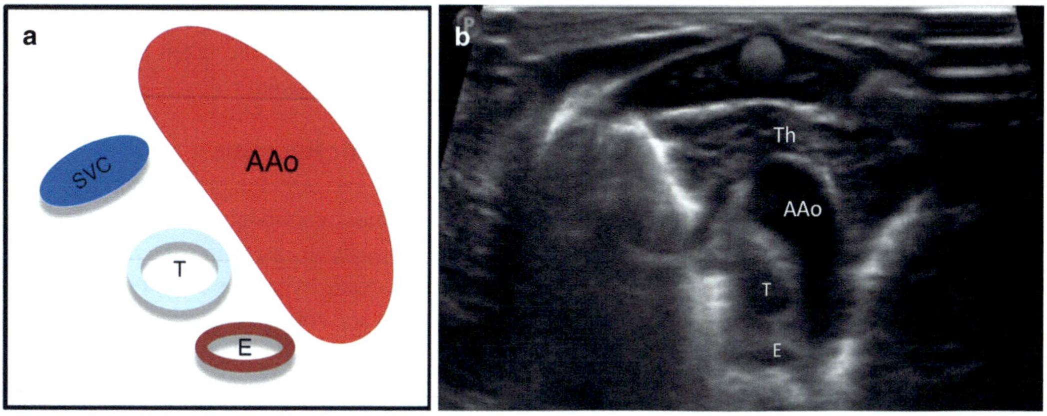

Fig. 5.16 Normal mediastinum at the level of the aortic arch. Also seen is the superior vena cava (SVC); Trachea (T); Esophagus (E); Thymus (Th). (**a**) Schematic diagram. (**b**) Ultrasound image

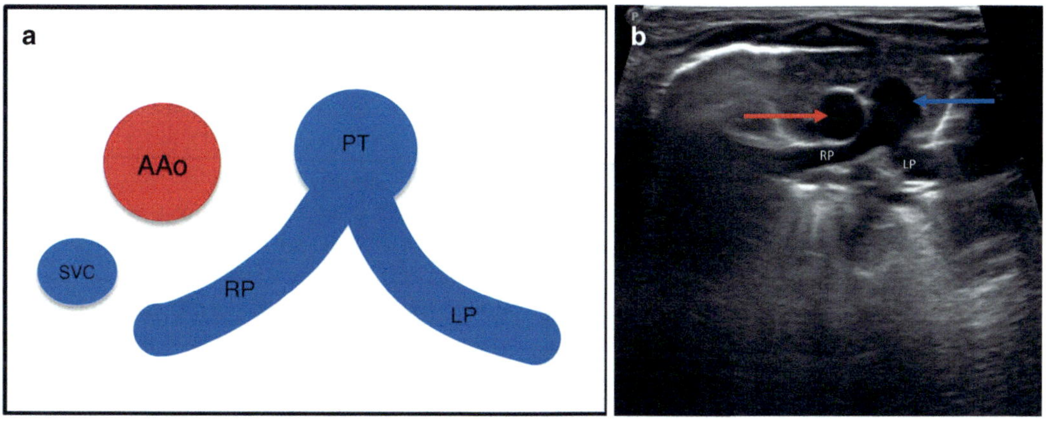

Fig. 5.17 Normal mediastinum, *PT* pulmonary trunk, *RP*, *LP* right and left pulmonary arteries, *SVC* superior vena cava, *AAo* ascending aorta. (**a**) Schematic diagram. (**b**) Transverse ultrasound image just below the suprasternal notch demonstrates Aorta (red arrow) and the pulmonary trunk (blue arrow)

thymus is a very pliable organ and does not cause compression of adjacent structures. This finding is useful as cardiac pulsations and respiratory movements affect thymic shape in contrast to mediastinal masses which are rigid (Fig. 5.18). This feature is best evaluated dynamically and therefore ultrasound is invaluable in differentiating enlarged thymus from masses.

5.4.15 Indications for Mediastinal Ultrasound

1. To evaluate mediastinal widening and rule out thymus as a cause.
2. To assist mediastinal biopsies.
3. Pneumomediastinum.

5.4.15.1 Pathologies

Mediastinal pathologies that can be evaluated on ultrasound include enlarged thymus, cystic hygroma and pneumomediastinum, to name a few. Other pathologies include vascular malformations and mediastinal masses.

5.4.15.2 Enlarged Thymus

Neonates are referred for ultrasound for evaluation of suspected mediastinal mass identified on radiograph and to differentiate an enlarged thymus from a true neoplasm. Thymus may be

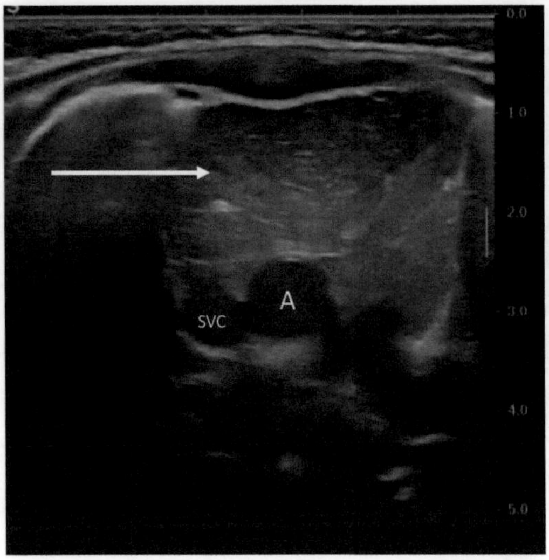

Fig. 5.18 Transverse images through the mediastinum at the level of the aorta showing the thymus as a hypoechoic structure showing a classical "stippled "appearance (arrow). *A* Aorta, *SVC* superior vena cava

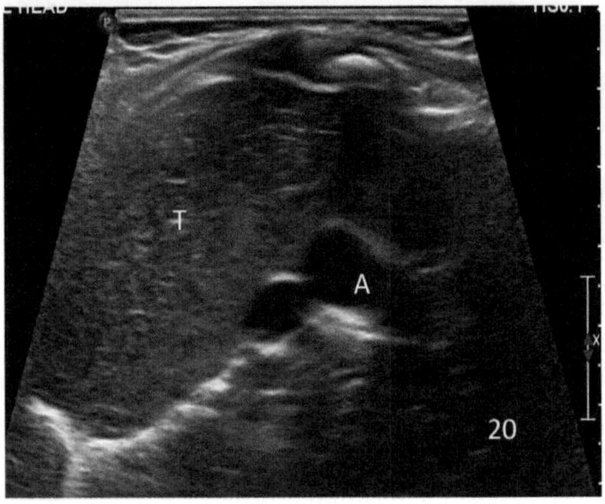

Fig. 5.19 Classic stippled appearance of the thymus in a neonate with mediastinal widening. This appearance confirms the mediastinal widening is due to the thymus

enlarged in neonates in response to stress. In case of true thymic enlargement, the thymus gland retains its homogeneous echotexture and starry-sky appearance. Change in its shape with cardiac pulsations or respiratory movement can also be assessed on USG as it is a dynamic imaging modality. As opposed to an enlarged thymus, mediastinal masses usually have a heterogeneous appearance and are rigid. Neonates with enlarged thymus identified on USG (Fig. 5.19) need not undergo further evaluation, whereas those with mediastinal neoplasms are taken up for further cross-sectional imaging.

5.4.15.3 Cystic Hygroma

Cystic hygromas are lymphatic malformations that occur most commonly in neck and axilla. About 10% of these extend into the mediastinum. Only 1% of cystic hygromas extend into the chest [54]. (They are soft in consistency and rarely cause compression of adjacent structures. But sometimes they may do so resulting in airway compromise). Other complications include infection, airway compromise, chylothorax and chylopericardium. Mediastinal ultrasound is indicated in neonates with cervical cystic hygromas to rule out mediastinal extension. Purely mediastinal hygromas can also be assessed on USG (Fig. 5.20). They appear as multi-locular cystic masses with echogenic septations. Vascularity is generally absent on colour Doppler evaluation. The lymphatic malformations with associated venous component show vascularity on Doppler evaluation and it is essential to differentiate cystic hygroma from a veno-lymphatic malformation. When complicated with chylothorax or chylopericardium, they appear as clear fluid without debris or septations.

5.4.15.4 Pneumomediastinum

Pneumomediastinum refers to air in the mediastinum. It occurs due to alveolar rupture with air dissecting through the interstitium into the hilum and finally into the mediastinum. Pneumomediastinum is often asymptomatic however neonates may present with respiratory symptoms, grunting or cyanosis [55] Pneumomediastinum is suspected when abnormal lucency is identified in the mediastinum on radiography. "Spinnaker sail" or "angel-wing" appearance may also be seen which occur due to lateral displacement of thymic lobes due to pneumomediastinum with their lateral margins lined by air. On ultrasound, it is identified as thick echogenic lines outlining the anterior and lateral margins of thymus with/without posterior acoustic shadowing. Echogenic line may also be seen posterior to the thymus anterior to the great ves-

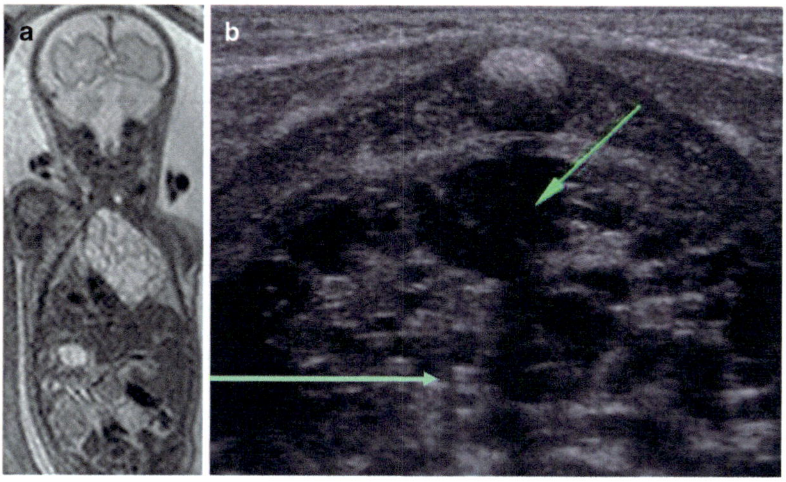

Fig. 5.20 (**a**) Fetal MR showing a multiloculated cystic anterior mediastinal mass consistent with cystic hygroma. (**b**) Ultrasound chest image acquired transternally and through the suprasternal notch confirming presence of a cystic hygroma (green arrows)

sels. Normally, only a thin echogenic line outlines thymus on USG; presence of thick hyperechoic line surrounding the thymus is the key to identify pneumomediastinum [55].

5.4.16 Challenges

Performing ultrasound on neonates can be challenging due to their small size and potential for movement. However, advancements in technology and specialized equipment have improved the accuracy and efficiency of neonatal mediastinal ultrasound.

Acknowledgement We would like to acknowledge the help of Dr. Isha Shah for the illustrations.

References

1. Kurepa D, et al. Neonatal lung ultrasound exam guidelines. J Perinatol. 2018;38(1):11–22.
2. Escourrou G, De Luca D. Lung ultrasound decreased radiation exposure in preterm infants in a neonatal intensive care unit. Acta Paediatr. 2016;105(5):e237–9.
3. Iovine E, Nenna R, Bloise S, et al. Lung ultrasound: its findings and new applications in neonatology and pediatric diseases. Diagnostics. 2021;11(4):652. https://doi.org/10.3390/diagnostics11040652.
4. O'Brien WD. Ultrasound-biophysics mechanisms. Prog Biophys Mol Biol. 2007;93(1–3):212–55. https://doi.org/10.1016/j.pbiomolbio.2006.07.010.
5. Bhalla D, Naranje P, Jana M, et al. Pediatric lung ultrasonography: current perspectives. Pediatr Radiol. 2022;52(10):2038–50. https://doi.org/10.1007/s00247-022-05412-9.
6. Verma A, Paul A, Tekleab AM, Lodha A, Lui K, Maheshwari A, et al. Lung ultrasound in neonates: an emerging tool for monitoring critically ill infants. Lung. 2023;2(1)
7. Gautam MS, Naren Satya SM, Prathyusha IS, Reddy KHC, Mayilvaganan KR, Raidu D. An atypical presentation of congenital pulmonary airway malformation (CPAM): a rare case with antenatal ultrasound findings and review of literature. Pol J Radiol. 2017;4(82):299–303. https://doi.org/10.12659/PJR.901447.
8. Ruoss JL, Bazacliu C, Cacho N, De Luca D. Lung ultrasound in the neonatal intensive care unit: does it impact clinical care? Children (Basel). 2021;8(12):1098. https://doi.org/10.3390/children8121098.
9. Bhoil R, Ahluwalia A, Chopra R, Surya M, Bhoil S. Signs and lines in lung ultrasound. J Ultrason. 2021;21(86):e225–33. https://doi.org/10.15557/JoU.2021.0036.
10. Lichtenstein DA, Mauriat P. Lung ultrasound in the critically ill neonate. Curr Pediatr Rev. 2012;8(3):217–23. https://doi.org/10.2174/157339612802139389.
11. Joshi P, Vasishta A, Gupta M. Ultrasound of the pediatric chest. Br J Radiol. 2019;92(1100):20190058.
12. Reuter S, Moser C, Baack M. Respiratory distress in the newborn. Pediatr Rev. 2014;35(10):417–28. https://doi.org/10.1542/pir.35-10-417.
13. Rachuri H, Oleti TP, Murki S, Subramanian S, Nethagani J. Diagnostic performance of point of care ultrasonography in identifying the etiology of respiratory distress in neonates. Indian J Pediatr. 2017;84:267–70.
14. Brusa G, Savoia M, Vergine M, Bon A, Copetti R, Cattarossi L. Neonatal lung sonography: interobserver agreement between physician interpreters with varying levels of experience. J Ultrasound Med. 2014;34:1549–54.

15. Autilo C, Echaide M, Benachi A, Marfaing-Koka A, Capoluongo ED, Pérez-Gil J, et al. A noninvasive surfactant adsorption test predicting the need for surfactant therapy in preterm infants treated with continuous positive airway pressure. J Pediatr. 2017;182:66–73.
16. Zong H, Huang Z, Zhao J, Lin B, Fu Y, Lin Y, et al. The value of lung ultrasound score in neonatology. Front Pediatr. 2022;11(10):791664. https://doi.org/10.3389/fped.2022.791664.
17. Mathai SS, Raju U, Kanitkar M. Management of respiratory distress in the newborn. Med J Armed Forces India. 2007;63(3):269–72. https://doi.org/10.1016/S0377-1237(07)80152-3.
18. Sawires HK, Ghany EAA, Hussein NF, Seif HM. Use of lung ultrasound in detection of complications of respiratory distress syndrome. Ultrasound Med Biol. 2015;41:2319–25.
19. Bouhemad B, Brisson H, Le-Guen M, Arbelot C, Lu Q, Rouby JJ. Bedside ultrasound assessment of positive end-expiratory pressure-induced lung recruitment. Am J Respir Crit Care Med. 2011;183(3):341–7. https://doi.org/10.1164/rccm.201003-0369OC.
20. Brat R, Yousef N, Klifa R, Reynaud S, Shankar Aguilera S, De Luca D. Lung ultrasonography score to evaluate oxygenation and surfactant need in neonates treated with continuous positive airway pressure. JAMA Pediatr. 2015;169(8):e151797. https://doi.org/10.1001/jamapediatrics.2015.1797.
21. Blank DA, Kamlin COF, Rogerson SR, Fox LM, Lorenz L, Kane SC, et al. Lung ultrasound immediately after birth to describe normal neonatal transition: an observational study. Arch Dis Child Fetal Neonatal Ed. 2018;103(2):F157–62. https://doi.org/10.1136/archdischild-2017-312818.
22. Volpicelli G, Skurzak S, Boero E, Carpinteri G, Tengattini M, Stefanone V, et al. Lung ultrasound predicts well extravascular lung water but is of limited usefulness in the prediction of wedge pressure. Anesthesiology. 2014;121:320–7.
23. Guglani L, Lakshminrusimha S, Ryan RM. Transient tachypnea of the newborn. Pediatr Rev. 2008;29(11):e59–65. https://doi.org/10.1542/pir.29.11.e59.
24. He L, Sun Y, Sheng W, Yao Q. Diagnostic performance of lung ultrasound for transient tachypnea of the newborn: a meta-analysis. PLoS One. 2021;16(3):e0248827. https://doi.org/10.1371/journal.pone.0248827.
25. Liu J, Wang Y, Fu W, Yang C-S, Huang J-J. Diagnosis of neonatal transient tachypnea and its differentiation from respiratory distress syndrome using lung ultrasound. Medicine (Baltimore). 2014;93:e197.
26. Sayad E, Silva-Carmona M. Meconium aspiration 2023 April 12. In: StatPearls. Treasure Island (FL): StatPearls Publishing. p. 2024.
27. Monfredini C, Cavallin F, Villani PE, Paterlini G, Allais B, Trevisanuto D. Meconium aspiration syndrome: a narrative review. Children (Basel). 2021;8(3):230. https://doi.org/10.3390/children8030230.
28. Mathur NB, Garg K, Kumar S. Respiratory distress in neonates with special reference to pneumonia. Indian Pediatr. 2002;39(6):529–37.
29. Liu J. Infectious pneumonia of the newborn. In: Neonatal lung ultrasonography. Dordrecht: Springer; 2018. p. 73–88.
30. Dietrich CF, Mathis G, Cui XW, Ignee A, Hocke M, Hirche TO. Ultrasound of the pleurae and lungs. Ultrasound Med Biol. 2015;41(2):351–65.
31. Barnes ME, Feeney E, Duncan A, Jassim S, MacNamara H, O'Hara J, et al. Pulmonary haemorrhage in neonates: systematic review of management. Acta Paediatr. 2022;111(2):236–44.
32. Liu J, Chi JH, Lu ZL, Fu W. The specific signs of lung ultrasound to diagnose pulmonary hemorrhage of the newborns: evidence from a multicenter retrospective case-control study. Front Pediatr. 2023;18(11):1090332.
33. Ali R, Ahmed S, Qadir M, Maheshwari P, Khan R. Pneumothoraces in a neonatal tertiary care unit: case series. Oman Med J. 2013;28(1):67–9. https://doi.org/10.5001/omj.2013.16.
34. Malek A, Afzali N, Meshkat M, Yazdi NH. Pneumothorax after mechanical ventilation in newborns. Iran J Pediatr. 2011;21(1):45–50.
35. Adekoya AO, Adekoya AO, Amosu LO, Olatunji AA, Olusola-Bello MA, Ashaolu OO. Primary spontaneous pneumothorax in a term neonate. Afr Health Sci. 2022;22(4):178–81. https://doi.org/10.4314/ahs.v22i4.21.
36. Dahmarde H, Parooie F, Salarzaei M. Accuracy of ultrasound in diagnosis of pneumothorax: a comparison between neonates and adults-a systematic review and meta-analysis. Can Respir J. 2019;2019:5271982. https://doi.org/10.1155/2019/5271982.
37. Łyźniak P, Świętoń D, Serafin Z, Szurowska E. Lung ultrasound in a nutshell. Lines, signs, some applications, and misconceptions from a radiologist's point of view. Polish J Radiol. 2023;88(1):294–310. https://doi.org/10.5114/pjr.2023.128866.
38. Husain LF, Hagopian L, Wayman D, Baker WE, Carmody KA. Sonographic diagnosis of pneumothorax. J Emerg Trauma Shock. 2012;5(1):76–81. https://doi.org/10.4103/0974-2700.93116.
39. Liu J, Cao HY. Pulmonary atelectasis of the newborn. In: Neonatal lung ultrasonography. Dordrecht: Springer; 2018. p. 89–102.
40. Durga D, Devi U, Gupta K, Maheshwari A, Suryawanshi P. Lung ultrasound as a novel tool to assess the severity and management of neonatal pneumonia. Lung. 2023, 2(4)
41. Liang HY, Liang XW, Chen ZY, Tan XH, Yang HH, Liao JY, Cai K, Yu JS. Ultrasound in neonatal lung disease. Quant Imaging Med Surg. 2018;8(5):535–46. https://doi.org/10.21037/qims.2018.06.01.
42. Blank DA, Rogerson SR, Kamlin COF, Fox LM, Lorenz L, Kane SC, et al. Lung ultrasound during the initiation of breathing in healthy term and late preterm infants immediately after birth, a prospective, observational study. Resuscitation. 2017;114:59–65.

43. Pezza L, Alonso-Ojembarrena A, Elsayed Y, Yousef N, Vedovelli L, Raimondi F, De Luca D. Meta-analysis of lung ultrasound scores for early prediction of bronchopulmonary dysplasia. Ann Am Thorac Soc. 2022;19(4):659–67. https://doi.org/10.1513/AnnalsATS.202107-822OC.
44. Lyle ANJ, Ohlsen TJD, Miller DE, Brown G, Waligorski N, Stark R, Taylor MR, Puia-Dumitrescu M. Congenital pleuropulmonary blastoma in a newborn with a variant of uncertain significance in DICER1 evaluated by RNA-sequencing. Matern Health Neonatol Perinatol. 2023;9(1):4. https://doi.org/10.1186/s40748-023-00148-2. Erratum in: Matern Health Neonatol Perinatol. 2023 May 25;9(1):7. PMID: 36922881; PMCID: PMC10018833
45. Ursini WP, Ponce CC. Congenital pulmonary airway malformation. Autops Case Rep. 2018;8(2):e2018022. https://doi.org/10.4322/acr.2018.022.
46. Migliaro F, et al. Is the double lung point an accurate diagnostic marker fir transient tachypnoea of the neonate? A prospective international study. J Pediatr Neonatal Individ Med. 2017;6:e060236.
47. Raimondi F, et al. Clinical data are essential to validate lung ultrasound. Chest. 2016;149:1575.
48. Wang D, Wheeler WB. A hybrid lesion of intralobar sequestration with mixed features of CPAM type I and type II unmasked following SARS-CoV-2 infection: case report and literature review. Int J Surg Case Rep. 2022;22(96):107336. https://doi.org/10.1016/j.ijscr.2022.107336.
49. Sperling JD, Sparks TN, Berger VK, Farrell JA, Gosnell K, Keller RL, et al. Prenatal diagnosis of congenital diaphragmatic hernia: does laterality predict perinatal outcomes? Am J Perinatol. 2018;35(10):919–24. https://doi.org/10.1055/s-0037-1617754.
50. Konstantinidi A, Liakou P, Kopanou Taliaka P, Lampridou M, Kalatzi N, et al. Congenital diaphragmatic Eventration in the neonatal period: systematic review of the literature and report of a rare case presenting with gastrointestinal disorders. Pediatr Rep. 2023;15(3):442–51. https://doi.org/10.3390/pediatric15030041.
51. Rea G, Sperandeo M, Di Serafino M, Vallone G, Tomà P. Neonatal and pediatric thoracic ultrasonography. J Ultrasound. 2019;1(22):121–30.
52. Coley BD. Pediatric chest ultrasound. Radiol Clin. 2005;43(2):405–18.
53. Wee T, Lee AF, Nadel H, Bray H. The paediatric thymus: recognising normal and ectopic thymic tissue. Clin Radiol. 2021;76(7):477–87.
54. Faul JL, Berry GJ, Colby TV, Ruoss SJ, Walter MB, Rosen GD, Raffin TA. Thoracic lymphangiomas, lymphangiectasis, lymphangiomatosis, and lymphatic dysplasia syndrome. Am J Respir Critical Care Med. 2000;161(3):1037–46.
55. Jung AY, Yang I, Go HS, Shin SM, Yoon HK, Woo JY, et al. Imaging neonatal spontaneous pneumomediastinum using ultrasound. J Med Ultrasonics. 2014;41:45–9.

Neonatal Liver and Gallbladder

6

Anmol Bhatia, Akshay Kumar Saxena,
and Kushaljit Singh Sodhi

6.1 Introduction

Early diagnosis and management are essential to reduce the morbidity in neonates with liver diseases [1]. The manifestations of liver diseases in neonates may differ from those in older children, and the most common presentation in neonates is cholestasis, irrespective of the underlying cause [1, 2]. Several disorders unique to neonates include cholestatic disorders, vascular abnormalities, tumors, and acquired conditions [1]. Radiologists need to be familiar with these etiologies as imaging has an important role to play in the diagnostic armamentarium, and early diagnosis is essential to reduce/prevent morbidity and mortality. Ultrasound (US) examination is the initial screening investigation for hepatobiliary pathologies in neonates. It is a quick, portable, and radiation-free modality, and thus, it is beneficial in the initial diagnostic workup. Sometimes, it is sufficient for assessing liver disorders and their follow-up, while further cross-sectional imaging modalities may be required in other conditions.

This chapter reviews the spectrum of hepatobiliary conditions that manifest in neonates and will help a general radiologist make the diagnosis of liver and gall bladder pathologies in neonatal population. Various categories of abnormalities that will be described include cholestatic disorders, tumors, vascular abnormalities, and a few other acquired miscellaneous conditions.

6.2 Imaging Technique and Probes

Curved or linear array transducers with frequencies ranging from 5.0 to 7.5 MHz are generally used for neonatal hepatobiliary imaging; however, transducers of higher frequency (5–20 MHz) may also be used because of their small size. Higher frequency scans help obtain more explicit images with a better spatial resolution.

A complete sonographic examination of the liver includes its assessment in longitudinal, axial, and oblique planes to evaluate the parenchyma, hepatic veins, portal veins, intrahepatic biliary tree, extrahepatic biliary tree, and gallbladder [3]. A standardized approach for scanning the liver should be followed: scanning in longitudinal and axial planes along the midline should be done for left lobe evaluation, followed

A. Bhatia (✉) · A. K. Saxena
Department of Radiodiagnosis and Imaging, Post Graduate Institute of Medical Education and Research, Chandigarh, India
e-mail: anmol_bhatia26@yahoo.co.in

K. S. Sodhi
Department of Radiodiagnosis and Imaging, Post Graduate Institute of Medical Education and Research, Chandigarh, India

Formerly: Mallinckrodt Institute of Radiology, St. Louis Children's Hospital, Washington University in St. Louis School of Medicine, St. Louis, Missouri, USA

K. S. Sodhi (ed.), *Neonatal Ultrasound*, https://doi.org/10.1007/978-981-97-8576-6_6

by scanning in longitudinal and oblique subcostal planes for right lobe evaluation.

The liver parenchyma in neonates is slightly hypoechoic or isoechoic relative to the cortex of the kidney. It is homogeneous in echotexture with uniformly distributed echoes of medium to low intensity (Fig. 6.1a). Within this homogeneous texture, anechoic linear structures are seen, which represent hepatic veins (HVs) (Fig. 6.1b, c) and intrahepatic portal vein (PV) branches (Fig. 6.1d, e). A hyperechoic rim representing periportal connective tissue is seen surrounding the branches of the PV [3].

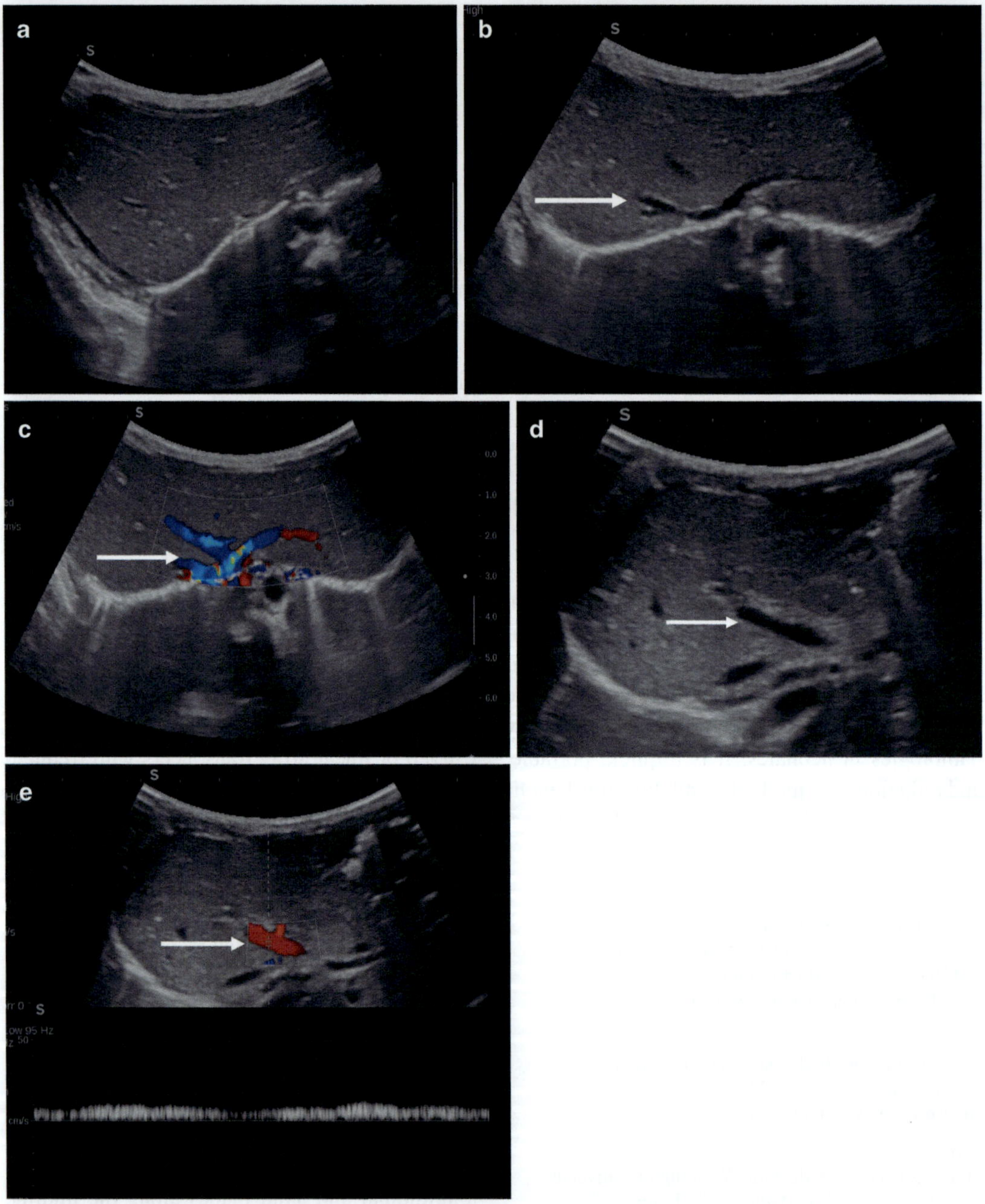

Fig. 6.1 Ultrasound images of a neonate show normal liver parenchyma (**a**), hepatic veins (arrows in **b** and **c**), and the portal vein (arrow in **d**). A pulse Doppler image (**e**) shows minimally phasic hepatopetal flow in the portal vein

A longitudinal scanning along the midclavicular line should be done to measure the span of the right lobe and evaluate the size of the liver [3]. The liver is relatively broader in neonates and extends much across the midline, with physiological hypertrophy of the left lobe. Subsequently, the right lobe volume increases more as compared to the left lobe [3]. The normal span of the right lobe of the liver in term neonates is 4–9.5 cm [3].

To evaluate the gallbladder (GB) and biliary ducts, the child needs to lie supine or, occasionally, on the right side. Scanning in the oblique and longitudinal planes is done with the transducer placed below the costal margin along the right hypochondrium, while the imaging is done in the epigastric region for scanning in the axial planes. Usually, intrahepatic bile ducts are not seen in US scans. However, the common hepatic duct (CHD) and common bile duct (CBD) can typically be seen at the porta. Right and left lobar biliary ducts join to form the CHD at the porta. The CBD starts from the junction of the CHD and the cystic duct. The GB is located along the inferior surface of the liver. It is piriform in shape and appears to be lengthened while scanning in the sagittal plane and round in the axial plane. GB can be divided into a proximal part (neck or infundibulum), body, and fundus. It joins the CHD through the cystic duct [4]. The length of a normal GB is 1.5–3 cm [3], and it should not exceed the span of the adjacent kidney, while a normal CBD measures up to 1–2 mm [1] (Fig. 6.2). Although there is no complete agreement in the literature about the normal caliber of CBD, it is said to be pathological if it is >7 mm [3].

Color Doppler and pulsed wave US determine the presence of flow and its direction in the PV and its intrahepatic branches, HVs, hepatic artery (HA), and intrahepatic inferior vena cava (IVC). The PV in newborns normally has a 3–5 mm diameter and shows a minimally phasic hepatopetal flow [3] (Fig. 6.2b). The HA has a continuous antegrade flow through the diastole (Fig. 6.3). HVs in neonates can show monophasic waveforms rather than the normal triphasic waveforms [1]. The presence of patent ductus venosus should also be evaluated in newborns, which is sometimes used for peripheral venous access through the umbilical vein (Fig. 6.4).

US elastography has emerged as a potentially promising tool in pediatric imaging to evaluate various conditions, especially for liver disorders such as biliary atresia (BA), and evaluate the degree of fibrosis [5]. The values of liver stiffness assessed by 2D shear wave elastography (SWE) have been shown to be significantly higher in patients with BA than in those with other chronic liver parenchymal diseases [6].

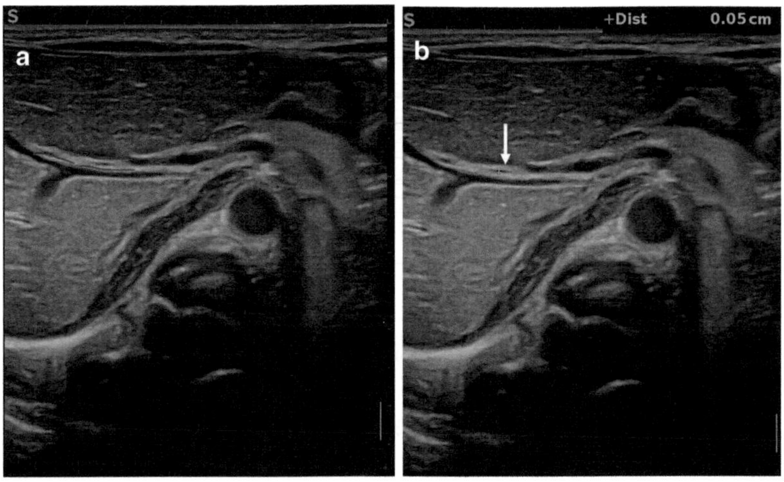

Fig. 6.2 Ultrasound images in a neonate show a normal common bile duct (outlined in red ink in **a** and measured using calipers in **b**)

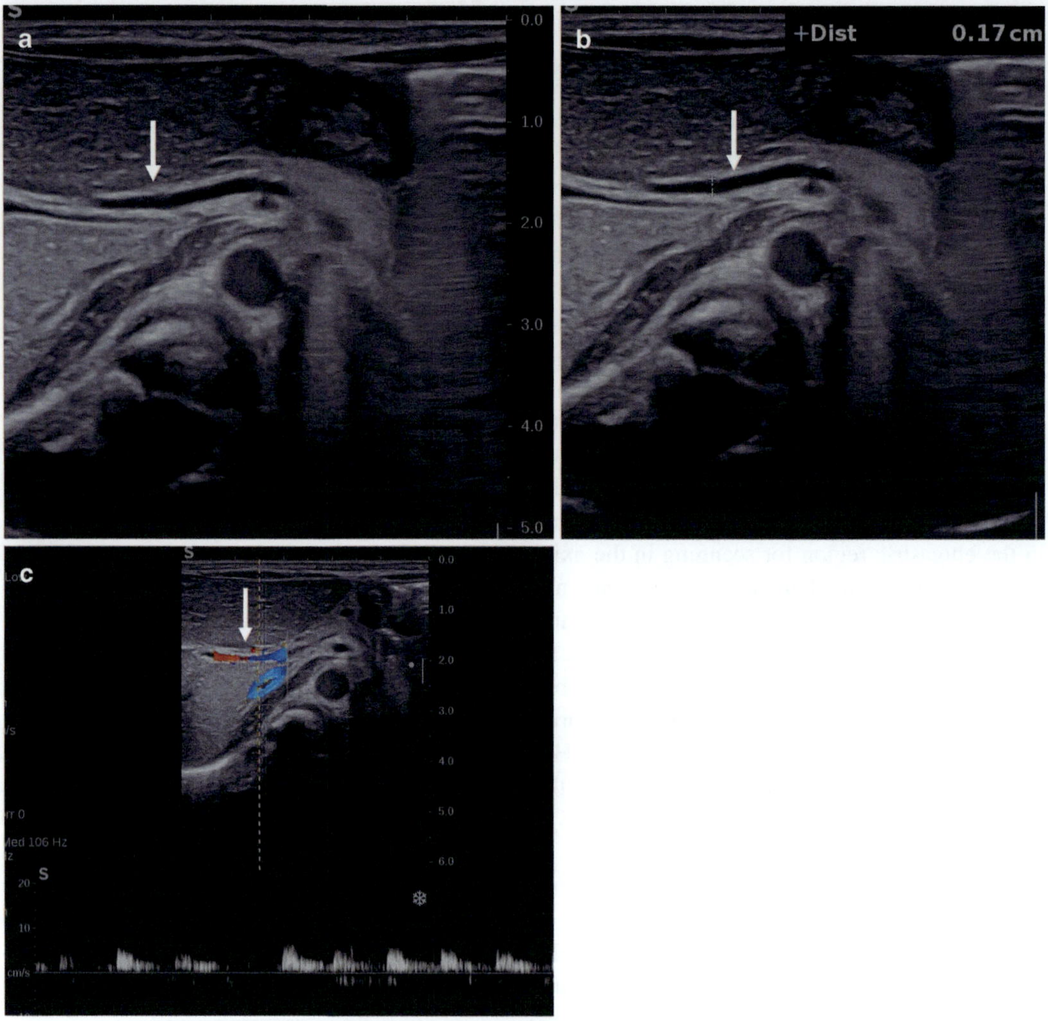

Fig. 6.3 Ultrasound images show a normal hepatic artery (arrows in **a** and **b**) measuring 1.7 mm in caliber. A continuous antegrade flow through the diastole is seen on the pulse Doppler image (**c**)

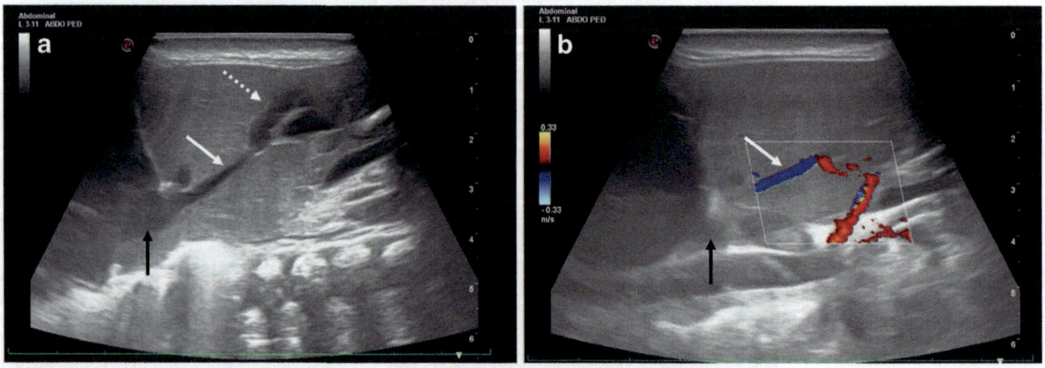

Fig. 6.4 Ultrasound images in a neonate show a patent ductus venosus (solid white arrow in **a** and **b**) between the umbilical vein (dotted white arrow in **a**) and the inferior vena cava (black arrows in **a** and **b**). Color Doppler image (**b**) shows color flow towards the inferior vena cava

6.3 Cholestatic Disorders

6.3.1 Biliary Atresia

Biliary atresia (BA) is characterized by the absence of or severely deficient biliary tree. It results due to progressive destruction, obliteration, and fibrosis of the biliary tree. The commonest mechanism proposed for the occurrence includes an immune-mediated inflammatory response induced by a viral agent in the biliary tree, resulting in progressive fibrosis and destruction of the biliary tract [7]. Other proposed mechanisms include pre-existing abnormal, small, fibrosed, or atretic ductal system that further worsens in the perinatal period, exposure to teratogens, or vascular insult [8].

BA results in progressive conjugated hyperbilirubinemia, and jaundice becomes evident in the immediate perinatal period. Liver in neonates with BA may progress to cirrhosis if left untreated [9]. Timely diagnosis in the neonatal period and an early surgical intervention (Kasai procedure) are warranted to improve the prognosis [7]. Children who do not do well with the post-surgery or are not surgical candidates need liver transplantation.

Most children (approximately 70–80%) present with isolated BA [8]. Two different variants of BA have also been described. The first one is BA with splenic malformation syndrome (BASM) [7, 8], in which multiple systemic anomalies are seen, like asplenia and polysplenia with situs ambiguus, situs inversus, absence of the IVC, preduodenal portal vein, and cardiac anomalies [10]. The second one is cystic BA, which manifests as a bile or mucus-containing cyst at the porta (Fig. 6.5), which does not communicate with the obliterated biliary tree [7, 11].

6.3.1.1 Ultrasonographic Findings

The liver echotexture is usually normal in the immediate neonatal period although an enlarged liver may be present. A GB ghost triad is seen, which consists of an absent or abnormal gallbladder showing a small length (<19–25 mm), an irregular shape, and a discontinuous or irregular echogenic wall (Fig. 6.6). Obliterated or the fibrotic remnant of CBD is seen as increased echogenicity (>4 mm) anterior to the right branch of the PV, which is called a triangular cord sign (Fig. 6.6) [12, 13].

On Doppler, the mean HA diameter and ratio of HA-to-PV diameter have been shown to be

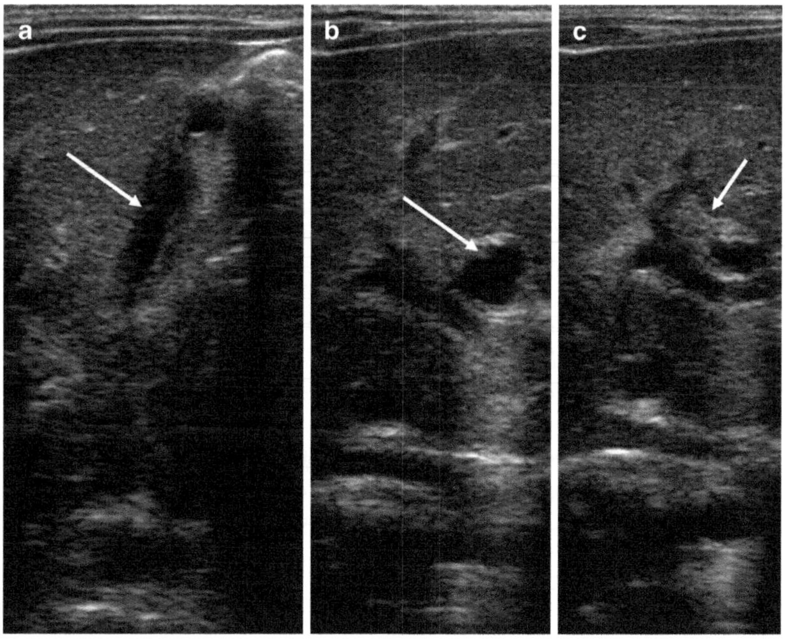

Fig. 6.5 Cystic biliary atresia (**a**–**c**). Grayscale ultrasound images show a small (measuring 12 mm in length) and contracted gallbladder (arrow in **a**), a small cystic structure at porta (arrow in **b**), and increased echogenicity anterior to the right portal vein (arrow in **c**)

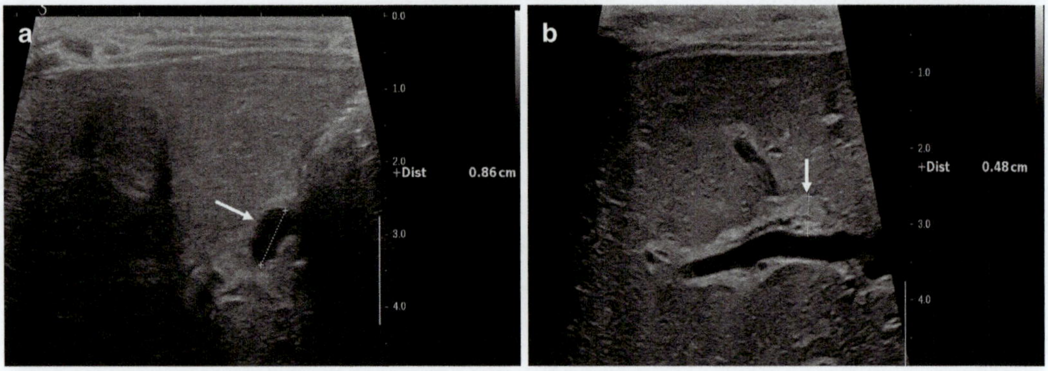

Fig. 6.6 Biliary atresia (**a** and **b**). Grayscale ultrasound images show a small-sized gallbladder (arrow in **a**) measuring 8.6 mm in length and increased echogenicity to the right portal vein (arrow in **b**) measuring 4.8 mm in thickness

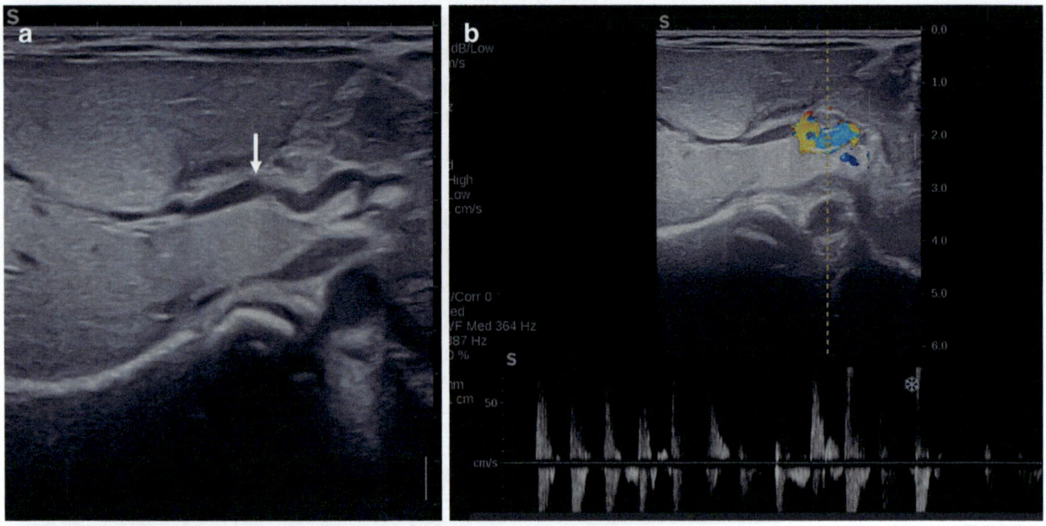

Fig. 6.7 Enlarged hepatic artery in biliary atresia (**a** and **b**). Grayscale ultrasound image (**a**) shows an enlarged hepatic artery (arrow in **a**) measuring 5 mm with turbulent flow and increased velocity on power Doppler image (**b**)

greater in BA patients (0.52 ± 0.12) (Fig. 6.7) than in normal children (0.40 ± 0.10) and neonatal hepatitis (0.40 ± 0.07) patients, with $P < 0.001$ [14]. Hepatic subcapsular flow, defined as an arterial flow that extends to the hepatic surface (Fig. 6.8), has also been described in children with BA [13].

The utility of SWE has been assessed to distinguish BA from hepatitis in recent years. Liver in neonates with BA show significantly higher SWE values (Fig. 6.9) than in infantile hepatitis [15, 16]. The mean SWE values ± SD in children with biliary atresia (20.46 ± 10.19 kPa) have been shown to be higher than in infantile hepatitis

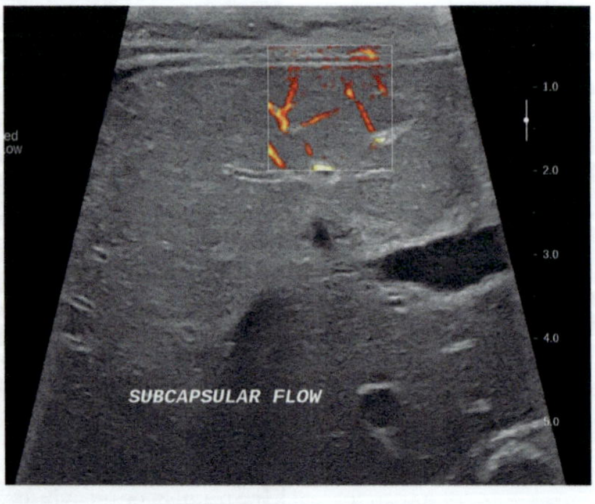

Fig. 6.8 Color Doppler image shows hepatic subcapsular flow in a neonate with biliary atresia

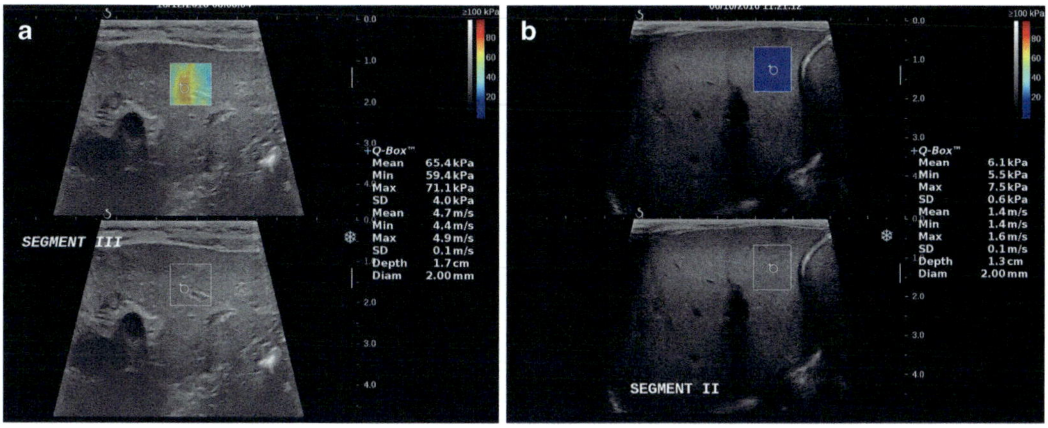

Fig. 6.9 The shear wave elastography image (**a**) shows a high elasticity value (65.4 kPa) of liver parenchyma in a neonate with biliary atresia, while the image (**b**) shows a low elasticity value (6.1 kPa) in a normal neonate

(6.29 ± 0.99 kPa) with $P < 0.01$ [16]. However, SWE is still not a universally accepted standard of care as an alternative biopsy.

6.3.2 Neonatal Hepatitis

Liver in neonatal hepatitis may be normal in US or enlarged with raised parenchymal echogenicity and a normal GB and biliary system. A small size GB may sometimes be seen due to a decreased volume of bile [4]. However, a reduction in the GB size would be seen after feeding the child with milk as the CBD is patent [17]. Further, as previously mentioned under BA, enlarged HA is a useful finding that will help to distinguish BA from neonatal hepatitis [12–14].

6.3.3 Progressive Familial Intrahepatic Cholestasis

Progressive Familial Intrahepatic Cholestasis (PFIC) constitutes a group of disorders with autosomal recessive inheritance related to bile production. The onset is in the immediate neonatal period, with the child presenting with deep jaundice, pruritus, and failure to thrive, and later, the child progresses to liver failure if untreated [18]. Imaging of PFIC is usually normal in neonates and is mainly helpful in excluding out other extrahepatic causes of cholestasis.

6.3.4 Gestational Alloimmune Liver Disease (GALD) and Neonatal Hemochromatosis

GALD occurs as a result of the production of maternal IgG antibodies against the fetal hepatocytes and is the commonest cause of neonatal acute liver failure. Neonatal hemochromatosis can result from any cause of liver failure in the neonatal period but is most often caused by GALD. It is the phenotypic expression of severe liver disease associated with extrahepatic siderosis [19]. Antenatal US shows features of intrauterine growth retardation (IUGR) and oligohydramnios, while liver failure and multiorgan dysfunction develop soon in the perinatal period [19]. A normal liver with a patent ductus venosus, which is a characteristic finding, is seen on US [20].

6.3.5 Alagille Syndrome

Alagille syndrome is an autosomal dominant cholestatic disease. It is diagnosed by the paucity of intrahepatic bile ducts on liver biopsy, in addi-

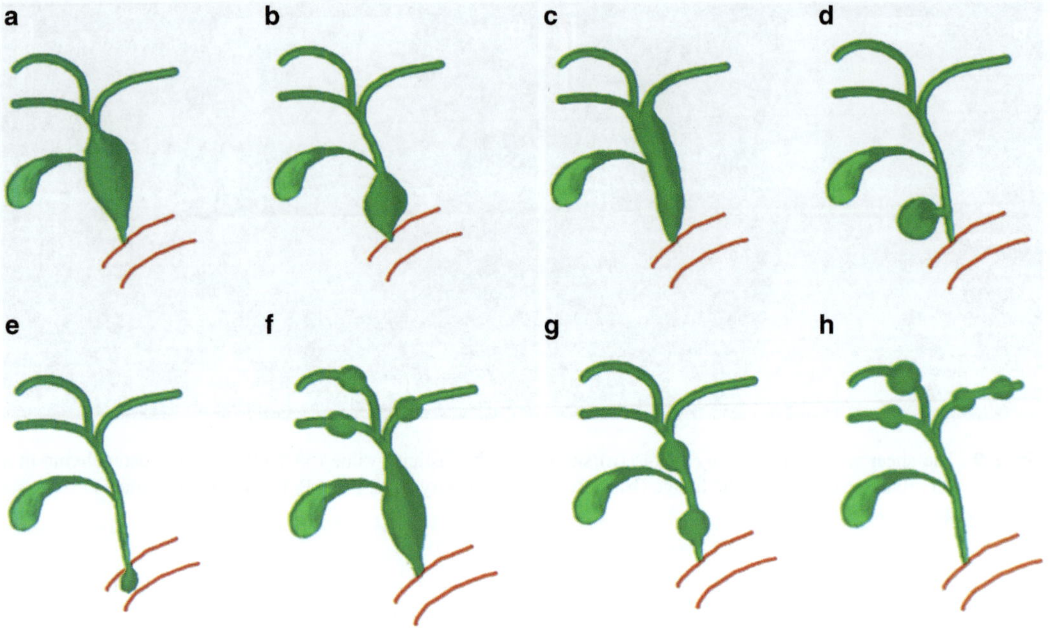

Fig. 6.10 Illustrative picture summarizing the Todani classification of choledochal cyst: Type I (6 **a–c**), type II (6**d**), type III (6**e**), type IVA (6**f**), type IVB (6**g**), and type V (6**h**). *Designed by:* Dr. *Harish Bhujade, Department of Radiodiagnosis and Imaging, PGIMER, Chandigarh, India*

tion to three of the following five clinical criteria: cholestasis, characteristic facies, vertebral anomalies, cardiac anomalies, and ocular abnormalities. It is an arteriohepatic dysplasia, and the vasculopathy can be seen as stenosis and aneurysms of intracranial and intra-abdominal arteries [21]. The diagnosis is primarily clinical, and findings in US may be like BA. Therefore, assessing the radiographs to look for bony anomalies in suspected Alagille syndrome, including butterfly vertebrae, is essential. On US, an abnormal shape and size of GB may be seen [22]. Triangular cord sign is absent in Alagille syndrome, while the hypertrophy of the HA is less often seen in Alagille syndrome as compared to BA [22].

6.3.6 Choledochal Cyst

Choledochal cyst is a fibropolycystic liver disorder and the most common congenital hepatobiliary anomaly. It is characterized by the dilatation of the intrahepatic and extrahepatic biliary tree and is classified into five types based on Todani classification (Fig. 6.10) as follows [23]:

- Type IA, IB, and IC (Fig. 6.10a–c): Cystic dilation, segmental dilation, and fusiform dilation, respectively.
- Type II (Fig. 6.10d): One or more diverticula of the CBD.

- Type III (Fig. 6.10e): Dilation of the intraduodenal portion of the CBD called choledochocele.
- Type IVA (Fig. 6.10f): Multiple intrahepatic and extrahepatic biliary dilatations.
- Type IVB (Fig. 6.10g): Multiple extrahepatic biliary cysts only.
- Type V (Fig. 6.10h): Intrahepatic ducts show saccular or fusiform dilatation. It is also known as Caroli disease.

Some authors describe a "type VI" cyst, which is an isolated cystic duct dilatation.

The exact etiology is unknown although the primary theory is related to anomalous pancreaticobiliary junction seen in many patients with a choledochal cyst. The long common presphincteric channel after the confluence of the CBD and the main pancreatic duct is a conduit for mixing and reflux of pancreatic enzymes and

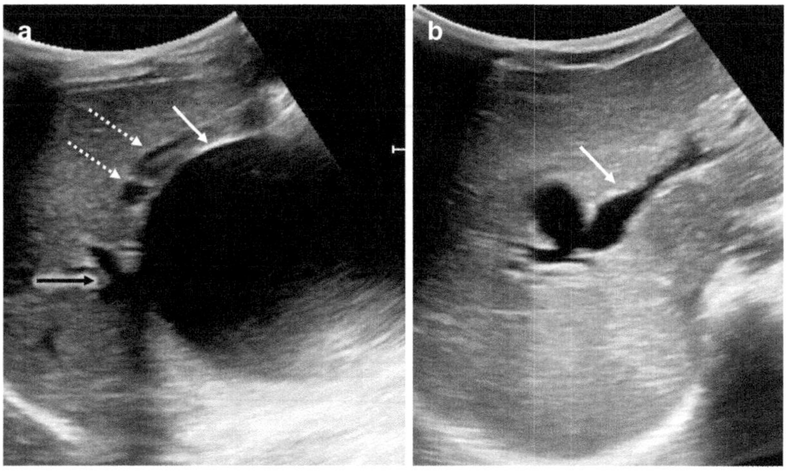

Fig. 6.11 Choledochal cyst. Grayscale ultrasound image shows cystic dilatation of common bile duct (solid white arrow in **a**) communicating with the intrahepatic biliary radicles (black arrow in **a**). The gallbladder was seen separate and compressed (dotted white arrows in **a**) by the dilated common bile duct. Dilated biliary radicles in the left lobe are seen (white arrow in **b**)

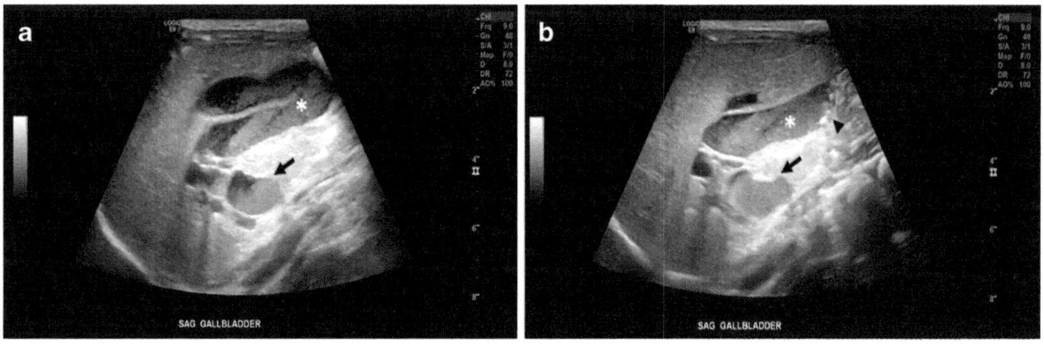

Fig. 6.12 Inspissated bile. Sagittal ultrasound images of the gall bladder (**a** and **b**) demonstrate a sludge-filled gallbladder (asterisk in **a** and **b**) with cholelithiasis (arrowhead in **b**) and a markedly dilated and debris-filled common bile duct (black arrow in **a** and **b**) up the level of the pancreatic head. *Image courtesy: Dr. Neha Kwatra, Department of Radiology, Boston Children's Hospital, Boston, USA*

bile, causing progressive weakness and dilatation of the CBD due to the destruction of the elastic fibers [24].

US easily makes the diagnosis, demonstrating the dilated biliary tree (Fig. 6.11) and a normal GB [4]. Magnetic resonance cholangiopancreatography (MRCP) may be done later, if required, for surgical management to demonstrate the extent and the type of biliary tree dilatation and the anatomy of the common channel.

6.3.7 Inspissated Bile Syndrome and Cholelithiasis

Inspissated bile syndrome, also known as bile-plug syndrome, is a condition in which the biliary tree is obstructed due to the impaction of sludge (viscous bile). Risk factors for sludge formation and cholelithiasis in neonates include prematurity, total parental nutrition, drugs like diuretics and cephalosporins, congenital heart disease, and hemolytic anemias [25, 26].

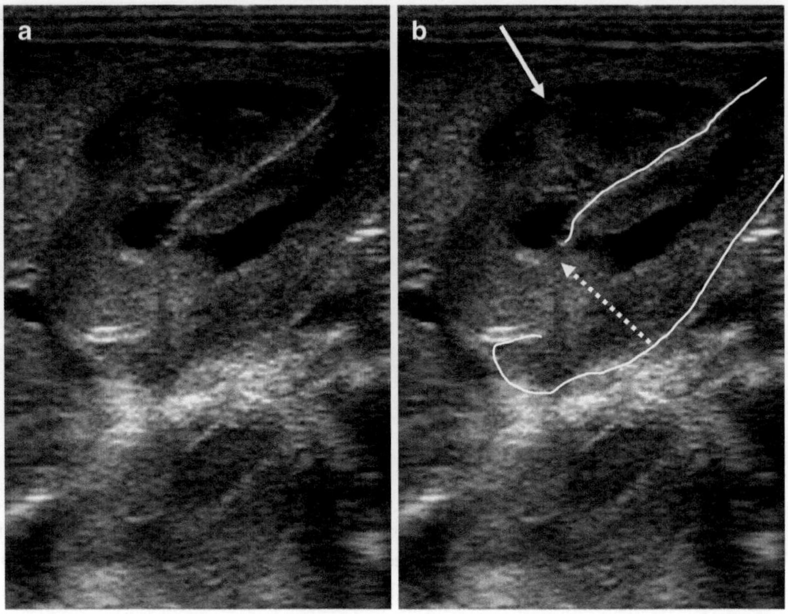

Fig. 6.13 Inspissated bile with gallbladder perforation. Grayscale ultrasound images (**a** and **b**) show a distended gallbladder filled with echogenic sludge (solid white arrow in annotated figure **b**). In addition, a rent is seen in the gallbladder wall (dotted white arrow in annotated figure **b**) along with a collection in the pericholecystic region (outlined in white in annotated figure **b**) which was tracking inferiorly

In inspissated bile syndrome, the GB and dilated CBD contain sludge, which is echogenic on US, but there is no posterior acoustic shadowing (Figs. 6.12 and 6.13) [4].

Neonatal cholelithiasis is seen as small echogenic foci on the US, which may not cause shadowing if <3 mm. Complications like choledocholithiasis and cholecystitis are known to occur with neonatal cholelithiasis [26].

6.4 Tumors

The most common liver lesions in neonates are hepatoblastoma, mesenchymal hamartoma, and hemangioma. Serum AFP levels help distinguish between these liver masses during the neonatal period. However, one must remember that the serum AFP level is usually elevated at birth (25,000–50,000 ng/mL) and does not reach adult levels (<25 ng/mL) until 6 months of age [27].

6.4.1 Hemangioma

Liver hemangiomas are the most common benign tumors in neonates and are the true vascular neoplasms. In the neonatal period, the two types that are known to be seen include infantile hepatic hemangioma (IHH) and congenital hepatic hemangioma (CHH).

IHHs develop within the first few weeks of life, thereby undergo proliferation during the initial few months of life, and gradually involute over the next few years [28]. They may be solitary, multifocal with normal intervening parenchyma, or diffuse type with multiple lesions replacing the entire parenchyma [29]. On histopathology, they are glucose transporter-1 protein (GLUT-1) positive. These hemangiomas are usually asymptomatic and often picked up in the US during the screening of children with cutaneous hemangiomas [29]. Hepatomegaly and occasionally high-output cardiac failure more commonly occur with diffuse patterns [29, 30]. These hemangiomas also express iodothyronine deiodinase (type 3), which inactivates thyroid hormone, thereby resulting in hypothyroidism [31].

CHHs are fully developed at birth and are usually seen as a single large mass. Based on the growth patterns, they may be classified as noninvoluting, partially involuting, and rapidly involuting. The rapidly involuting CHHs begin to involute soon after birth, and the involution is completed by around 14 months of life [32]. Noninvoluting CHHs may grow proportionately

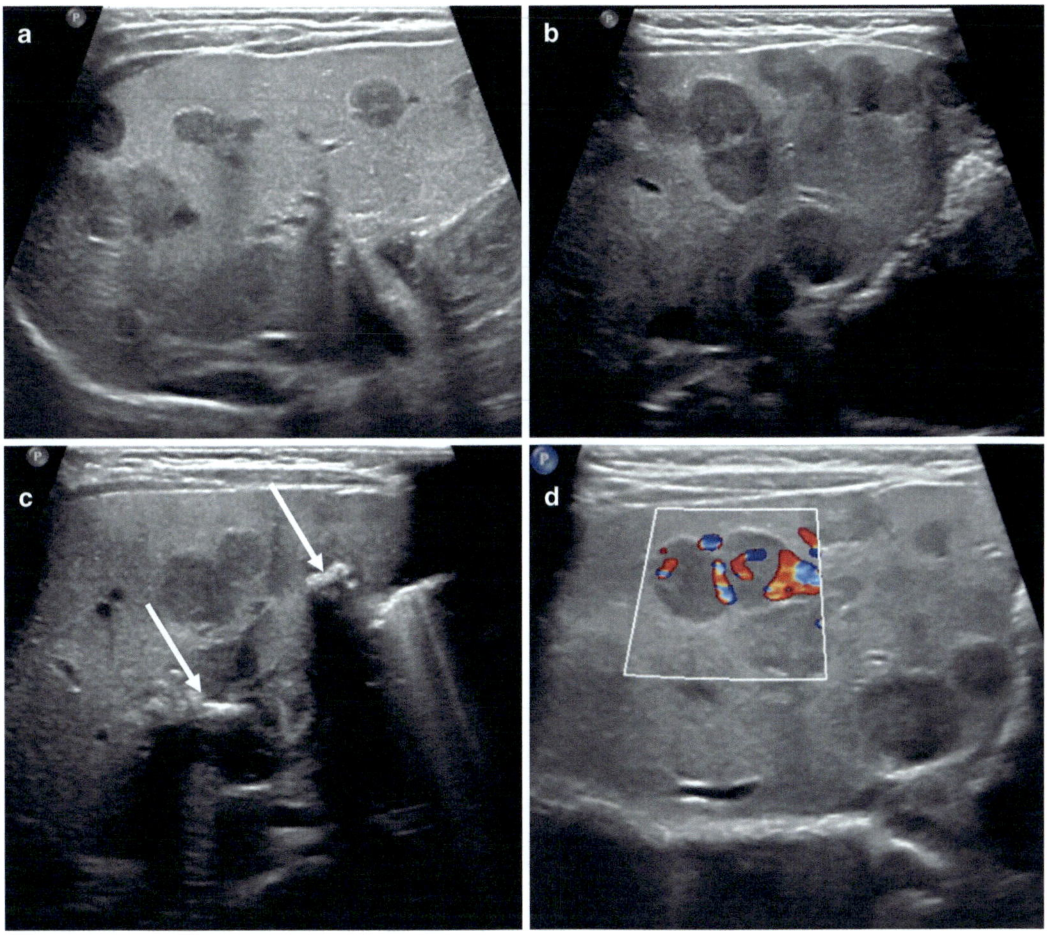

Fig. 6.14 Congenital hepatic hemangiomas. Grayscale ultrasound images (**a**–**c**) show multiple scattered lesions in the liver showing variable echogenicity with foci of calcification (showing distal acoustic shadowing) in a few of them (arrows in **c**). Color Doppler image (**d**) shows focal areas of vascularity within the lesions

to the child's growth. Consumptive coagulopathy or high-output cardiac failure can be seen in children with large lesions similar to that in diffuse type IHHs [28, 29].

US is the initial screening investigation for imaging hepatic hemangiomas. Variable echogenicity and vascularity patterns are seen on US (Fig. 6.14). CHHs show heterogeneous echotexture due to necrosis, hemorrhage, fibrosis, and calcification [29]. Calcifications are often seen in involuting CHHs. However, normal levels of AFP help to differentiate the hemangiomas with calcifications from hepatoblastoma.

6.4.2 Mesenchymal Hamartoma

Mesenchymal hamartoma is a benign tumor that is characterized by the presence of immature mesenchymal tissue and abnormal bile ducts on histopathology [30]. They are usually large tumors (size more than 10 cm) and are predominantly cystic (Fig. 6.15) in appearance but may be partially or completely solid (Fig. 6.16) sometimes, usually beyond the neonatal age group [31, 32]. Serum AFP levels are normal or only mildly raised, which helps to differentiate it from hepatoblastoma [33]. They do not show vascularity on color Doppler [33, 34].

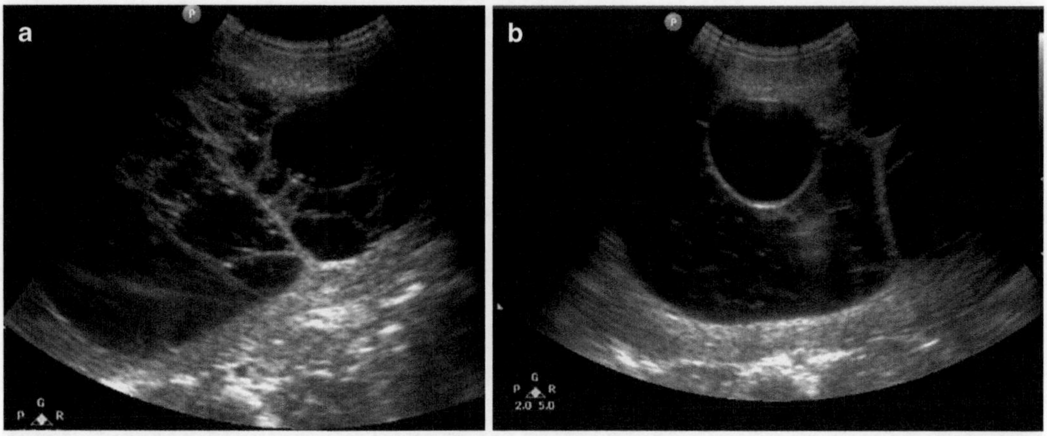

Fig. 6.15 Mesenchymal hamartoma. Grayscale ultrasound images (**a** and **b**) show a multiseptated cystic lesion within the liver

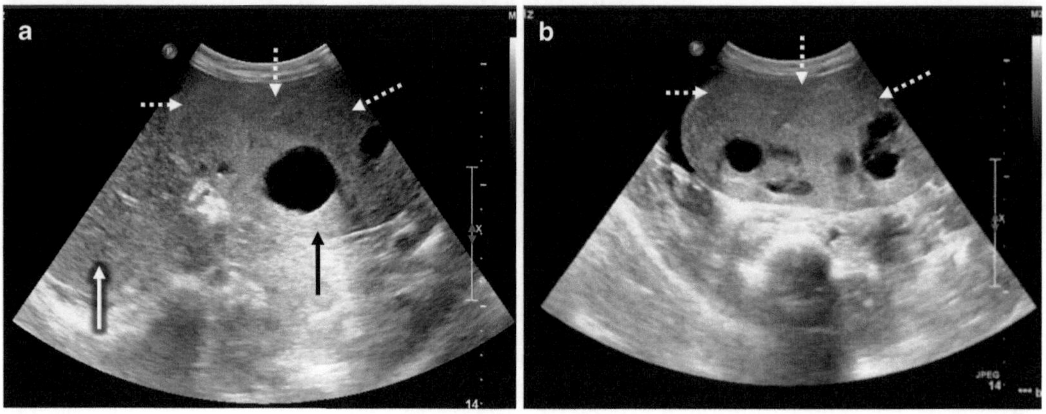

Fig. 6.16 Mesenchymal hamartoma. Grayscale ultrasound images (**a** and **b**) show an exophytic lesion (black arrow in **a**) arising from the liver (solid white arrow in **a**). The lesion is predominantly solid (dotted white arrows in **a** and **b**), with few cystic areas within

6.4.3 Hepatoblastoma

Hepatoblastoma is the most common primary malignant neoplasm of the liver. Children present with abdominal distension with a palpable mass on clinical examination. Serum AFP is markedly elevated in up to 90% of cases [35]. 4% of these tumors are congenital [35]. Predisposing conditions include Beckwith-Wiedemann syndrome, Wilms tumor, type 1A glycogen storage disease, familial adenomatous polyposis, fetal alcohol syndrome, Gardner syndrome, and trisomy 18. Hepatoblastoma has been reported in low birth-weight neonates, premature neonates, and neonates born to females taking oral contraceptives. A strong association has been shown between low birth weight and hepatoblastoma, which has raised the issue of a potential contribution caused by different iatrogenic exposures that happen in the newborn intensive care unit [34, 35].

Hepatoblastoma is usually seen as a well-defined solid mass on US. It is often hyperechoic compared to the adjacent parenchyma (Fig. 6.17) but can show a heterogeneous echogenicity due to necrosis and hemorrhage. 50% of these tumors

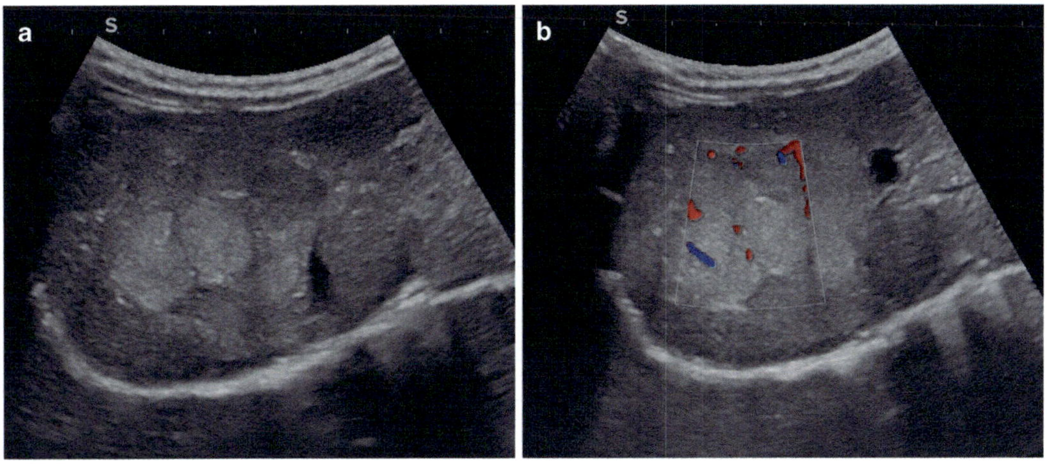

Fig. 6.17 Hepatoblastoma. Grayscale ultrasound image (**a**) shows a predominantly echogenic lesion in the right lobe of the liver. Color Doppler image (**b**) shows focal areas of vascularity within the lesion. Serum AFP was more than 10,000 ng/mL

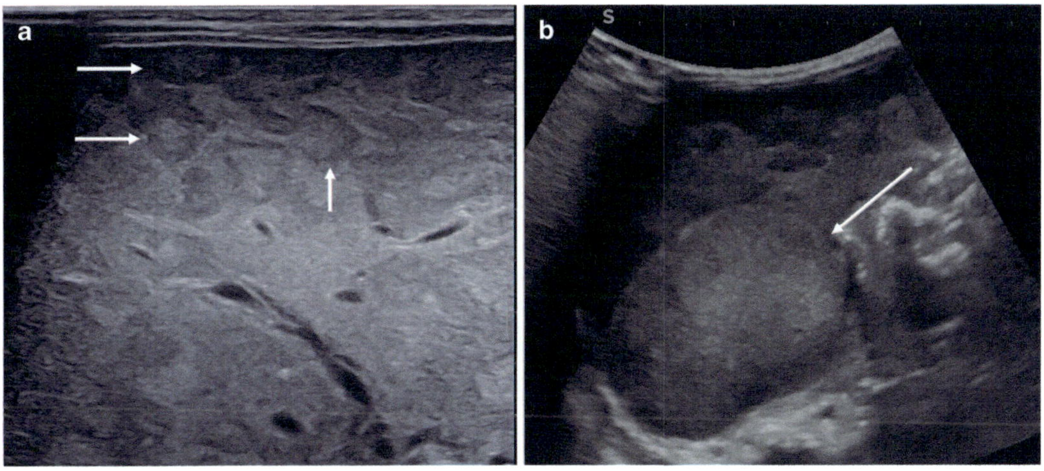

Fig. 6.18 Metastases. Grayscale ultrasound image (**a**) shows ill-defined isoechoic to hyperechoic small lesions (white arrows placed on a few of the lesions) diffusely infiltrating the liver parenchyma. A large suprarenal mass (arrow in **b**) was also seen on the right side, suggestive of neuroblastoma with liver metastases

show calcification [35, 36]. On color Doppler, a variable degree of vascularity is seen within the tumor. However, it is often hypovascular. Tumor thrombus may involve the hepatic and portal veins. On color Doppler, flow within the thrombus helps to distinguish the tumor thrombus from the bland thrombus [35, 37].

Cross-sectional imaging is further required and is important for staging using the pretreatment extent of the disease (PRETEXT) system, which is important for determining the surgical resectability of the tumor before as well as after chemotherapy [38]. The PRETEXT number is assigned depending on the sections of the liver involved, along with the assessment of various annotation factors.

6.4.4 Metastases

Hepatic metastases in neonates can be seen in neuroblastoma. The appearance is highly variable, ranging from one or more focal lesions showing variable echogenicity and vascularity to a diffuse infiltrative pattern with loss of normal hepatic architecture and hepatomegaly (Fig. 6.18). The latter pattern is most often seen in stage IV-S neuroblastoma.

6.5 Vascular Diseases: Portosystemic Shunts

A portosystemic shunt (PSS) diverts the blood in the portal venous system to a systemic vein, bypassing the liver. It can either be intrahepatic or extrahepatic, depending on whether the shunt occurs within or outside the liver. PSS may be identified antenatally or manifest immediately after birth in neonates with persistent hyperbilirubinemia, abnormality on galactosemia screening, hyperammonemia, and abnormal liver function tests [39].

Intrahepatic PSS can be solitary or multiple and have abnormal communications between the intrahepatic branches of PV and hepatic veins. On US, these are seen as dilated and tortuous vas-

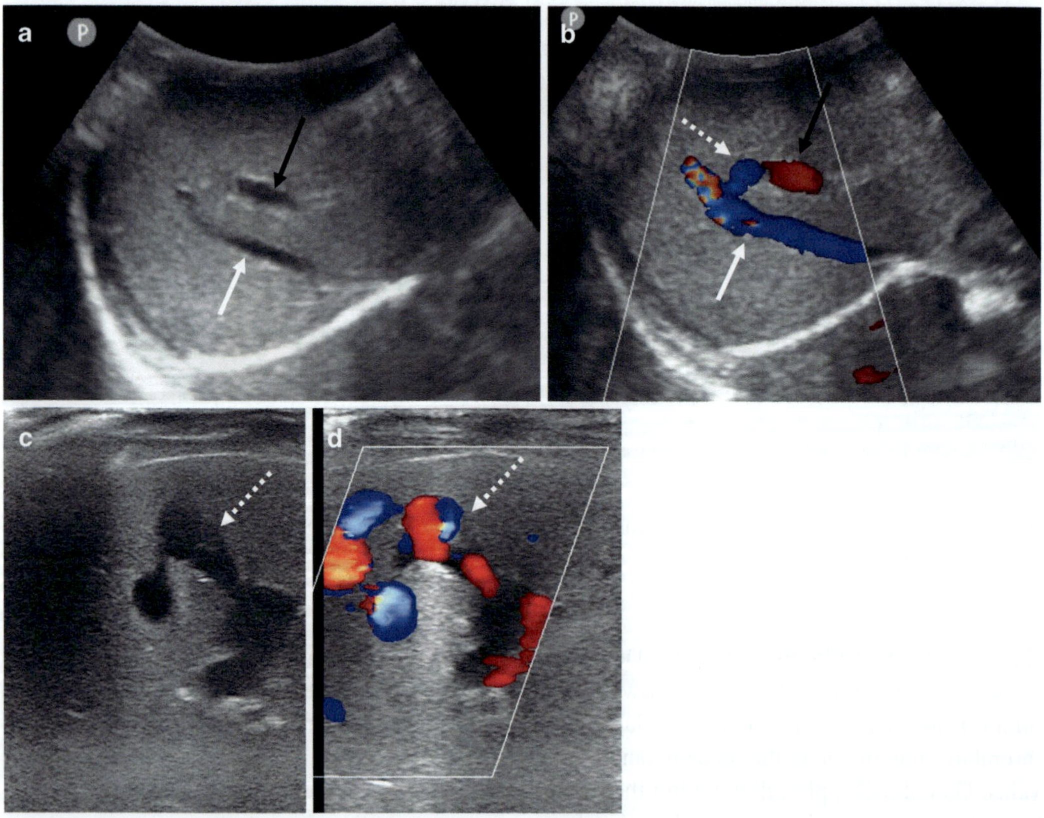

Fig. 6.19 Intrahepatic portosystemic shunt (**a**–**d**). A dilated hepatic vein is seen (solid white arrow in **a** and **b**) with an abnormal tortuous vascular channel (dotted white arrows in **b**, **c**, and **d**) coursing from the portal vein (black arrow in **a** and **b**) towards the dilated hepatic vein. *Image courtesy: Dr. Sreedhara BC, Department of Radiodiagnosis and Imaging, PGIMER, Chandigarh, India*

cular channels which are joining the intrahepatic branches of the PV and hepatic veins (Fig. 6.19) [39, 40]. Turbulent biphasic or triphasic waveforms are seen on color Doppler in the PV due to presence of the hepatic venous flow pattern showing cardiac pulsations. The branches of PV may become attenuated and show slow or reversal of the direction of the flow when large shunts are present. While findings on US in cases of intrahepatic PSS are usually diagnostic, further cross-sectional angiography studies can demonstrate the detailed anatomy of the abnormal vasculature. Endovascular interventions are performed for therapeutic occlusion [40, 41].

Extrahepatic PSS, also known as Abernethy malformation, is of two types. In type 1, the main PV is absent, and all the portal circulation blood is diverted into the systemic circulation through the IVC from the level of the superior mesenteric vein or splenic vein. Whereas in type 2, the main PV is intact, and there is only a partial flow diversion of the blood in the portal circulation through a side-to-side extrahepatic anastomosis. Extrahepatic PSS is usually difficult to diagnose on US and should be suspected in neonates with small-sized livers, attenuated main PV and its intrahepatic branches, and increased blood flow in HA [39]. Further cross-sectional contrast-enhanced studies can be done to define the exact anatomy of extrahepatic PSS [39, 40].

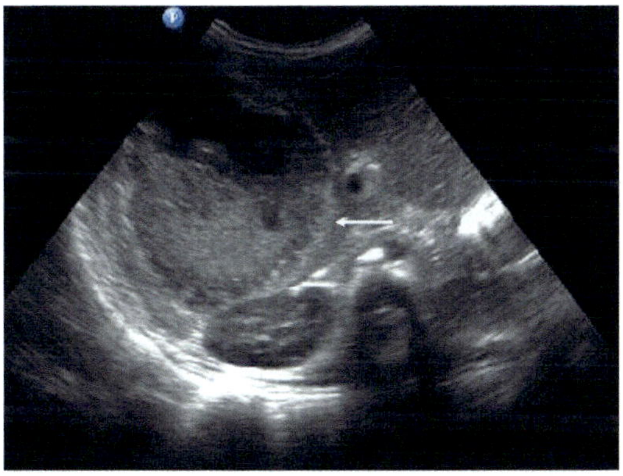

Fig. 6.20 Hepatic abscess. Grayscale ultrasound image shows a well-defined lesion (arrow) with irregular echogenic shaggy walls and diffuse internal echoes and fluid-debris level within

6.6 Some Miscellaneous Acquired Conditions

6.6.1 Abscess

Causes of hepatic abscess in neonates include bacteremia, necrotizing enterocolitis (NEC), and malpositioned umbilical venous catheter (UVC) [42]. Due to a relatively immunocompromised state, preterm neonates are probably more susceptible [43]. US can help in the initial diagnosis as well as follow-up. It is typically seen as a complex, heterogeneous, avascular hypoechoic lesion with an echogenic wall (Fig. 6.20) on US [44].

6.6.2 Portal Venous Air

In the neonatal period, the most common causes resulting in the portal venous air are NEC and UVC placement. Portal venous air is seen as branching linear lucent structures overlying the liver on a plain radiograph. US is more sensitive for detecting air in portal venous system, which is seen as discrete punctate or linear echogenic

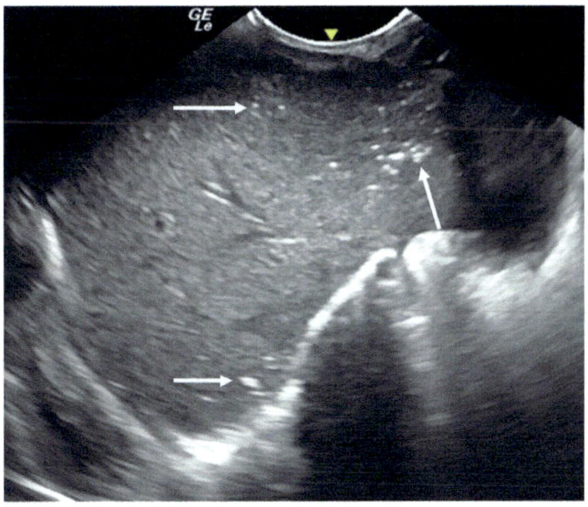

Fig. 6.21 Portal venous gas. Ultrasound image in a neonate with necrotising enterocolitis shows tiny echogenic foci (arrows) within the portal vein branches indicative of air. *Image courtesy: Dr. CV Kanimozhi, Kanchi Kamakoti CHILDS Trust Hospital, Chennai, India*

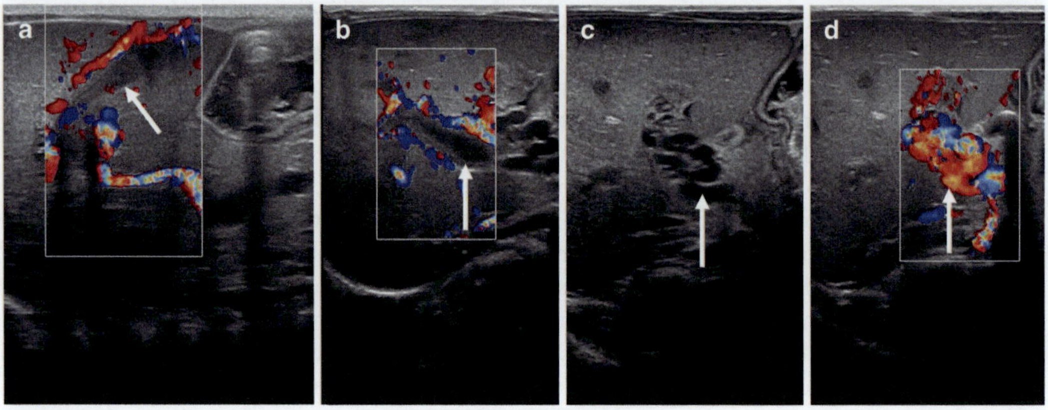

Fig. 6.22 Portal vein thrombosis following omphalitis (**a**–**d**). Color Doppler images (**a** and **b**) show thrombosed umbilical vein (arrow in **a**) and portal vein (arrow in **b**). Grayscale (**c**) and Color Doppler (**d**) images show portal cavernoma at porta (arrows in **c** and **d**)

foci (Fig. 6.21) extending up to the liver periphery [41].

6.6.3 Portal Vein Thrombosis

The major risk factors for portal vein thrombosis (PVT) in neonates are UVC placement for prolonged periods or ascending infection after omphalitis [45]. UVC-related or omphalitis-related PVT may be nonocclusive or occlusive and usually involve the left branch of the PV at its junction with the umbilical vein. PVT is seen as echogenic intraluminal content without Doppler flow in the vessel (Fig. 6.22).

References

1. Shamir SB, Kurian J, Kogan-Liberman D, Taragin BH. Hepatic imaging in neonates and young infants: state of the art. Radiology. 2017;285:763–77.
2. Bezerra JA, Balistreri WF. Cholestatic syndromes of infancy and childhood. Semin Gastrointest Dis. 2001;12:54–65.
3. Di Serafino M, Severino R, Gioioso M, Rossi E, Vezzali N, Pelliccia P, et al. Paediatric liver ultrasound: a pictorial essay. J Ultrasound. 2020;23:87–103.
4. Di Serafino M, Gioioso M, Severino R, Esposito F, Vezzali N, Ferro F, et al. Ultrasound findings in paediatric cholestasis: how to image the patient and what to look for. J Ultrasound. 2020;23:1–12.
5. Dong B, Duan Y, Wang H, Chen Y, Lyu G. Performance of two-dimensional shear wave elastography for detecting advanced liver fibrosis and cirrhosis in patients with biliary atresia: a systematic review and meta-analysis. Pediatr Radiol. 2023;53:2642–50.
6. Ding C, Wang Z, Peng C, Pang W, Tan SS, Chen Y. Diagnosis of liver cirrhosis with two-dimensional shear wave elastography in biliary atresia before Kasai portoenterostomy. Pediatr Surg Int. 2022;38:209–15.
7. Verkade HJ, Bezerra JA, Davenport M, Schreiber RA, Mieli-Vergani G, Hulscher JB, et al. Biliary atresia and other cholestatic childhood diseases: advances and future challenges. J Hepatol. 2016;65:631–42.
8. Lakshminarayanan B, Davenport M. Biliary atresia: a comprehensive review. J Autoimmun. 2016;73:1–9.
9. Hartley JL, Davenport M, Kelly DA. Biliary atresia. Lancet. 2009;374:1704–13.
10. Davenport M, Tizzard SA, Underhill J, MieliVergani G, Portmann B, Hadzić N. The biliary atresia splenic malformation syndrome: a 28-year single-center retrospective study. J Pediatr. 2006;149:393–400.
11. Caponcelli E, Knisely AS, Davenport M. Cystic biliary atresia: an etiologic and prognostic subgroup. J Pediatr Surg. 2008;43:1619–24.
12. Humphrey TM, Stringer MD. Biliary atresia: US diagnosis. Radiology. 2007;244:845–51.
13. Lee MS, Kim MJ, Lee MJ, Yoon CS, Han SJ, Oh J-T, et al. Biliary atresia: color Doppler US findings in neonates and infants. Radiology. 2009;252:282–9.
14. Kim WS, Cheon JE, Youn BJ, Yoo S-Y, Kim WY, Kim I-O, et al. Hepatic arterial diameter measured with US:adjunct for US diagnosis of biliary atresia. Radiology. 2007;245:549–55.
15. Raizner A, Shillingford N, Mitchell PD, Harney S, Raza R, Serino J, et al. Hepatic inflammation may influence liver stiffness measurements by transient

elastography in children and young adults. J Pediatr Gastroenterol Nutr. 2017;64:512–7.

16. Wang X, Qian L, Jia L, Bellah R, Wang N, Xin Y, et al. Utility of shear wave elastography for differentiating biliary atresia from infantile hepatitis syndrome. J Ultrasound Med. 2016;35:1475–9.
17. Ikeda S, Sera Y, Akagi M. Serial ultrasonic examination to differentiate biliary atresia from neonatal hepatitis: special reference to changes in size of the gallbladder. Eur J Pediatr. 1989;148:396–400.
18. Srivastava A. Progressive familial intrahepatic cholestasis. J Clin Exp Hepatol. 2014;4:25–36.
19. Whitington PF. Gestational alloimmune liver disease and neonatal hemochromatosis. Semin Liver Dis. 2012;32:325–32.
20. Tsai A, Paltiel HJ, Sena LM, Kim HB, Fishman SJ, Alomari AI. Neonatal hemochromatosis and patent ductus venosus: clinical course and diagnostic pitfalls. Pediatr Radiol. 2009;39:823–7.
21. Saleh M, Kamath BM, Chitayat D. Alagille syndrome: clinical perspectives. Appl Clin Genet. 2016;9:75–82.
22. Cho HH, Kim WS, Choi YH, Cheon J-E, Lee SM, Kim I-O, et al. Ultrasonography evaluation of infants with Alagille syndrome: in comparison with biliary atresia and neonatal hepatitis. Eur J Radiol. 2016;85:1045–52.
23. Todani T, Watanabe Y, Narusue M, Tabuchi K, Okajima K. Congenital bile duct cysts: classification, operative procedures, and review of thirty-seven cases including cancer arising from choledochal cyst. Am J Surg. 1977;134:263–9.
24. Babbitt DP. Congenital choledochal cysts: new etiological concept based on anomalous relationships of the common bile duct and pancreatic bulb [in French]. Ann Radiol (Paris). 1969;12:231–40.
25. Bollu BK, Dawrant MJ, Thacker K, Thomas G, Chenapragadda M, Gaskin K, et al. Inspissated bile syndrome: safe and effective minimally invasive treatment with percutaneous cholecystostomy in neonates and infants. J Pediatr Surg. 2016;51:2119–22.
26. Jeanty C, Derderian SC, Courtier J, Hirose S. Clinical management of infantile cholelithiasis. J Pediatr Surg. 2015;50:1289–92.
27. Koklu E, Gunes T, Akcakus M, Ozturk MA, Kurtoglu S. Alpha-fetoprotein levels in the neonatal period. Eur J Pediatr. 2008;167:961–2.
28. Merrow AC, Gupta A, Patel MN, Adams DM. 2014 revised classification of vascular lesions from the International Society for the Study of Vascular Anomalies: radiologic-pathologic update. Radiographics. 2016;36:1494–516.
29. Kulungowski AM, Alomari AI, Chawla A, Christison-Lagay ER, Fishman SJ. Lessons from a liver hemangioma registry: subtype classification. J Pediatr Surg. 2012;47:165–70.
30. Kuroda T, Kumagai M, Nosaka S, et al. Critical infantile hepatic hemangioma: results of a nationwide survey by the Japanese Infantile Hepatic Hemangioma Study Group. J Pediatr Surg. 2011;46:2239–43.
31. Huang SA, Tu HM, Harney JW, et al. Severe hypothyroidism caused by type 3 iodothyronine deiodinase in infantile hemangiomas. N Engl J Med. 2000;343:185–9.
32. Roebuck D, Sebire N, Lehmann E, Barnacle A. Rapidly involuting congenital haemangioma (RICH) of the liver. Pediatr Radiol. 2012;42:308–14.
33. Ros PR, Goodman ZD, Ishak KG, et al. Mesenchymal hamartoma of the liver: radiologic-pathologic correlation. Radiology. 1986;158:619–24.
34. Pugmire BS, Towbin AJ. Magnetic resonance imaging of primary pediatric liver tumors. Pediatr Radiol. 2016;46:764–77.
35. Chung EM, Cube R, Lewis RB, Conran RM. From the archives of the AFIP: pediatric liver masses—radiologic-pathologic correlation. I. Benign tumors. Radiographics. 2010;30:801–26.
36. Duigenan S, Anupindi SA, Nimkin K. Imaging of multifocal hepatic lesions in pediatric patients. Pediatr Radiol. 2012;42:1155–68.
37. Towbin AJ, Meyers RL, Woodley H, et al. 2017 PRETEXT: radiologic staging system for primary hepatic malignancies of childhood revised for the paediatric hepatic international tumour trial (PHITT). Pediatr Radiol. 2018;48:536–54.
38. Bernard O, Franchi-Abella S, Branchereau S, Pariente D, Gauthier F, Jacquemin E. Congenital portosystemic shunts in children: recognition, evaluation, and management. Semin Liver Dis. 2012;32:273–87.
39. Lee WK, Chang SD, Duddalwar VA, et al. Imaging assessment of congenital and acquired abnormalities of the portal venous system. Radiographics. 2011;31:905–26.
40. Corness JAG, McHugh K, Roebuck DJ, Taylor AM. The portal vein in children: radiological review of congenital anomalies and acquired abnormalities. Pediatr Radiol. 2006;36:87–96.
41. Simeunovic E, Arnold M, Sidler D, Moore SW. Liver abscess in neonates. Pediatr Surg Int. 2009;25:153–6.
42. Tan NW, Sriram B, Tan-Kendrick AP, Rajadurai VS. Neonatal hepatic abscess in preterm infants: a rare entity? Ann Acad Med Singap. 2005;34:558–64.
43. Hagerott HE, Kulkarni S, Restrepo R, Reeves-Garcia J. Clinical-radiologic features and treatment of hepatic lesions caused by inadvertent infusion of parenteral nutrition in liver parenchyma due to malposition of umbilical vein catheters. Pediatr Radiol. 2014;44:810–5.
44. Williams S, Chan AK. Neonatal portal vein thrombosis: diagnosis and management. Semin Fetal Neonatal Med. 2011;16:329–39.
45. Woodward PJ, Sohaey R, Kennedy A, Koeller KK. From the archives of the AFIP: a comprehensive review of fetal tumors with pathologic correlation. Radiographics. 2005;25:215–42.

7 Neonatal Gastrointestinal Tract

Caroline Rutten and Govind B. Chavhan

7.1 Introduction

Various conditions can affect the neonatal bowel, mostly congenital. Most of these conditions require imaging for diagnosis and management. While plain radiography and fluoroscopy have traditionally been considered the gold standard modalities for many conditions such as malrotation and necrotizing enterocolitis, the ability of ultrasound to provide information on bowel wall thickness, real-time assessment of perfusion and peristalsis, without radiation exposure, makes it a highly useful modality to investigate a broad array of neonatal gastrointestinal tract conditions. This chapter discusses and illustrates neonatal bowel conditions in which ultrasound plays an important role in management. Some conditions such as bowel atresia, meconium ileus, Hirschsprung's disease, and small left colon syndrome are not addressed in this chapter since ultrasound does not play a significant role in their assessment.

C. Rutten · G. B. Chavhan (✉)
Department of Diagnostic Imaging, The Hospital for Sick Children, Toronto, ON, Canada
e-mail: govind.chavhan@sickkids.ca

7.2 Technical Aspects

The challenges in performing bowel ultrasound in the neonatal population are manifold. The bowel content, particularly bowel gas, is the most significant barrier for ultrasound wave transmission and can hamper the evaluation of bowel significantly. Variability in the degree of gaseous distention of bowel in neonates affects the success of ultrasound in the evaluation of bowel. Other factors include motion and abdominal distension, which may be exacerbated by respiratory support. Techniques to enhance bowel visibility include gentle compression of the abdominal wall using the transducer, exploring different acoustic windows, different positioning to displace bowel gas, and aspirating gastric air when a gastric tube is present. For assessment of the pylorus, turning the infant slightly on the right can displace gas towards the fundus and move the gastric fluid in the antrum, creating a more favorable acoustic window (Fig. 7.1).

As for any ultrasound examination, creating a tranquil, comforting setting for the baby is crucial. Administration of a glucose solution, using warmed ultrasound gel or scanning the patient in the caregiver's arms can be beneficial to decrease crying and motion. Most of the bowel loops in neonates can be scanned using high-frequency linear probes. Optimal imaging is achieved with high-resolution linear probes, usually ranging from 12 to 20 MHz. A color Doppler velocity

K. S. Sodhi (ed.), *Neonatal Ultrasound*, https://doi.org/10.1007/978-981-97-8576-6_7

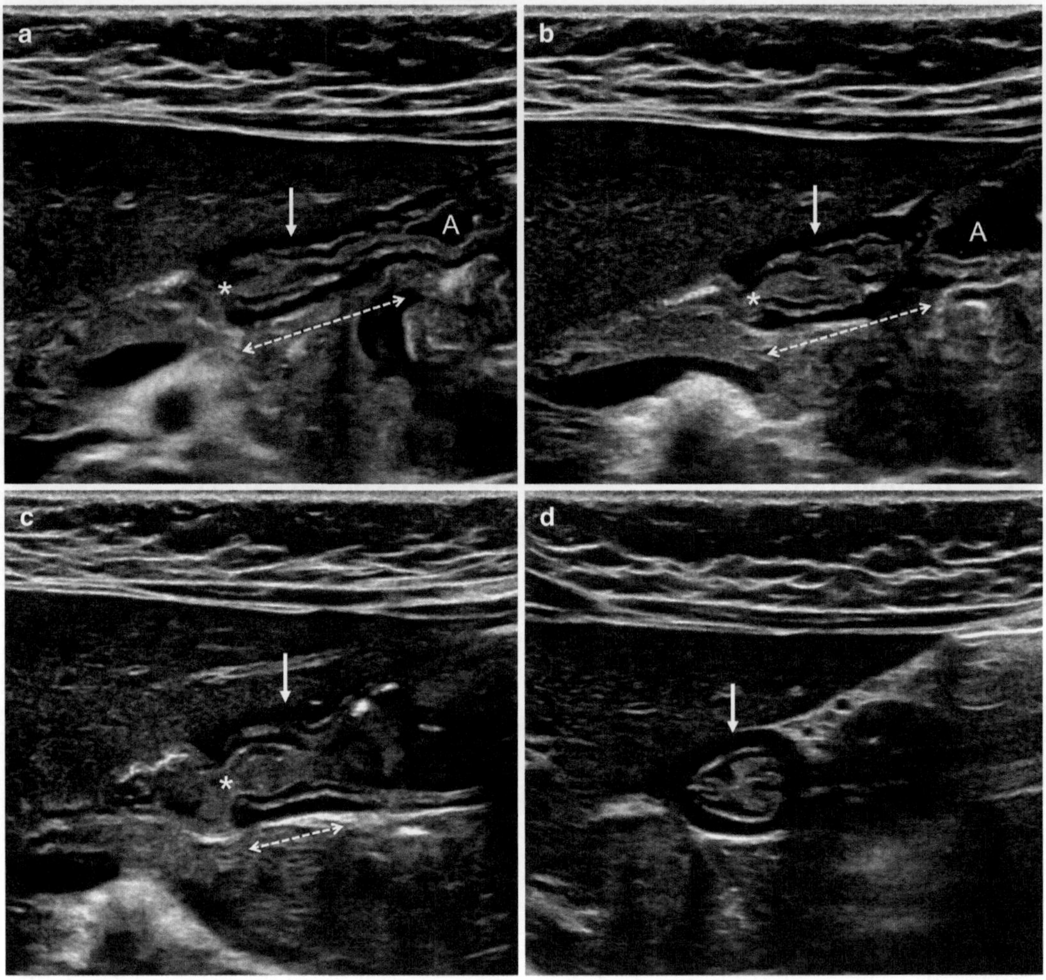

Fig. 7.1 Normal pyloric muscle in a 10-week-old female infant with (**a**–**c**) longitudinal and (**d**) transverse ultrasound views. The antral fluid content is outlining proximal part of pyloric channel (**a** and **b**). The morphology and length of the muscle (arrow) and pyloric channel (<-->) vary with contraction, as does the size of the pyloric orifice (asterisk)

scale in the 5–10 cm/s range is usually adequate to assess mural vascularity of the bowel.

7.3 Normal Bowel Appearance

The normal sonographic appearance of the bowel is that of alternating hyperechoic and hypoechoic layers, reflecting its different histological layers, often referred to as the "gut signature" [1, 2]. These layers, from inside to outside, include: the mucosa (echogenic); muscularis mucosa (hypoechoic); submucosa (echogenic); muscularis propria (hypoechoic); and the serosa (echogenic). Although there are five layers, only three layers are usually identifiable on ultrasound, especially in a normal bowel. It is often not possible to separate the innermost mucosa from the luminal content and the outermost serosa from the surrounding fat (Fig. 7.2).

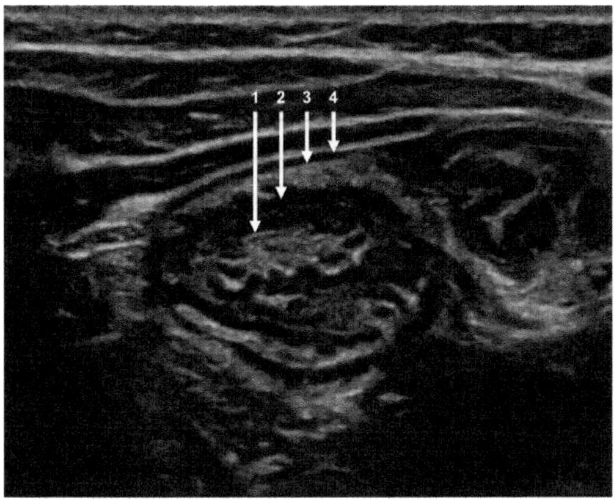

Fig. 7.2 Bowel layers from inside to outside: (*1*) echogenic mucosa; (*2*) hypoechoic muscularis mucosa; (*3*) echogenic submucosa; (*4*) hypoechoic muscular propria. The outermost serosa is too thin to be visualized)

Diseased thickened bowel wall is often easier to image than normal bowel wall. Factors such as reduced motility, mural thickening, adjacent fluid, or increased echogenicity of the surrounding fat usually make the bowel wall assessment easier.

In neonates, the right colon and cecum are often not fixed to the retroperitoneum [3] since the colonic haustra have not yet developed. As such, it is often not possible to discriminate between small and large bowel, particularly in the right flank and lower quadrants. A study found that normal colon diameter in newborns without gastrointestinal problems ranges from 0.80 to 1.35 cm, with a caliber <0.65 cm suggestive of microcolon [4]. However, it is important to note that normal bowel caliber varies with gestational age, making it more difficult to define strict values in the neonatal population [5]. In our experience, a bowel caliber above 1.5 cm in a newborn is usually suggestive of dilation.

The normal thickness of the bowel wall has been reported to range from 1 to 2–3 mm [6, 7]. In our experience, subjective assessment of the bowel loops in comparison to others within the same patient appears to be the best approach. The actual vessels within bowel wall may not be seen in many neonates with normal collapsed bowel loops. The presence of mesenteric flow in such situations indicates normal bowel vascularity. Vascular assessment of the neonatal bowel is usually done quadrant wise.

7.4 Hypertrophic Pyloric Stenosis

Hypertrophic pyloric stenosis (HPS) is a common acquired condition in which the pyloric sphincter becomes thickened, resulting in gastric outlet obstruction. The etiology is unknown, but it is postulated to result from failure of muscle relaxation or hypertrophy of the mucosa resulting in hypertrophy of pyloric muscles. Usage of prostaglandin and erythromycin has been reported to be associated with HPS in some cases. It usually presents between 2 weeks and 3 months of age with the median age of presentation being 6 weeks. It affects males more commonly. Infants typically present with projectile, non-bilious, vomiting. Severe cases may lead to dehydration and hypochloremic alkalosis, requiring prompt correction before surgical intervention.

Ultrasound is the modality of choice to diagnose hypertrophic pyloric stenosis. It allows direct visualization of its features, which include a thickened pyloric muscle and an elongated pyloric canal, and the absence of passage of gastric content through it (Fig. 7.3).

In our experience, the morphology of the pyloric sphincter and real-time dynamics hold

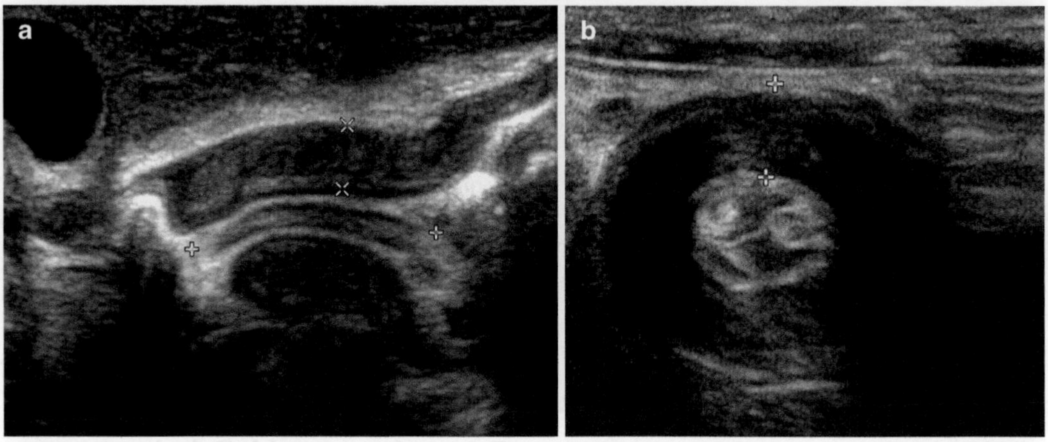

Fig. 7.3 Typical hypertrophic pyloric stenosis in a 6-week-old baby with projectile vomiting. (**a**) Sagittal and (**b**) transverse ultrasound images through the pyloric channel demonstrate thickened hypoechoic muscle layer measuring 4.5 mm (marked by xx) and elongated pyloric channel measuring 19 mm (marked by ++). Also note closed lumen with a thickened echogenic mucosa

more significance than numerical values since measurements in patients with pyloric spasm may overlap with those of hypertrophic pyloric stenosis [8] and threshold values vary by study, with age and weight [9]. However, the numbers may help to increase confidence in diagnosis. Commonly presented threshold values include: a thickened pyloric muscle with a cut-off value of 3 mm; elongation of the pyloric canal greater than 12–15 mm in length; and a pyloric transverse diameter > 13 mm [10]. The pyloric muscle may still open in hypertrophic pyloric stenosis, and a few air bubbles may be seen passing through the pyloric canal, which shouldn't rule out the diagnosis. However, the contraction pattern of the muscle in this scenario is abnormal, with muscle layers remaining parallel to one another. This is contrary to the opening of pylorus in the pyloric spasm, which will open with bend/wavy pyloric muscles.

Ultrasound may also be useful in the postoperative setting if vomiting persists following pyloromyotomy. However, it must be known that the pyloric muscle thickness may take up to 5 months to completely normalize after surgery (Fig. 7.4) [11].

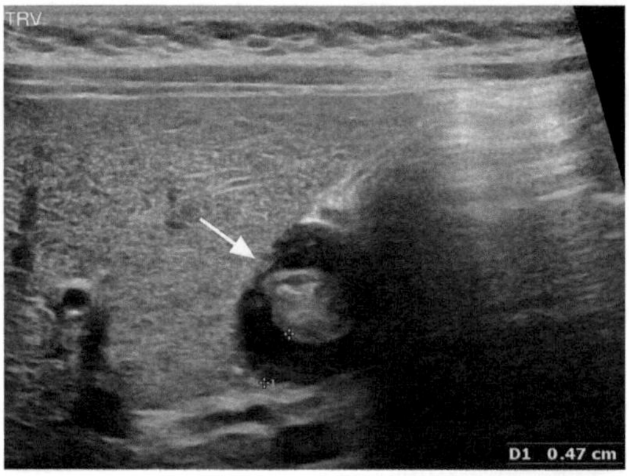

Fig. 7.4 Post-pyloromyotomy appearance of the pyloric muscle in a 3-month-old male with recurrent symptoms. Transverse ultrasound image of the pylorus shows persistent concentric hypoechoic muscular thickening (marked by ++) and a focal anterior mural defect (arrow) corresponding to the pyloromyotomy site

7.5 Malrotation and Midgut Volvulus

Midgut volvulus is a life-threatening surgical emergency in a neonate. Most cases are identified in the neonatal period in association with midgut malrotation. It is characterized by clockwise twisting of the small bowel, its mesentery, and the superior mesenteric vein (SMV) around the superior mesenteric artery (SMA), leading to bowel obstruction and possible vascular compromise. Most infants present with bilious vomiting.

Traditionally, upper GI contrast study has been considered the gold standard for the diagnosis of malrotation and midgut volvulus. However, more recently most centers, including ours, are using US with Doppler as the first modality for assessment of suspected midgut volvulus [12] with contrast study reserved for cases equivocal on US. Obscuration of midline structure by excess of bowel gas is the commonest cause for equivocal US. In our experience, demonstrating a parallel course of the SMA and SMV for a length up to the level of umbilicus excludes volvulus and may obviate need for upper GI contrast study in correlation with clinical features. In normal rotation, the SMV lies to the right of the SMA, and more specifically to the right of the axis formed between the aorta and SMA, and the third part of the duodenum has a retroperitoneal course between the aorta and SMA. While an abnormal orientation of the superior mesenteric vessels (SMV located anteriorly or to the left of the aorta-SMA axis) (Fig. 7.5) can be indicative of

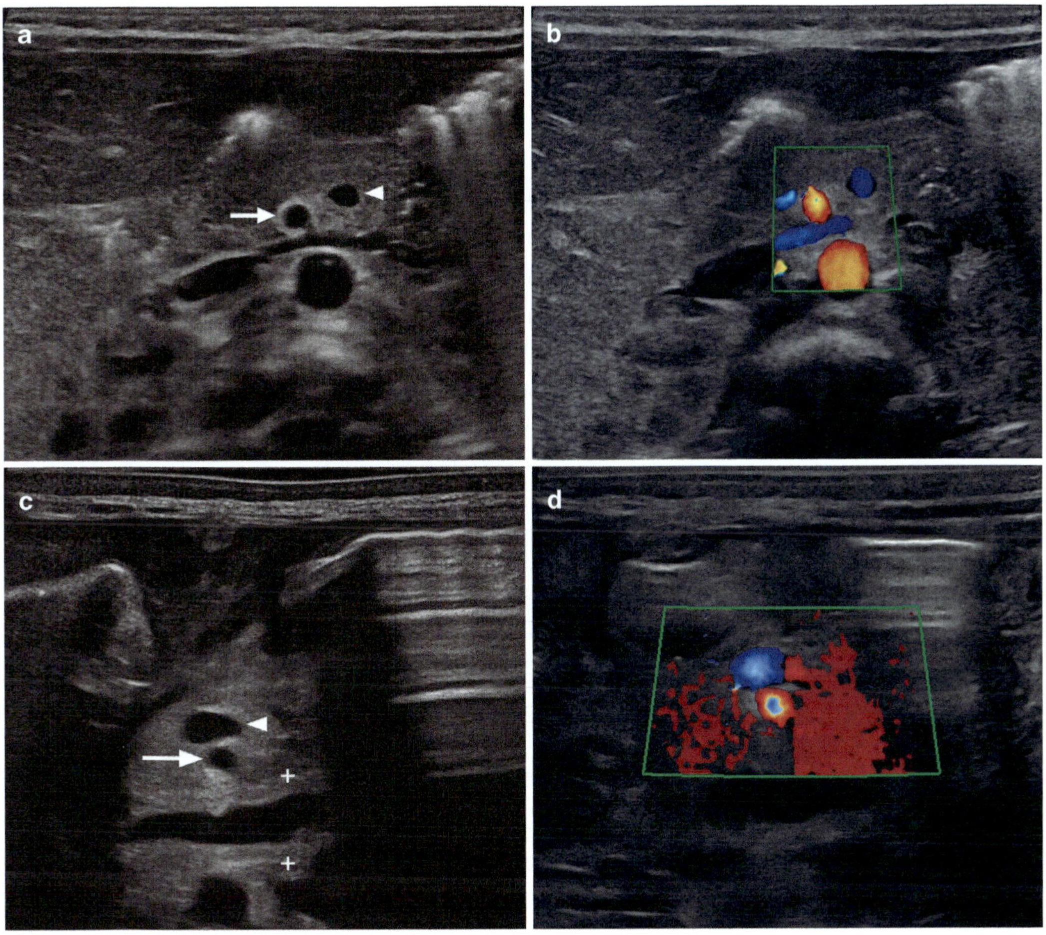

Fig. 7.5 Abnormal orientation of the superior mesenteric vessels, without associated midgut volvulus. Gray-scale (**a**) and color Doppler (**b**) ultrasound images show reversed orientation of the superior mesenteric vessels. Gray-scale (**c**) and color Doppler (**d**) ultrasound images show anterior-posterior orientation of the superior mesenteric vessels. SMA (arrow) typically shows thicker and more echogenic wall as compared to SMV (arrowhead). The third duodenum (marked by ++) is seen crossing the midline between the aorta and SMA (**d**)

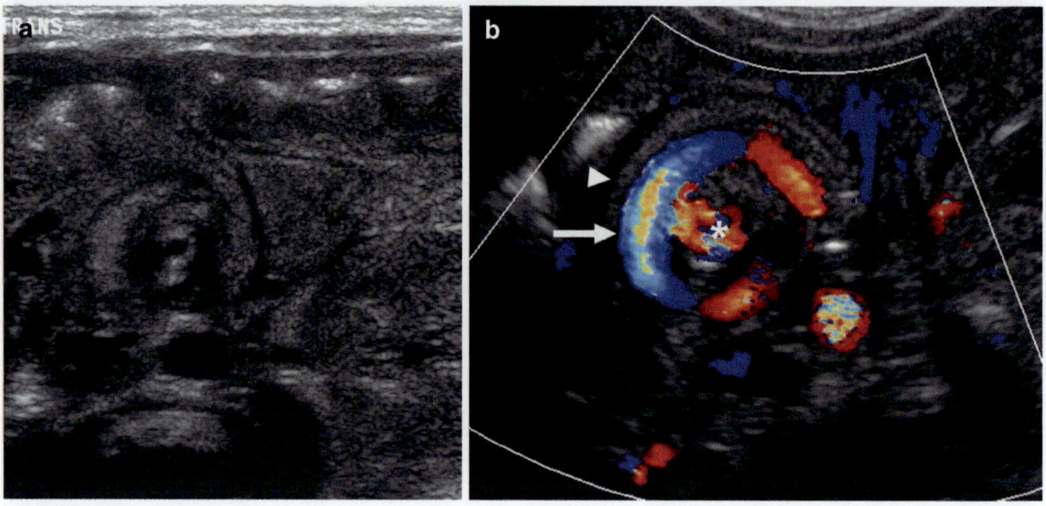

Fig. 7.6 Midgut volvulus in a 9-day-old newborn with bilious emesis. Transverse gray-scale (**a**) and color Doppler (**b**) ultrasound images of the mid-abdomen demonstrate a classic "whirlpool sign" with twisting of the superior mesenteric vein (arrow) and bowel (arrowhead) around the superior mesenteric artery (asterisk)

malrotation, not all abnormalities correlate with malrotation [13]. The sensitivity and specificity of these findings varies according to the studies.

On ultrasound, the diagnosis of midgut volvulus is based on identifying clockwise swirling of the SMV, its branches, and surrounding bowel around the SMA when scanning in the craniocaudal direction, also known as the whirlpool sign [12] (Fig. 7.6). The whirlpool sign is highly specific (100%), and its presence should result in prompt surgical repair without further imaging test. The sensitivity of whirlpool sign ranges 94% [12]. Visualization of the twisting of the bowel loops is essential to confidently diagnose a volvulus. Focusing too much on color Doppler to look for twisting of the vessels or abnormal flow direction may be a source of error. One of the most common pitfalls of this sign is the counterclockwise swirling of the jejunal branches of the SMV around the SMA, which is a normal finding, but may mimic a whirlpool sign and be mistaken for a volvulus (it has been named "pseudovolvulus"). The first jejunal branch of the SMV can usually be easily seen. It may course anteriorly or posteriorly to the SMA [14].

The whirlpool sign may also be associated with segmental volvulus which is unrelated to malrotation and usually seen in the lower abdomen or peripherally, contrary to the midline upper abdominal location of midgut volvulus. This phenomenon may be an isolated finding or associated with intestinal atresia, duplication cyst, or meconium pseudocyst [15]. The upper gastrointestinal series are usually of limited yield in this entity since they are usually limited to evaluating the stomach and duodenum.

7.6 Bowel Obstruction

Ultrasound is frequently utilized at our institution when there is a suspicion of neonatal bowel obstruction, primarily to rule out midgut volvulus or to assess for anomalies associated with a suspected pathology. In this setting, ultrasound can sometimes provide useful information complementing the findings from radiographs and fluoroscopy. Meconium within the bowel typically presents as heterogeneous, echogenic material, and its marked heterogeneity may sometimes be surprising (Fig. 7.7). Furthermore, ultrasound can sometimes help to identify the precise location of the obstruction which is helpful for planning appropriate intervention.

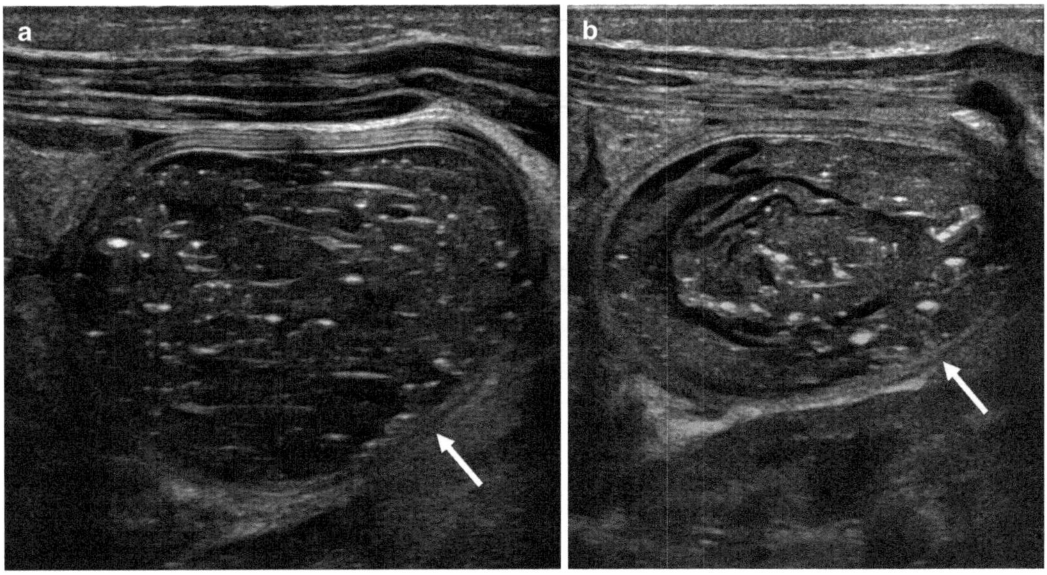

Fig. 7.7 Bowel obstruction in a 2-day-old term newborn male with Hirschsprung's disease. Transverse gray-scale ultrasound images through the left flank (**a**, **b**) show a distended, meconium-filled left colon measuring up to 1.5 cm in diameter (arrows)

7.7 Necrotizing Enterocolitis

Necrotizing Enterocolitis (NEC) is a common serious gastrointestinal condition affecting newborns with mortality rates up to 40% [16]. It predominantly affects premature babies but approximately 10% of NEC cases are term babies [16]. Predisposing factors include low-birth-weight, formula-fed babies, and congenital cardiac disease. The etiology of NEC is unknown, but it is thought to be due to complex interaction of factors including prematurity, mucosal damage, infection resulting into ischemia, necrosis, and ultimately bowel perforation. NEC is treated with stoppage of enteral feed, nasogastric tube, and broad-spectrum antibiotics. Bowel necrosis and perforation are treated surgically.

In this condition, imaging serves two main purposes: assisting in diagnosis when there is clinical uncertainty and assessing for potential complications. Abdominal radiographs have traditionally been the mainstay of imaging, both for initial assessment and follow-up. Recently, many studies have demonstrated that ultrasound can be a valuable adjunct to assess for radiographically occult necrosis or perforation. The radiographic signs include gaseous intestinal distension, pneumatosis intestinalis, portal venous gas, and free air. Ultrasound can also capture these findings but offers the additional advantage of assessing bowel wall thickness, echogenicity, vascularity, peristalsis, free fluid, and collections.

In earlier stages, increased mural vascularity may be seen with variable blood flow patterns, such as the zebra, ring, and Y-shaped patterns [16]. In later stages, reduced or absent perfusion ensue. Identifying pneumatosis intestinalis on ultrasound can be challenging as gas trapped between bowel wall and luminal content can exhibit a similar appearance (Fig. 7.8). In contrast to intraluminal gas, intramural gas will not change position with peristalsis. Careful observation for several seconds can help to make the distinction.

Thinning of the bowel wall and lack of perfusion on ultrasound are highly suggestive of severely ischemic or necrotic bowel loops [16]. Signs of bowel perforation include complex intraperitoneal fluid and free intraperitoneal air. The direct visualization of a breach in the bowel wall is possible but has rarely been reported (Fig. 7.9). Pneumoperitoneum, walled-off fluid

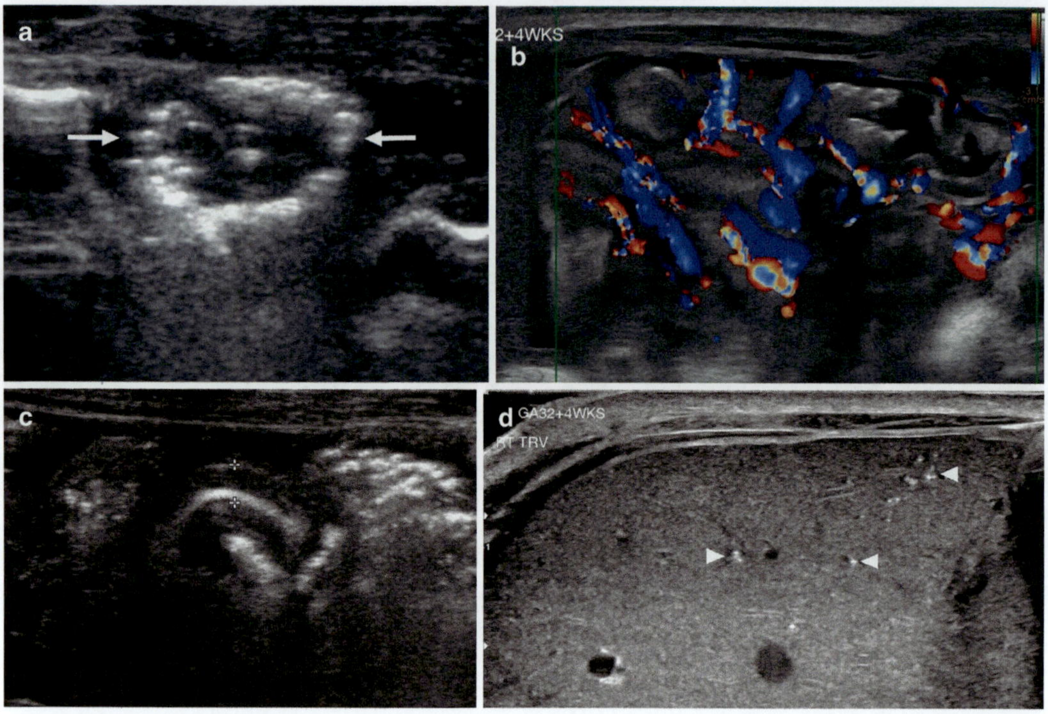

Fig. 7.8 Necrotizing enterocolitis in a 12-day-old preterm newborn. (**a**–**c**) Transverse gray-scale and color Doppler ultrasound images through the right lower quadrant demonstrate (**a**) extensive, circumferential pneumatosis intestinalis (arrows), (**b**) marked mural hyperemia, and (**c**) bowel wall thickening (marked by ++). (**d**) Transverse image through the liver showing echogenic foci of portal venous gas (arrowheads)

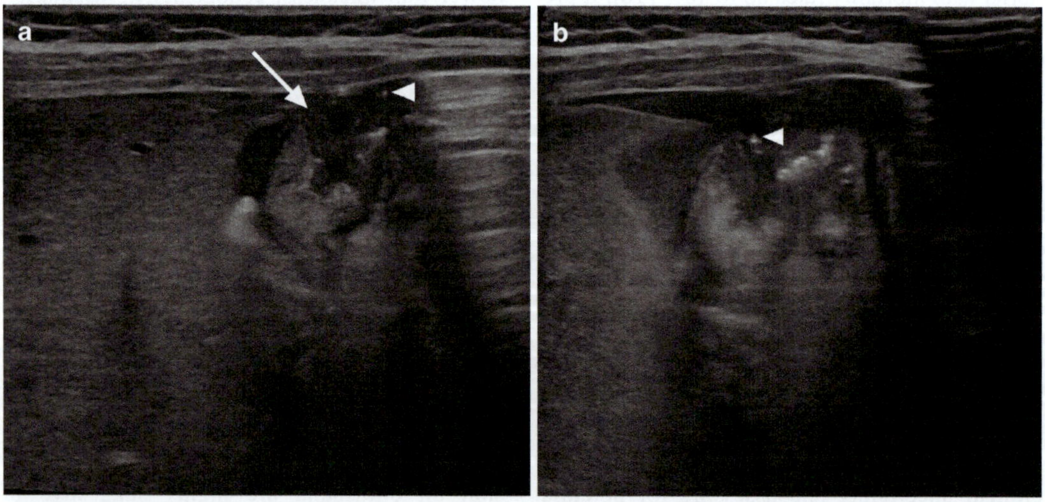

Fig. 7.9 Bowel perforation in a 6-month-old baby girl with a history of necrotizing enterocolitis. (**a**) Transverse and (**b**) longitudinal ultrasound images show a focal discontinuity of the bowel wall in the right upper quadrant (arrow) with adjacent echogenic foci of free air (arrowhead). An isolated perforation of the transverse colon and copious feculent ascites were found at surgery

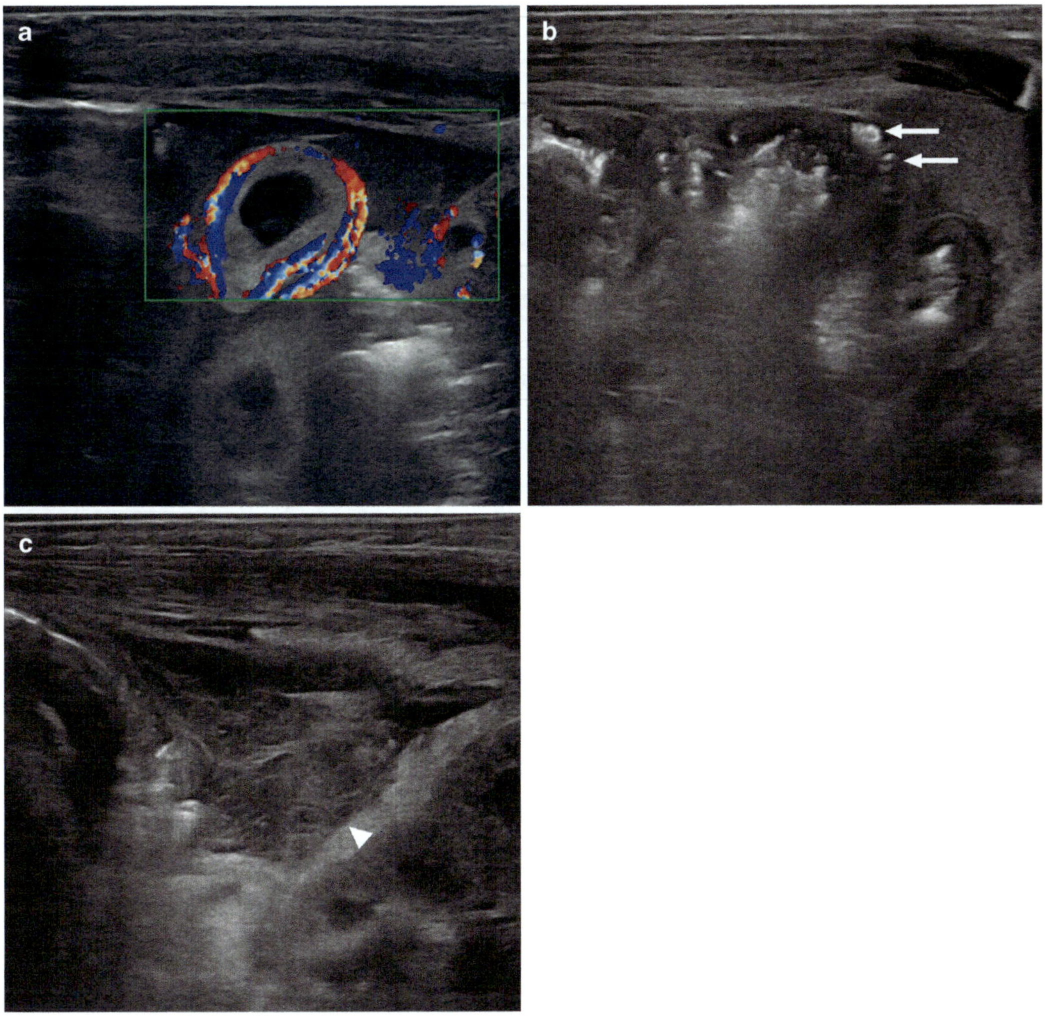

Fig. 7.10 Necrotizing enterocolitis complicated with sigmoid perforation in a 3-day-old preterm newborn. (**a**) Transverse color Doppler (scale 3.1 cm/s) ultrasound view through the left flank showing a thickened small bowel loop (mural thickness 2.1 mm) with loss of normal mural stratification and hyperemia, surrounded by turbid fluid. (**b**) Transverse ultrasound at the level of the splenic flexure showing pneumatosis intestinalis (arrows). (**c**) Transverse left upper quadrant image showing a complex fluid collection (arrowhead)

collection, and complex-free fluid are considered high-risk findings on ultrasound and have been correlated with worse outcomes/need for surgery [17] (Fig. 7.10).

7.8 Duplication Cyst

Enteric duplication cysts are rare congenital gastrointestinal cysts formed during the embryonic development of the GI tract. They may be an incidental finding or be diagnosed secondary to complications such as bowel obstruction (intrinsic, extrinsic, or intussusception) or gastrointestinal bleeding. They are usually detected prenatally or during the first year of life [18]. They can occur anywhere along the GI tract with the distal ileum being the commonest site.

Ultrasound is an excellent modality for the assessment of duplication cysts. The cysts may be spherical or tubular and are outlined by a stratified wall. The classical finding of duplication

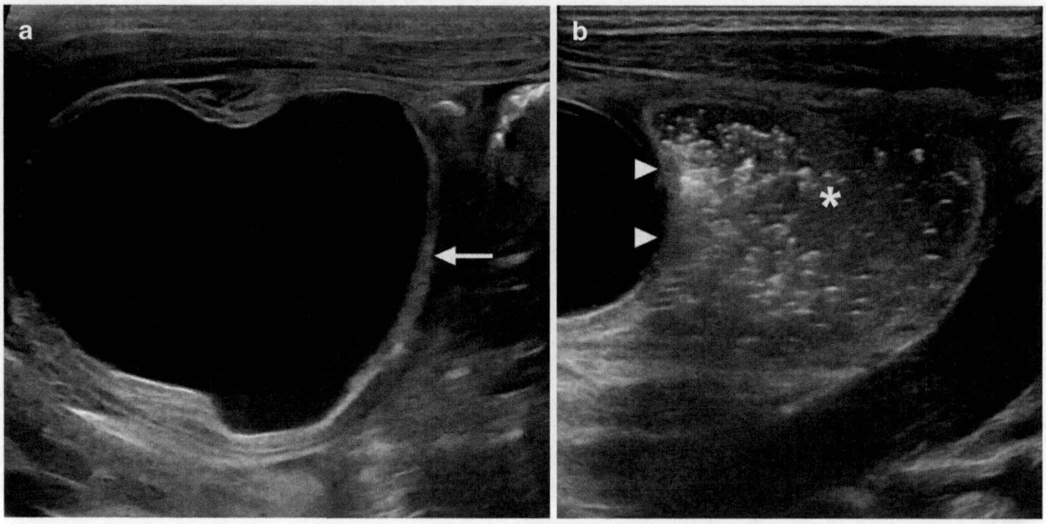

Fig. 7.11 Right upper quadrant colonic duplication cyst in a 5-day-old male causing secondary bowel obstruction with a distended ascending colon. (**a**) Transverse and (**b**) sagittal ultrasound images show a well-defined cyst with gut signature and anechoic content (arrow). It shares a muscular wall (arrowheads) with the adjacent, content-filled, colon (asterisk)

cyst on ultrasound includes a cyst in relation to GI tract with "double-wall" or "gut-signature" (Fig. 7.11). In most cases, inner hyperechoic mucosa and outer hypoechoic smooth muscle layer constitute the "double-wall." Most duplication cysts do not communicate with the bowel lumen though many share a common wall with muscular layer continuous between the cyst and the adjacent bowel loop (Fig. 7.10). Their content may be purely anechoic, but some may contain echogenic debris or septations [18].

It is important to note that double-wall sign is not specific to duplication cyst and can be seen with other cystic lesions derived from bowel including Meckel's diverticulum. Other abdominal cystic lesions seen in neonates including mesenteric cyst and ovarian cyst in baby girls need to be considered in the differential as false double-wall sign may be seen in these lesions.

7.9 Hernias

7.9.1 Inguinal

A congenital inguinal hernia occurs when intra-abdominal content passes into the scrotal cavity or labia through an incompletely obliterated processus vaginalis, which normally closes spontaneously during the first year of life [19]. These are more common in premature infants and male infants with a male:female ratio of approximately 6:1 [20]. The herniated sac may contain omental fat, intestines (Fig. 7.12), fluid, bladder, ovaries (Fig. 7.13), fallopian tubes, and, very rarely, the uterus. The hernia can become incarcerated when its content cannot be reduced.

Most inguinal hernias are diagnosed clinically. Ultrasound is indicated when clinical

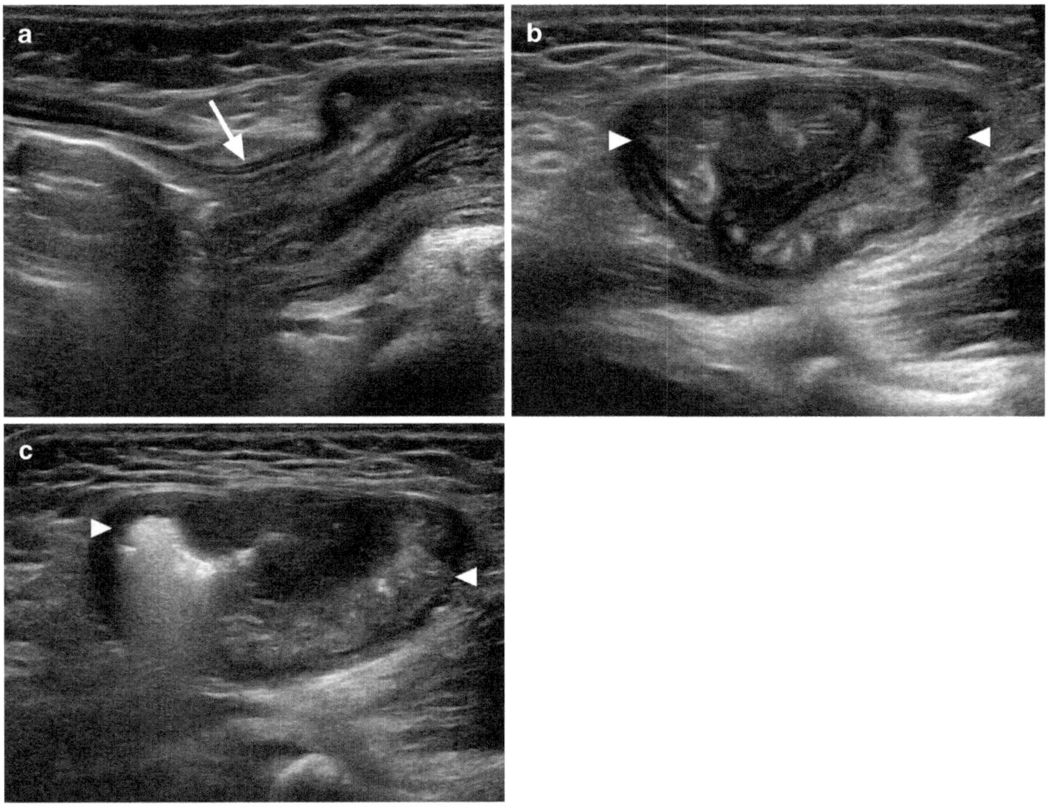

Fig. 7.12 Inguinal hernia in a 4-week-old male with (**a**) longitudinal and (**b**, **c**) transverse images through the left inguinoscrotal region. There are several loops of bowel (arrowheads) herniating into the left inguinal canal (arrow)

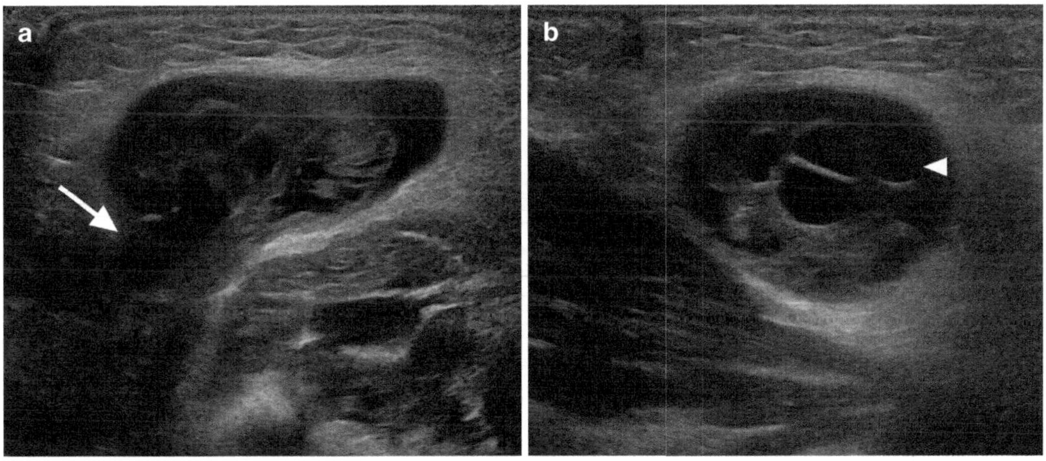

Fig. 7.13 Inguinal hernia in a 5-week-old female presenting with right labial swelling with (**a**) longitudinal and (**b**) transverse images through the right inguinal region. The ovary is seen herniating through the inguinal canal (arrow) with multiple normal follicles (arrowhead)

examination is inconclusive and in the setting of acute findings. Analyzing the content of the hernial sac and its vascularity on color Doppler is also important in preoperative planning. Examination of the inguinal canal at rest may or may not show the hernia. It is essential to assess the inguinal canal with straining, which can be elicited with crying or pressing the lower abdomen. It is also important to examine the contralateral inguinal canal as patency of processus vaginalis is often bilateral.

7.9.2 Umbilical

A congenital umbilical hernia occurs due to incomplete closure of the umbilical ring fascia allowing intra-abdominal content to protrude through a patent umbilical ring. It is a common condition seen in approximately 15–23% of newborns [21, 22]. It is significantly more prevalent in premature and low-birth-weight babies [21]. It occurs in boys and girls equally. The herniated sac may contain omental fat, intestines, or fluid (Fig. 7.14).

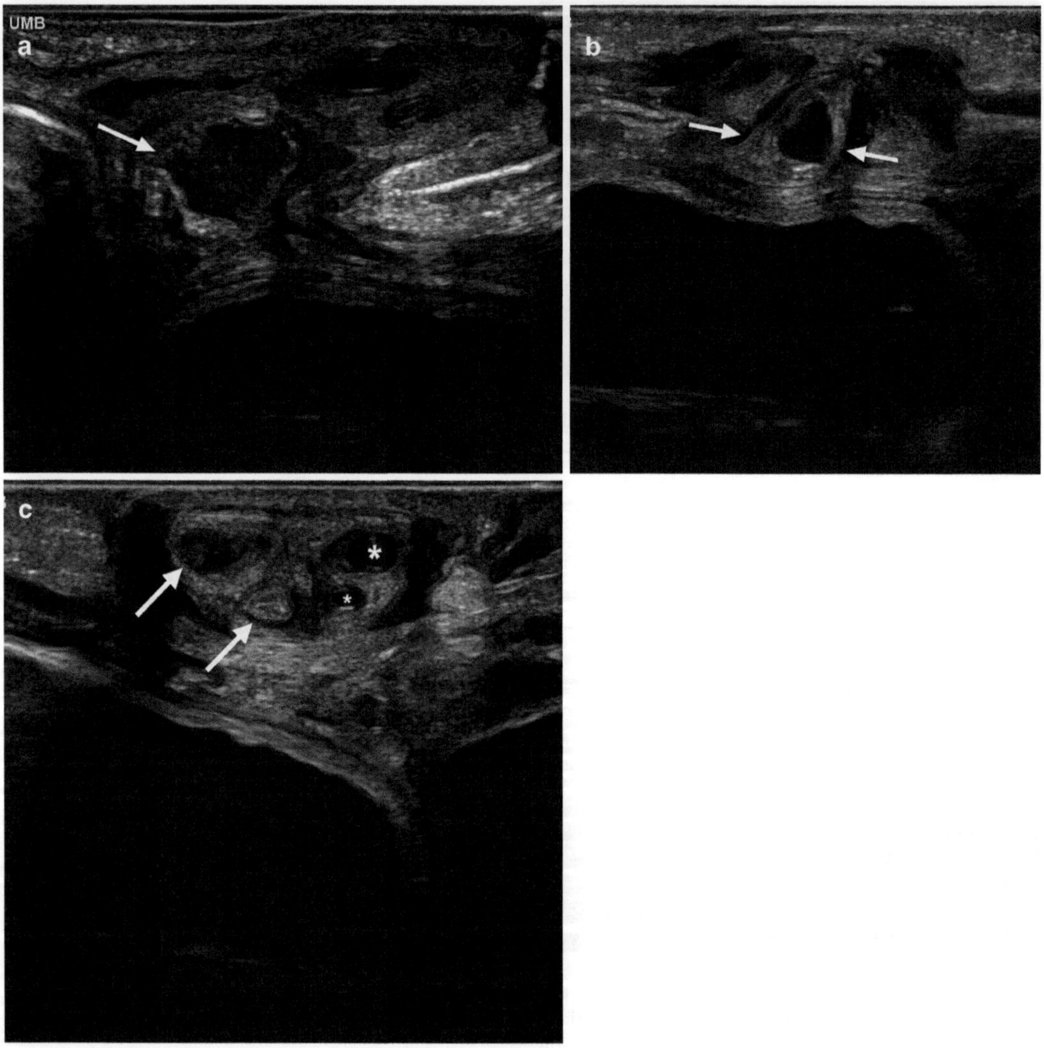

Fig. 7.14 Umbilical hernia in a 1-day-old male with longitudinal (**a**) and transverse (**b**, **c**) images showing bowel loops herniating through the umbilical ring (arrows) adjacent to the umbilical cord with cord vessels (asterisks)

Most umbilical hernias occur in otherwise normal babies, but rarely umbilical hernias can be associated with trisomies, metabolic disorders like hypothyroidism, and mucopolysaccharidoses, and some syndromes like Beckwith-Wiedemann, Down, and Ehlers-Danlos syndrome.

Diagnosis is clinical and ultrasound is rarely required for the diagnosis. Ultrasound will demonstrate the defect size and contents within the hernia. Complications are uncommon and most umbilical hernias seen in neonates close spontaneously within 2 years [22].

7.10 Meconium Peritonitis

Meconium peritonitis is a result of intrauterine bowel perforation and meconium leakage into the peritoneal cavity. Conditions like small bowel atresia, meconium ileus, usually in the setting of cystic fibrosis, volvulus, and imperforate anus are among the causes of prenatal bowel perforation [23]. Intra-abdominal calcification is the hallmark of meconium peritonitis (Fig. 7.15). There may be secondary development of a meconium pseudocyst from the leakage of peritoneal content. Ultrasound is the modality of choice to assess for a pseudocyst which will present as an intraperitoneal cyst of variable size, outlined by a rim of calcification. These cysts may be quite large, with resulting mass effect on the adjacent organs (Fig. 7.16).

Ultrasound helps to differentiate peritoneal distribution of calcification in meconium peritonitis from other causes. Imaging findings including radiographs and ultrasound could help to predict the need for surgery in neonates with meconium peritonitis by showing intestinal obstruction, ascites, volvulus, and pneumoperitoneum [24].

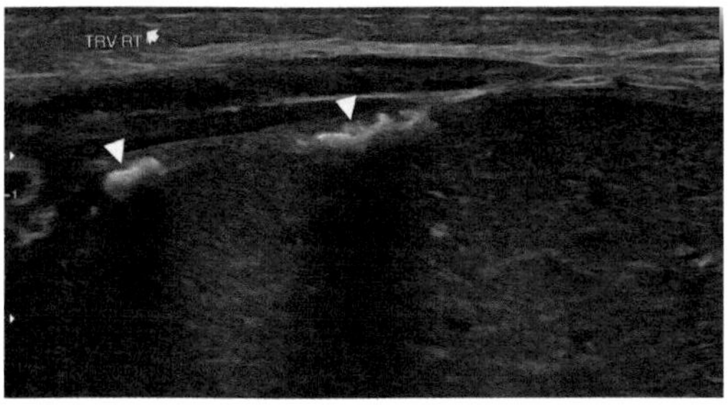

Fig. 7.15 Transverse ultrasound image of the right upper quadrant demonstrates plaque-like peritoneal calcifications (arrowheads) on the liver surface in a 4-day-old-baby boy with meconium peritonitis

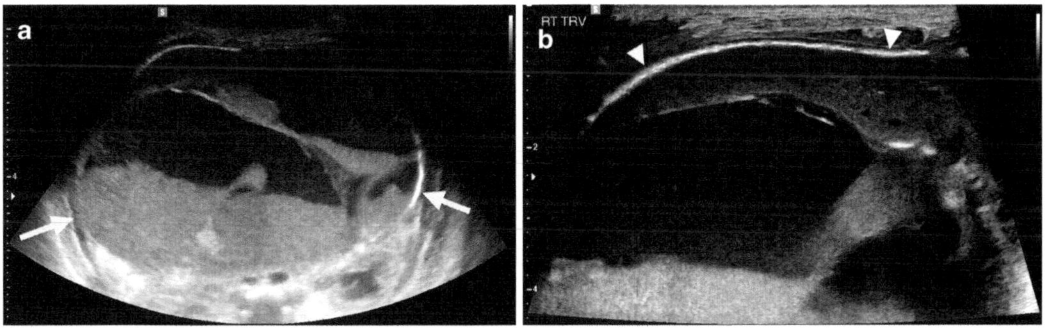

Fig. 7.16 Meconium pseudocyst in a 1-day-old-baby girl occupying most of the abdominal cavity. Transverse curvilinear (**a**) and linear (**b**) transducer ultrasound images show a large complex cyst with multiple septations and dependent echogenic debris (arrows), outlined by a thin, calcified rim (arrowheads)

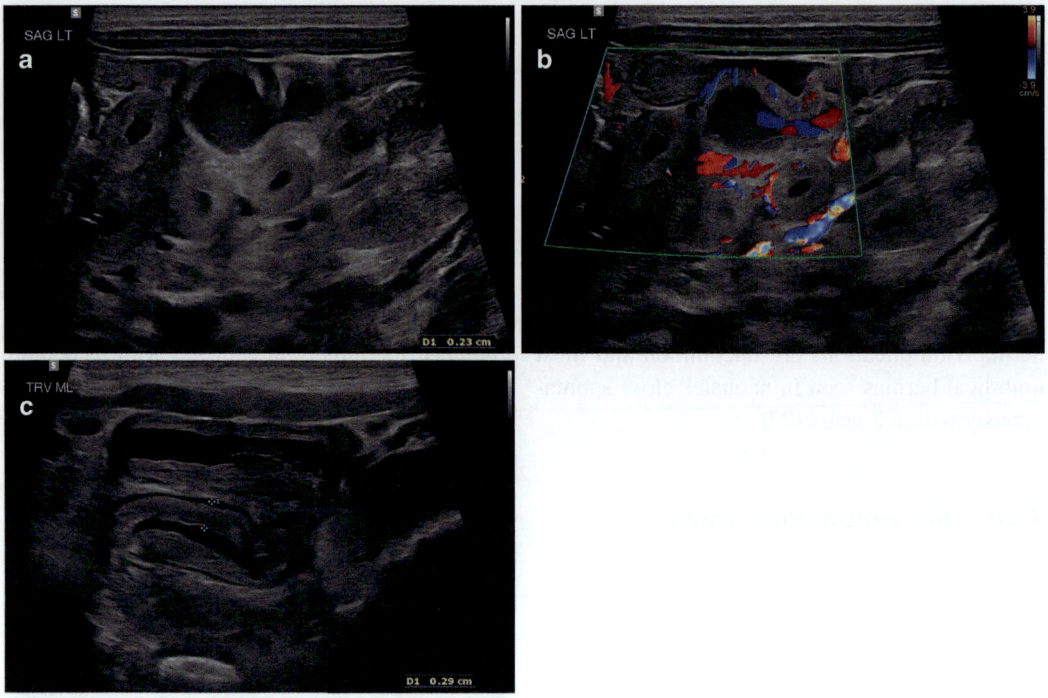

Fig. 7.17 Food protein-induced enterocolitis syndrome in an 8-day-old male term newborn with bloody stool. (**a**–**c**) Gray-scale and color Doppler ultrasound images show circumferential, edematous wall thickening (2.9 mm; marked by ++) and hyperemia throughout most of the small bowel loops and colon, with markedly reduced peristalsis. No other cause was found for the symptoms, which improved with dietary management

7.11 Food Protein-Induced Enterocolitis Syndrome

Food protein-induced enterocolitis syndrome (FPIES) is a gastrointestinal hypersensitivity disorder induced by food, with cow's milk and soy allergy being the commonest cause in neonates [25]. Most cases of FPIES resolve by the age of 3 years. This condition can mimic other diseases, like necrotizing enterocolitis, both in clinical presentation and imaging findings. Clinical symptoms may include nonspecific symptoms such as abdominal distension, blood stool, and feeding intolerance, which can overlap with other conditions. Imaging findings can include intestinal dilatation, bowel wall thickening, reduced peristalsis, pneumatosis intestinalis, and portal venous gas (Fig. 7.17) [26]. It may be valuable to consider this diagnosis when encountering enterocolitis in a term neonate when the clinical presentation doesn't align with necrotizing enterocolitis.

7.12 Conclusion

Many conditions affect neonatal bowel, most of which are congenital or developmental. Imaging plays an important role in their assessment and treatment. Ultrasound is an excellent, radiation-free, imaging modality for neonatal bowel assessment that can be utilized at the bedside. It is the modality of choice for assessment of pyloric stenosis, duplication cysts, hernias, and meconium peritonitis. Ultrasound has recently become the first modality of assessment in neonates with suspected malrotation and volvulus. It plays an important role in the assessment of neonates with necrotizing enterocolitis alongside plain radiographs.

References

1. Siegel MJ. Pediatric sonography. Lippincott Williams & Wilkins; 2011.
2. Rumack CM, Levine D. Diagnostic ultrasound: diagnostic ultrasound. Elsevier Health Sciences; 2017.
3. Veyrac C, Baud C, Prodhomme O, Saguintaah M, Couture A. US assessment of neonatal bowel (necrotizing enterocolitis excluded). Pediatr Radiol. 2012;42(Suppl. 1):S107–14. https://doi.org/10.1007/s00247-011-2173-5.
4. Ju H, Feng S, Huang Y. Diagnostic value of the microcolon using ultrasonography in small bowel atresia. BMC Pediatr. 2022;22:576. https://doi.org/10.1186/s12887-022-03629-z.
5. Lap C, Voskuilen C, Pistorius L, Mulder E, Visser G, Manten G. Reference curves for the normal fetal small bowel and colon diameters; their usefulness in fetuses with suspected dilated bowel. J Matern Neonatal Med. 2018;33:1–11. https://doi.org/10.1080/14767058.2018.1498837.
6. Priyadarshi A, Rogerson S, Hinder M, Tracy M. Neonatologist performed point-of-care bowel ultrasound: is the time right? Australas J Ultrasound Med. 2019;22:15–25. https://doi.org/10.1002/ajum.12114.
7. Bohnhorst B. Usefulness of abdominal ultrasound in diagnosing necrotising enterocolitis. Arch Dis Child Fetal Neonatal Ed. 2013;98:F445–50. https://doi.org/10.1136/archdischild-2012-302848.
8. Cohen HL, Zinn HL, Haller JO, Homel PJ, Stoane JM. Ultrasonography of pylorospasm: findings may simulate hypertrophic pyloric stenosis. J Ultrasound Med. 1998;17:705–11. https://doi.org/10.7863/jum.1998.17.11.705.
9. Said M, Shaul DB, Fujimoto M, Radner G, Sydorak RM, Applebaum H. Ultrasound measurements in hypertrophic pyloric stenosis: don't let the numbers fool you. Perm J. 2012;16:25–7.
10. Costa Dias S, Swinson S, Torrão H, Gonçalves L, Kurochka S, Vaz CP, et al. Hypertrophic pyloric stenosis: tips and tricks for ultrasound diagnosis. Insights Imaging. 2012;3:247–50. https://doi.org/10.1007/s13244-012-0168-x.
11. Yoshizawa J, Eto T, Higashimoto Y, Saitou T, Maie M. Ultrasonographic features of normalization of the pylorus after pyloromyotomy for hypertrophic pyloric stenosis. J Pediatr Surg. 2001;36:582–6. https://doi.org/10.1053/jpsu.2001.22287.
12. Nguyen HN, Navarro OM, Bloom DA, Feinstein KA, Guillerman RP, Munden MM, et al. Ultrasound for Midgut Malrotation and Midgut volvulus: AJR expert panel narrative review. Am J Roentgenol. 2022;218:931–9. https://doi.org/10.2214/AJR.21.27242.
13. Son J, Lee S, Kim W, Jung S-M, Jeon TY, Yoo S-Y, et al. Abnormal orientation of the superior mesenteric vessels detected in asymptomatic infants: what is its destiny? Front Pediatr. 2021;9:665448. https://doi.org/10.3389/fped.2021.665448.
14. Papavasiliou P, Arrangoiz R, Zhu F, Chun YS, Edwards K, Hoffman JP. The anatomic course of the first jejunal branch of the superior mesenteric vein in relation to the superior mesenteric artery. Int J Surg Oncol. 2012;2012:538769. https://doi.org/10.1155/2012/538769.
15. Garel J, Daneman A, Rialon K, Zani A, Fecteau A, Piero A. The role of sonography for depiction of a whirlpool sign unrelated to midgut malrotation in neonates. Pediatr Radiol. 2020;50:46–56. https://doi.org/10.1007/s00247-019-04508-z.
16. Epelman M, Daneman A, Navarro OM, Morag I, Moore AM, Kim JH, et al. Necrotizing enterocolitis: review of state-of-the-art imaging findings with pathologic correlation. Radiographics. 2007;27:285–305. https://doi.org/10.1148/rg.272055098.
17. Silva CT, Daneman A, Navarro OM, Moore AM, Moineddin R, Gerstle JT, et al. Correlation of sonographic findings and outcome in necrotizing enterocolitis. Pediatr Radiol. 2007;37:274–82. https://doi.org/10.1007/s00247-006-0393-x.
18. Sangüesa Nebot C, Llorens Salvador R, Carazo Palacios E, Picó Aliaga S, Ibañez Pradas V. Enteric duplication cysts in children: varied presentations, varied imaging findings. Insights Imaging. 2018;9:1097–106. https://doi.org/10.1007/s13244-018-0660-z.
19. Saguintaah M, Eulliot J, Bertrand M, Prodhomme O, Béchard N, Bolivar-Perrin J, et al. Canal of Nuck abnormalities in Pediatric female patients. Radiographics. 2022;42:541–58. https://doi.org/10.1148/rg.210145.
20. Anon. Inguinal hernias and hydroceles in infancy and childhood: a consensus statement of the Canadian association of paediatric surgeons. Paediatr Child Health. 2000;5:461–2. https://doi.org/10.1093/pch/5.8.461.
21. Zendejas B, Kuchena A, Onkendi EO, Lohse CM, Moir CR, Ishitani MB, et al. Fifty-three-year experience with pediatric umbilical hernia repairs. J Pediatr Surg. 2011;46:2151–6. https://doi.org/10.1016/j.jpedsurg.2011.06.014.
22. Zens T, Nichol PF, Cartmill R, Kohler JE. Management of asymptomatic pediatric umbilical hernias: a systematic review. J Pediatr Surg. 2017;52:1723–31. https://doi.org/10.1016/j.jpedsurg.2017.07.016.

23. Shinar S, Agrawal S, Ryu M, Van Mieghem T, Daneman A, Ryan G, et al. Fetal meconium peritonitis—prenatal findings and postnatal outcome: a case series, systematic review, and meta-analysis. Ultraschall Med. 2022;43:194–203. https://doi.org/10.1055/a-1194-4363.
24. Caro-Domínguez P, Zani A, Chitayat D, Daneman A. Meconium peritonitis: the role of postnatal radiographic and sonographic findings in predicting the need for surgery. Pediatr Radiol. 2018;48:1755–62. https://doi.org/10.1007/s00247-018-4198-5.
25. Nowak-Wegrzyn A, Muraro A. Food protein-induced enterocolitis syndrome. Curr Opin Allergy Clin Immunol. 2009;9:371–7. https://doi.org/10.1097/ACI.0b013e32832d6315.
26. Guo Y, Si S, Jia Z, Lv X, Wu H. Differentiation of food protein-induced enterocolitis syndrome and necrotizing enterocolitis in neonates by abdominal sonography. J Pediatr. 2021;97:219–24. https://doi.org/10.1016/j.jped.2020.03.001.

8 Neonatal Retroperitoneum

Amit Gupta, Devasenathipathy Kandasamy, and Sumera Ali

8.1 Introduction

A myriad of pathologies can affect the retroperitoneum in neonates [1–3]. Aside from the kidneys, these pathologies majorly arise from or are related to the adrenal glands. These include congenital, metabolic, traumatic, vascular, and neoplastic etiologies. They can have a highly variable clinical presentation including asymptomatic incidental findings on abdominal imaging, upper abdominal mass detected on prenatal imaging, multiple systemic metastases from malignancy, and neonatal hypovolemic shock. Ultrasound (US) is an ideal modality to image the adrenal glands in neonates as it allows high-resolution visualization of these organs without the need for sedation or anesthesia and can be performed easily at the patient's bedside. Ultrasound is often the initial imaging modality used to identify and diagnose neonatal adrenal pathologies [1].

A. Gupta
All India Institute of Medical Sciences, New Delhi, India

D. Kandasamy (✉)
Radiodiagnosis and interventional Radiology, All India Institute of Medical Sciences, New Delhi, India

S. Ali
Department of Radiology, Emory University School of Medicine, Atlanta, GA, USA

In this chapter, we review the US appearances of normal neonatal adrenal glands as well as the role of the US in diagnosing various neonatal adrenal pathologies and their mimics. Thrombosis of the major retroperitoneal vessels and rare primary retroperitoneal masses in the neonatal age group are also discussed.

8.2 Adrenal US Technique in Neonates

Transducer: It is necessary to use a linear high-frequency transducer, preferably in the range of 10–15 MHz for visualizing the neonatal adrenals with the required anatomical detail [2]. It is essential to use a clean ultrasound probe with warmed jelly and short scan times, especially in a neonatal intensive care unit setting.

Probe position: The adrenal US is usually performed as a part of an abdominal or renal US. The adrenal glands are visualized in bilateral flanks using the liver as the acoustic window for the right adrenal and spleen for the left adrenal. The right adrenal gland can be visualized in 97–100% of newborns, while the left adrenal gland is only visible in 83–96% of newborns, often due to interference from gas in the stomach or bowel [3]. Keeping the patient in a decubitus or prone position can aid visualization in case of shadowing by overlying bowel gas.

K. S. Sodhi (ed.), *Neonatal Ultrasound*, https://doi.org/10.1007/978-981-97-8576-6_8

8.3 Normal Adrenal Anatomy

Location: The adrenal glands, which are dual endocrine organs, are situated in the retroperitoneum, at the upper edge of the perirenal fascia, and are separated from the kidneys by perirenal fat. The two adrenals differ slightly in their location and relationship with adjacent structures. The right adrenal gland is located anterior and superior to the right kidney, adjacent to the lateral side of the right diaphragmatic crus, medial to the right lobe of the liver, and behind the inferior vena cava (IVC). Conversely, the left adrenal gland is positioned anterior and medial to the left kidney, adjacent to the lateral side of the aorta and left diaphragmatic crus, and medial to the spleen [4].

Size: The adrenal gland is discernible via obstetric ultrasound as early as 13–14 weeks of gestation, during which it appears large, globular, and approximately half the length of the kidney [5]. Upon birth, the adrenal gland is notably large, with a length of about one-third that of the kidney. This dimension diminishes to one-thirtieth of the kidney's size by adulthood and adrenals are seldom visualized on the US in adults [6]. Post-birth, the gland undergoes atrophy, with serial sonographic examinations indicating a reduction in size by up to 50% within the first 6 weeks postnatally. Beginning from the second year of life, the gland gradually enlarges, reaching its adult dimensions by puberty. The adrenal body and two limbs are also well discernible on the US in neonates. Ultrasound measurements can accurately assess the gland, with normal neonatal adrenal length ranging from 0.9 to 3.6 cm (average 1.5–1.7 cm) and limb thickness from 0.2 to 0.5 cm (average 0.3 cm) [2].

Shape: The shape of normal adrenal glands is highly variable; however, the right adrenal is mostly triangular or pyramidal and the left adrenal is semilunar in shape. On the US, adrenal glands can assume an L, V, or Y shape according to the viewing plane [4] (Fig. 8.1). The surface of the gland should be smooth without any focal nodules; however, a mild wavy contour to the gland is normal.

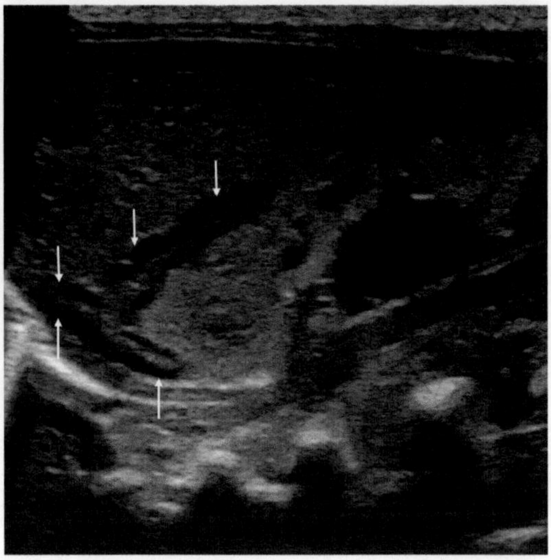

Fig. 8.1 Normal US appearance of the neonatal adrenal gland (arrows). The adrenal gland shows a Y shape and prominent thick hypoechoic outer cortex and a thin hyperechoic central medulla

US appearance: The sonographic characteristics of the normal adrenal gland evolve with age. The gland is composed of a central medullary layer that is hyperechoic, originating from neuroendocrine tissue responsible for catecholamine production. The cortex, derived from coelomic mesoderm, appears hypoechoic [6]. In neonates, the adrenal gland shows prominent corticomedullary differentiation with a prominent thick hypoechoic outer cortex and a thin hyperechoic central medulla (Fig. 8.1). The hypoechoic neonatal adrenal cortex consists of a substantial transient inner fetal zone that gradually atrophies, alongside a slender outer zone that matures into the adult cortex. This cortex undergoes differentiation into three zones, which produce aldosterone, glucocorticoids, and androgens. By around 5–6 months of age, the gland may appear hyperechoic due to the atrophy of most of the hypoechoic fetal zone and its replacement by fibrous tissue. As this fibrous tissue diminishes, the gland's appearance shifts to hypoechoic, and by the age of 1 year, it mirrors the adult gland's hypoechoic appearance, encased by hyperechoic fat [2].

8.4 Adrenal Pathologies in Neonates

Various conditions affecting neonatal adrenal glands and their mimics are classified in Table 8.1.

8.4.1 Congenital Adrenal Anomalies

Discoid adrenal: The term "discoid adrenal gland" derives from its distinctive shape and is also referred to as a straight or pancake adrenal gland. This morphology is typically associated with congenital renal anomalies, occurring when the corresponding kidney is absent or ectopically positioned, leading to an unoccupied renal fossa. A kidney's presence is essential for the adrenal gland to develop its standard triangular or Y configuration. Without the normal upward pressure from the developing kidney on the same side, the adrenal gland assumes a flattened or discoid form [2] (Fig. 8.2). Despite this altered shape, the normal echogenic medulla and the surrounding hypoechoic cortex remain visible and should not be confused with an atrophic kidney. No medical intervention is necessary for a discoid adrenal gland.

Horseshoe adrenal: A horseshoe adrenal gland represents an uncommon congenital anomaly, manifested by the fusion of the medial aspects of each adrenal gland [7]. This condition frequently occurs in conjunction with asplenia syndrome (the most prevalent association), neural tube defects, renal anomalies, and

Table 8.1 Various adrenal gland pathologies and their mimics affecting neonates

Etiology	Pathology
Congenital	Discoid adrenal gland Horseshoe adrenal gland Adrenal epithelial cysts
Traumatic/vascular	Adrenal hemorrhage
Metabolic	Congenital adrenal hyperplasia
Neoplastic	Neuroblastoma
Adrenal lesion mimics	Extralobar sequestration Exophytic renal and hepatic tumors

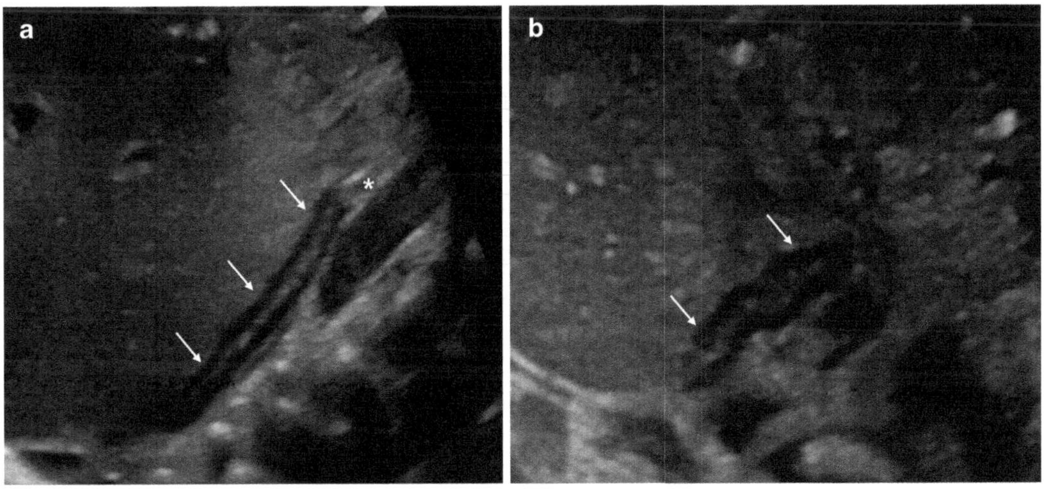

Fig. 8.2 (**a**) Longitudinal and (**b**) transverse US images show a discoid adrenal gland (arrows) in a neonate with empty renal fossa (asterisk). A note is made of normal corticomedullary echotexture of the adrenal gland

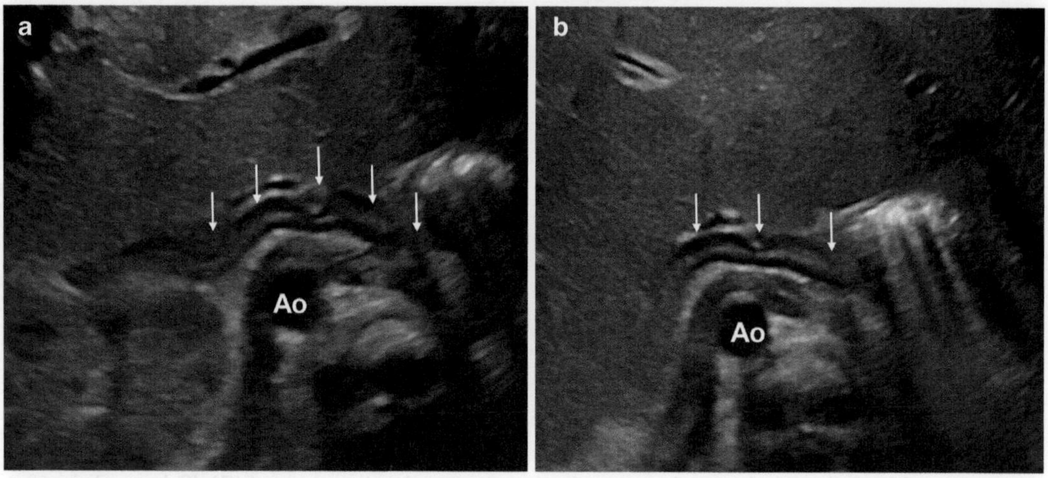

Fig. 8.3 (**a**, **b**) US sections show a single centrally located horseshoe adrenal gland (arrows) with fusion of the medial aspects of the glands anterior to the aorta (Ao). A note is made of normal corticomedullary echotexture of the adrenal gland

Cornelia de Lange syndrome. Asplenia syndrome, also known as right isomerism, is typified by the presence of bilateral trilobed lungs, duplicated right atria, a liver positioned along the midline, absence of the spleen, malrotation, and congenital heart defects [8]. Renal anomalies correlated with a horseshoe adrenal gland encompass bilateral renal agenesis and a horseshoe kidney. US is beneficial for evaluating a horseshoe adrenal gland in neonates and infants, revealing a single adrenal gland centrally located with the fused section extending anteriorly to the aorta (Fig. 8.3). It is crucial to investigate any associated renal and spinal cord anomalies [8]. Most individuals with a horseshoe adrenal gland exhibit no clinical or biochemical signs of adrenal dysfunction. Nonetheless, the accompanying abdominal, renal, cardiac, and spinal anomalies require medical attention.

Adrenal epithelial cysts: True epithelium-lined adrenal cysts are rare incident findings in infants. On the US, these are characteristically well-defined, thin-walled, anechoic lesions showing posterior acoustic enhancement and absence of Doppler flow [3]. However, the presence of any septations, mural nodules, or calcifications should lead to consideration of other differentials including post-hemorrhagic pseudocyst, lymphatic cyst, or cystic neuroblastoma.

8.4.2 Adrenal Hemorrhage

Adrenal hemorrhage is the most common cause of adrenal masses in neonates, frequently manifesting within the initial days of life. Occurring in two out of every 1000 neonates, adrenal hemorrhages are almost four times as prevalent as neuroblastomas [3]. The relatively large size and high vascularity of the neonatal adrenal gland are believed to increase its vulnerability to hemorrhage. Bilateral cases account for 10% of occurrences, with a 70% likelihood of being on the right side. The rationale for the increased incidence of adrenal hemorrhage on the right side remains speculative though it may occur secondary to the compression of the right adrenal between the liver and the right kidney [9]. Notably, adrenal hemorrhage linked to renal vein thrombosis predominantly occurs on the left side, attributed to the left adrenal vein's drainage into the renal vein, in contrast to the right adrenal vein's direct drainage into the inferior vena cava.

Adrenal hemorrhages in neonates may be detected incidentally during ultrasound examinations, especially in those with a history of complicated deliveries, birth trauma, sepsis, perinatal hypoxia, or bleeding disorders. Clinical manifestations can vary, including palpable masses, anemia, jaundice, abdominal discomfort, and shock. Infants born to diabetic mothers exhibit a higher incidence of renal vein thrombosis and adrenal hemorrhage. Additionally, approximately 1% of children may experience adrenal hemorrhage following blunt abdominal trauma, often alongside other visceral injuries. Waterhouse-Friderichsen syndrome can lead to severe bilateral adrenal hemorrhage and subsequent adrenal insufficiency.

The imaging appearance of adrenal hemorrhage varies with the age of the hemorrhage and the patient. Serial ultrasound is preferred for monitoring adrenal hemorrhage, initially presenting as a slightly echoic to isoechoic mass, which may be homogeneous or heterogeneous [3] (Fig. 8.4). The lesion might only affect part of the gland, with possible visualization of a normal adrenal section adjacent to the hemorrhage. The absence of internal flow is confirmed through color Doppler ultrasound, given the avascular nature of the mass [10]. Over time, adrenal hemorrhages undergo cystic transformation and resolution. The hemorrhage may liquefy into a more complex mass with a central hypoechoic region and internal debris, eventually becoming completely cystic—the so-called adrenal pseudocyst (Fig. 8.5). Early calcification within 1–2 weeks may show punctate or curvilinear echogenicity. Ultimately, the hemorrhage resolves, allowing the adrenal gland to revert to its normal size and shape.

Neuroblastoma simulates adrenal hemorrhage in 50% of the cases and stands as the primary differential diagnosis, necessitating short-term follow-up ultrasounds due to the generally favorable prognosis of neonatal neuroblastoma. A neuroblastoma, usually, either remains the same or size increases and develops more heterogeneous echogenic solid elements with time. Rarely, even congenital neuroblastoma can show a size reduction which makes the distinction from adrenal hemorrhage even more difficult [3].

While most adrenal hemorrhage cases resolve without clinical consequences, severe bilateral hemorrhages causing adrenal insufficiency

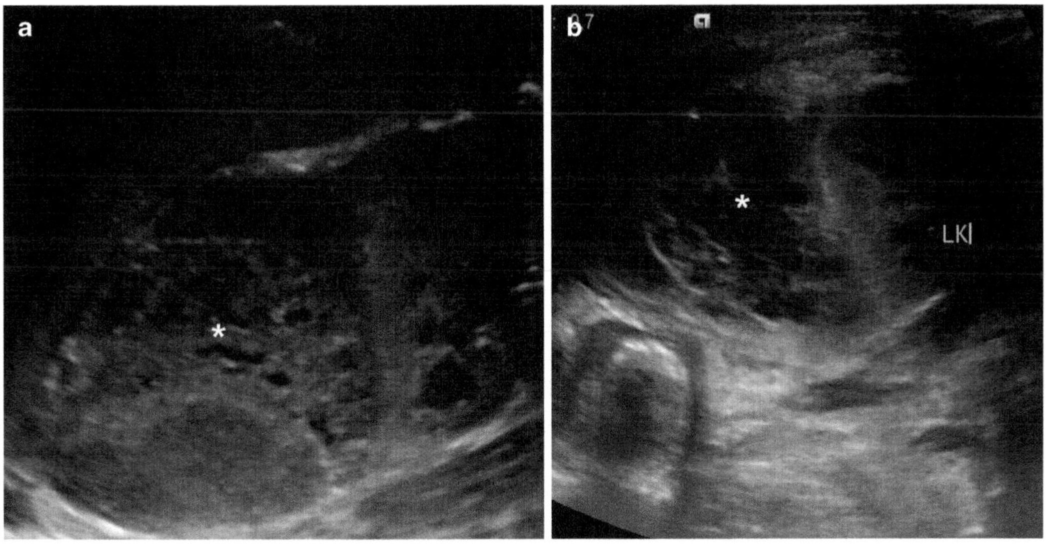

Fig. 8.4 Incidentally detected subacute adrenal hemorrhage in a 3-week-old neonate. (**a**, **b**) Grayscale US images show a heterogeneous, predominantly hyperechoic left suprarenal lesion (asterisk) with few internal cystic areas. *LK* left kidney

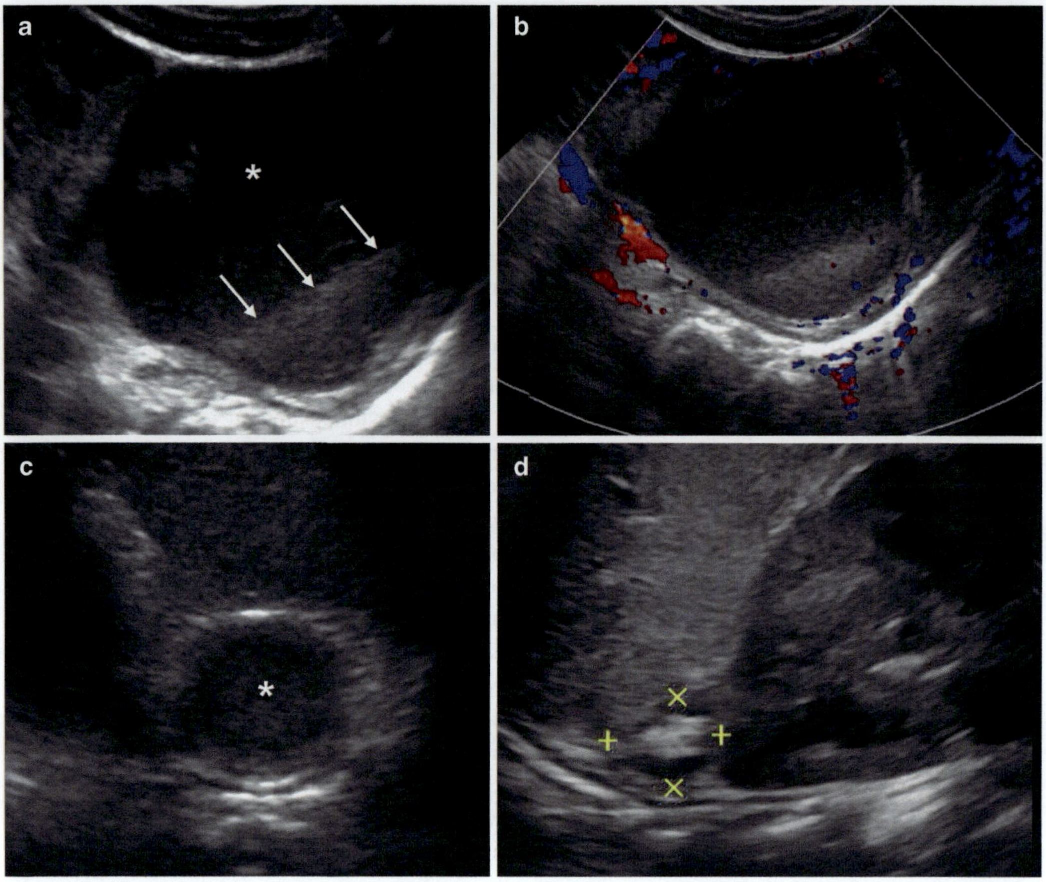

Fig. 8.5 Incidentally detected adrenal hemorrhage in a 40-day-old infant showing resolution on follow-up US. (**a**) Initial scan at the age of 40 days shows a well-defined cystic lesion (asterisk) in the right suprarenal location with internal debris and layering of contents (arrows). (**b**) Color Doppler shows no internal vascularity. (**c**) Follow-up US after 4 weeks shows a significant reduction in the size of the lesion (asterisk). (**d**) Follow-up US after 8 weeks shows complete resolution of the cystic adrenal lesion with residual calcification (markers) in the adrenal gland

necessitate glucocorticoid and possibly mineralocorticoid and androgen replacement therapies.

Adrenal calcifications: On the US, calcifications are usually seen as echogenic foci causing posterior acoustic shadowing (Fig. 8.6). However, small foci may not show shadowing. Although adrenal calcifications are relatively nonspecific and carry a wide range of differential diagnoses, a few calcific patterns, and associated abdominal findings may point towards a more specific diagnosis [11, 12]. As discussed, resolving adrenal hemorrhage shows punctate calcifications with normal-sized adrenal gland. Post-hemorrhagic pseudocysts show peripheral curvilinear calcific foci. Infrequently, disseminated viral infections, including neonatal herpes simplex and cytomegalovirus infections, can lead to adrenal calcifications [11]. A solid suprarenal mass showing calcific foci within is highly suggestive of a neuroblastoma. Wolman disease is a peculiar autosomal recessive enzyme deficiency disorder that shows dense calcifications with enlargement of bilateral adrenals. The presence of associated hepatosplenomegaly and enlarged abdominal lymph nodes due to lipid deposition in the presence of bilateral adrenal calcifications points towards this rare diagnosis [13].

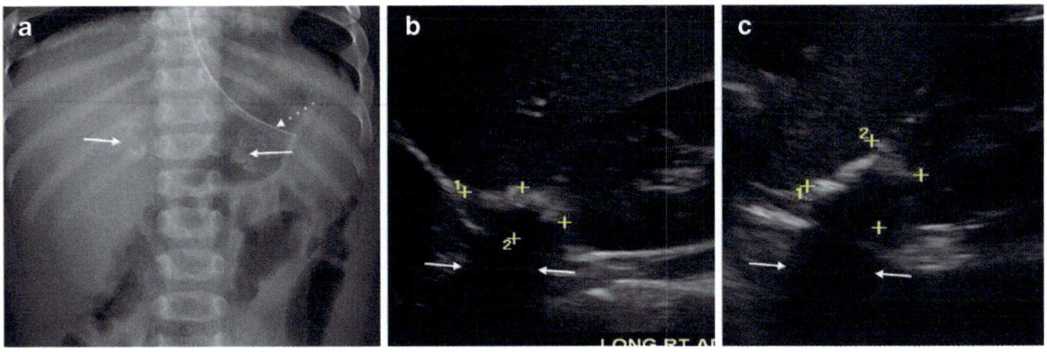

Fig. 8.6 Incidentally detected bilateral adrenal calcifications in a 1 month old infant. (**a**) The abdominal radiograph shows bilateral paravertebral calcifications (arrows). Note made of orogastric tube in situ (dotted arrow). (**b, c**) US images show echogenic calcifications (markers) in bilateral adrenal glands with posterior acoustic shadowing (arrows)

8.4.3 Congenital Adrenal Hyperplasia (CAH)

CAH, also referred to as adrenogenital syndrome, represents a group of autosomal recessive metabolic disorders characterized by a deficit in the enzymes necessary for the production of cortisol and aldosterone in the adrenal cortex. The predominant cause, accounting for 90–95% of cases, is a deficiency in 21-hydroxylase, attributed to a non-functional mutation in the CYP21A2 gene. Another, albeit rarer, cause is a deficiency in 11-β-hydroxylase [14]. The lack of adequate cortisol production triggers an excessive release of adrenocorticotropic hormone (ACTH) from the pituitary gland due to disrupted negative feedback mechanisms. This excess ACTH prompts the adrenal cortex to enlarge and produce more steroid precursors, which are then converted into androgens, leading to the masculinization of external genitalia.

Females with CAH, particularly those with a 21-hydroxylase deficiency, often exhibit ambiguous genitalia at birth, such as clitoral enlargement and fused labial folds, while males may experience early isosexual puberty. In girls, CAH is a leading cause of ambiguous genitalia [15]. Approximately 75% of these cases also exhibit reduced aldosterone synthesis, resulting in a severe salt-wasting crisis marked by low sodium levels, high potassium levels, and low blood pressure, typically manifesting within the first few weeks of life [14]. Early identification of CAH is crucial for appropriate gender assignment in girls with ambiguous genitalia and to avert the life-threatening salt-wasting crisis. Additionally, boys with CAH may develop testicular adrenal rest tumors due to prolonged ACTH stimulation, leading to the growth of adrenal-like tissue in the testes, which typically present as bilateral, small, and numerous growths [16].

US is preferred for evaluating suspected CAH in newborns and infants, with specific measurements of the adrenal gland indicating the condition. Features such as a limb length of 20 mm or more, a mean width of 4 mm or more, and normal differentiation between the cortex and medulla suggest CAH [17]. However, a normal size of the adrenal glands does not rule out CAH. On the other hand, a characteristic "cerebriform" appearance of adrenals with maintained corticomedullary differentiation is considered specific for CAH even with normal adrenal size. The "cerebriform" morphology refers to an abnormally lobulated and unfolded contour of the adrenals (much like the cerebral gyral folds) (Fig. 8.7). The stippled echogenic appearance of the adrenals is another US feature described in CAH [18].

US also facilitates the visualization of normal uterus and ovaries in females with ambiguous genitalia [18]. For testicular adrenal rest tumors, ultrasound reveals bilateral, multifocal masses within the testis, typically hypoechoic in com-

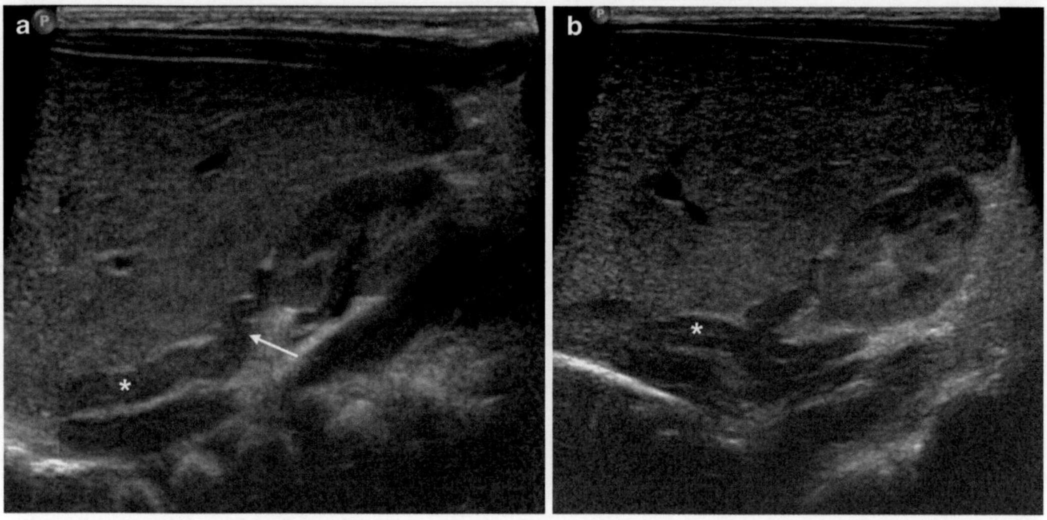

Fig. 8.7 Congenital adrenal hyperplasia in a female neonate presenting with ambiguous genitalia at birth. (**a**, **b**) US images show a diffusely enlarged adrenal gland (asterisk) with a typical lobulated "cerebriform appearance" (arrow)

parison to the surrounding testicular tissue. These masses are generally avascular or display reduced vascularization on color Doppler US [19].

Elevated serum levels of 17-hydroxy-progesterone confirm CAH, with differences in 11-deoxycortisol and deoxycorticosterone levels helping to distinguish between 11-β-hydroxylase and 21-hydroxylase deficiencies [15]. The treatment regimen for classical CAH involves glucocorticoid and mineralocorticoid replacement although it requires monitoring for long-term side effects like reduced bone density, early bone maturation, obesity, and fertility issues. Testicular adrenal rest tumors are benign and tend to stabilize or diminish with glucocorticoid treatment [16].

8.4.4 Neuroblastoma

Neuroblastoma is the most common extracranial solid malignancy of infancy [20]. These heterogeneous tumors originate from pluripotent neural crest cells, found in the neuronal ganglia within the peripheral nervous system. Congenital neuroblastoma accounts for 5% of cases of neuroblastomas. Within the context of congenital neuroblastoma, about 20% of cases are identified before birth in the antenatal US, and 16% are recognized within the first month of life [21]. Generally, infants under 12 months old diagnosed with neuroblastoma have a favorable outlook, with a 5-year survival rate estimated at 90% [22].

Most antenatal neuroblastomas are discovered incidentally on the US without any maternal or fetal signs of distress. The clinical presentation of neuroblastoma in neonates varies widely, as symptoms are influenced by the primary tumor's location and the presence of metastases. The most common sites for these tumors, in descending order of frequency, are the adrenal gland, paravertebral retroperitoneum, posterior mediastinum, neck, and pelvis [23]. In instances where congenital neuroblastoma is not detected before birth, the newborn may show no symptoms, potentially leading to a scenario where the tumor regresses spontaneously without ever being clinically identified. Since the adrenal gland is the most prevalent location for congenital neuroblastoma, 65% of affected neonates present with a unilateral retroperitoneal mass in the abdomen [21]. This can cause hypertension due to the compression of the renal artery, activating the renin-angiotensin-aldosterone system, or from catecholamine release by the tumor. Spinal cord compression by the tumor may rapidly lead to neurological emergencies, including permanent leg paralysis and loss of bowel or bladder control in neonates [23]. Additionally, these infants may exhibit pallor, rapid breathing, lethargy, and distinctive "blueberry muffin" skin nodules, indicative of neuroblastoma metastases to the skin. Interestingly, the characteristic paraneoplastic opsoclonus-myoclonus syndrome associated with neuroblastomas does not occur below one year of age due to the time required for the antibody formation responsible for these symptoms [23].

US is the initial modality of choice for the work-up of neonates with suspected neuroblastoma [23]. Of the antenatally detected neuroblastomas, about 75% are localized to the adrenal glands, more commonly in the right adrenal gland [22]. These adrenal neuroblastomas display diverse ultrasonographic morphologies, including solid masses, hypoechoic cystic masses, and cystic masses with mixed echogenicity [21]. Neuroblastoma characteristically displaces the ipsilateral kidney inferiorly without invading it, affecting the positioning of the aorta and the inferior vena cava. The sonographic characteristics of neuroblastomas vary, including increased echogenicity, necrosis, hemorrhage, and occasionally calcifications [24] (Fig. 8.8). Doppler imaging techniques, such as power and color Doppler, are pivotal for assessing blood flow and are particularly sensitive to detecting flow. Neuroblastomas most often encase, rather than invade the adjacent blood vessels. Nonetheless, it is important to look for the presence of vascular invasion in cases of neuroblastoma and Doppler US can aid in differentiating between bland and tumor thrombi and enhancing the detection of vascular invasion and liver metastases [25]. Doppler has also proven useful for the accurate detection and monitoring of tumor characteristics and hemodynamic activity, significantly improving the accuracy of prenatal and postnatal diagnosis of neuroblastoma [25, 26].

Cystic neuroblastoma: A unique pathological neuroblastoma variant identified during the perinatal period is distinguished by the presence of one or several cysts, either macroscopic or microscopic, within the tumor (Fig. 8.9). It is believed to either represent a precursor to neuroblastoma or develop from the bleeding and necrosis within a pre-existing tumor [20]. Several studies suggest that this form of neuroblastoma is generally nonmalignant and may decrease on its own, similar to other types of neuroblastoma found in newborns. The spontaneous regression of cystic neuroblastomas has a reported incidence of 2% [27]. Clinically, cystic neuroblastoma is noteworthy for being detectable before birth, having a lower likelihood of metastasis, and exhibiting reduced levels of tumor markers [28]. US plays a critical role in identifying and assessing these tumors,

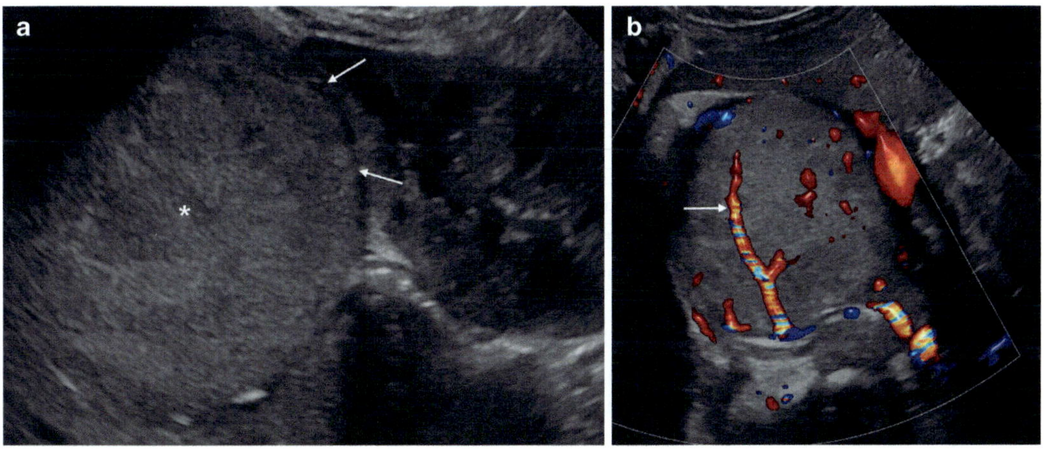

Fig. 8.8 Right adrenal neuroblastoma in a 4-week-old neonate. (**a**) The grayscale US image shows a well-defined homogeneous hyperechoic mass lesion (asterisk) in the right suprarenal location causing displacement and slight buckling of the right kidney (arrows). (**b**) Color Doppler image shows internal vascularity within the mass (arrow)

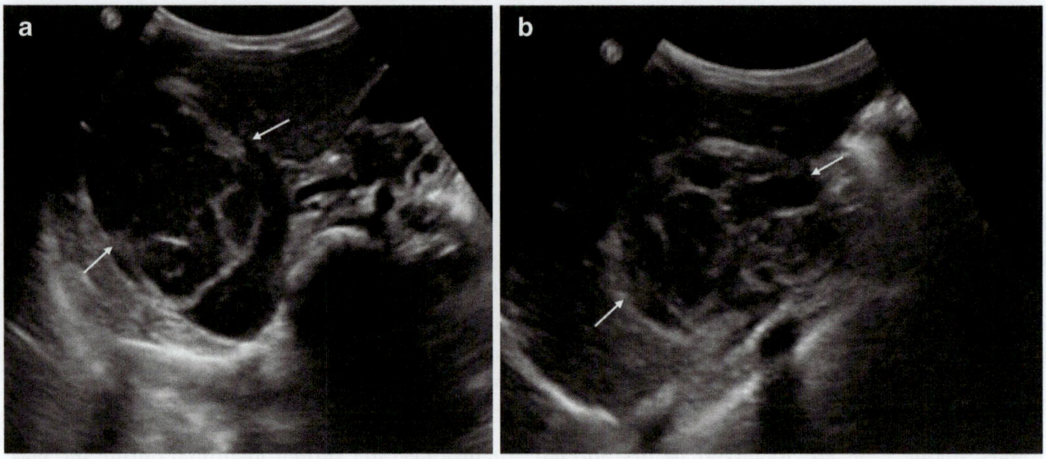

Fig. 8.9 Surgically proven case of cystic neuroblastoma in a 6-week-old infant. Transverse (**a**) and longitudinal (**b**) US images show a well-defined predominantly cystic right suprarenal mass (arrows) with a thick wall and multiple internal septations (Image courtesy: Dr. Ishan Kumar, Banaras Hindu University, Varanasi)

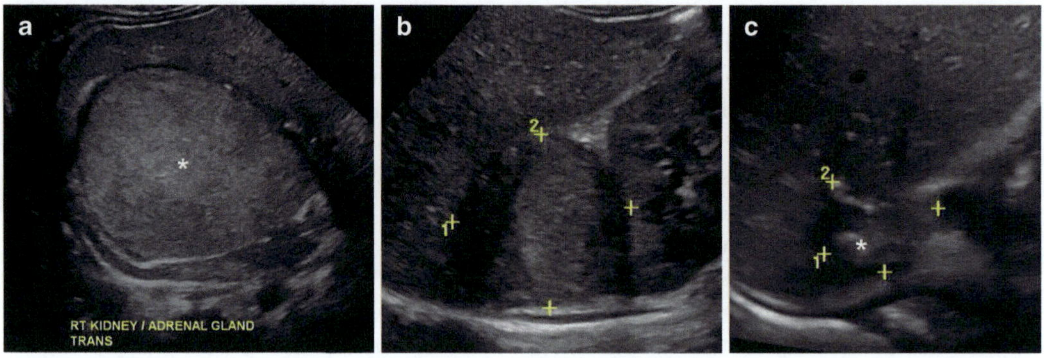

Fig. 8.10 Post-chemotherapy resolution of neuroblastoma on follow-up (same patient as in Fig. 8.8). (**a**) The initial US shows a large hyperechoic mass (asterisk) in the right suprarenal location. (**b**) A follow-up US shows a significant reduction in the size of the mass (markers). (**c**) A later follow-up US shows almost complete resolution of the mass with few echogenic calcifications (asterisk)

particularly in distinguishing cystic changes in congenital adrenal neuroblastoma, and has shown to be more effective than CT scans in this capacity. It has been suggested that a thorough ultrasound examination is often adequate for determining the disease extent in individuals with cystic congenital adrenal neuroblastoma, pointing out the limited additional diagnostic benefit of CT and MRI [28]. Thus, it is recommended that US be the primary method for initial and subsequent evaluations of this rare neuroblastoma variant. Furthermore, testing for urinary catecholamine levels and MIBG scintigraphy shows a low success rate in detecting cystic congenital adrenal neuroblastoma, underscoring the significance of US in its diagnosis. US is also useful for follow-up of infants who are on chemotherapy for neuroblastoma (Fig. 8.10).

Cystic neuroblastoma versus adrenal hemorrhage: Adrenal hemorrhage with cystic transformation is a primary differential for these cases. Perinatal adrenal hemorrhage frequently happens in the presence of risk factors like bleeding tendency and sepsis, but it may also manifest without any known predisposing conditions. Distinguishing between the two categories of neonatal adrenal cystic lesions often presents a challenge. Additionally, perinatal neuroblastomas may also develop components of bleeding, and often show normal urinary catecholamine metabolite levels, further complicating the differentiation process [28].

Although prenatally detected adrenal cysts favor neuroblastoma, the possibility of adrenal hemorrhage cannot be ruled out [29]. The sonographic appearance of adrenal hemorrhage changes over time and may liquefy within several days. At this stage, differentiation from cystic neuroblastoma is extremely difficult. Over time, serial sonographic monitoring typically shows adrenal hemorrhages decreasing in size, eventually disappearing or turning into small calcifications. However, the literature reports that regression in size of congenital neuroblastoma is also not an uncommon phenomenon [27]. However, cystic neuroblastomas tend to evolve into more complex solid and cystic structures, indicating a decrease in cystic components and an increase in solid tissue on follow-up US [29]. This suggests a distinct progression pattern for cystic neuroblastomas. Considering this, it has been suggested that neuroblastoma should be suspected if an adrenal mass does not resolve within 3 months, with the median resolution time for hemorrhages being 90 days [29]. While calcifications may emerge later in hemorrhages, their presence in the neonatal period is rare, making calcifications at initial diagnosis more indicative of neuroblastomas. Color Doppler US showing vascularization within neuroblastoma highlights its well-perfused capsule, aiding in differentiating it from adrenal hemorrhages [25]. The presence of hemorrhagic areas within the mass is not particularly helpful for the differentiation between neonatal adrenal cystic masses as neuroblastomas have also been noted to have areas of bleeding. Although hepatic metastasis strongly points to neuroblastoma, they are rarely observed in the neonatal age group. In summary, while congenital cystic neuroblastomas and adrenal hemorrhages exhibit many overlapping imaging characteristics, factors such as prenatal detection, initial calcification, vascularity on color Doppler US, and evolution into a more complex mass within 90 days, tend to support a diagnosis of neuroblastoma over hemorrhage. Hence, serial US follow-up is essential to differentiate between cystic congenital adrenal neuroblastoma and adrenal hemorrhage when opting for a watchful waiting approach to managing a suprarenal cystic lesion in newborns. Biopsy of a suprarenal mass in a neonate is usually deferred as it is an invasive technically challenging procedure and also because congenital neuroblastomas are associated with an excellent prognosis without any surgical intervention and a high rate of spontaneous resolution [29].

The features useful for differentiation between neuroblastoma and adrenal hemorrhage in a neonate are summarized in Table 8.2.

Other primary adrenal neoplasms like pheochromocytoma, adrenocortical carcinoma, and adrenal teratoma are more common in young children of adolescent age; but can rarely present in infancy [30] (Fig. 8.11).

8.4.5 Adrenal Lesion Mimics

Extralobar sequestration: Pulmonary sequestration refers to a type of bronchopulmonary foregut malformation that contains non-functioning lung tissue with no communication with the bronchial tree [31]. Although sequestrations mostly occur in the left lower lobe of the lungs, they can be present in a subdiaphragmatic location (around 8–10% of cases), typically on the left [32]. Most subdiaphragmatic sequestrations are extralobar with an anomalous systemic arterial supply and systemic venous drainage. On the US, the subdiaphragmatic sequestration is seen as a heterogeneous echogenic mass, usually pyramidal in shape in the left suprarenal location. Color Doppler is highly useful to demonstrate the anomalous feeding artery arising from the aorta or its branches like the celiac and superior mesenteric artery (Fig. 8.12). Normal adrenal gland may be visualized separately from the suprarenal mass, and this finding should raise a possibility for a non-adrenal lesion [32]. Surgical resection is the treatment of choice for subdiaphragmatic pulmonary sequestration with an excellent prognosis in the absence of other associated congenital anomalies like diaphragmatic hernia, vertebral, or cardiac malformations [32].

Table 8.2 Differential diagnosis between cystic neuroblastoma and adrenal hemorrhage in neonates

Feature	Cystic neuroblastoma	Adrenal hemorrhage	Significance for differential diagnosis
Risk factors for adrenal hemorrhage	Absent	Frequent	++
Elevated urine catecholamine levels	Infrequent	Absent	–
Prenatal detection	More common	Uncommon	+
Change in size on follow-up US	Remains stable or size increases. But, can show a decrease in size	Typically show a decrease in size, gradually disappearing (median resolution time: 90 days)	++
Changes in morphology on follow-up US	Becomes more heterogeneous with solid components (even if decrease in size due to resorption of cystic areas)	Develops more cystic component ± residual calcifications	+++
Calcifications	More common at initial diagnosis	Develop later with the resolution of the mass	++
Doppler findings	Vascularity present	No vascularity	+
Hepatic metastases on the US	Strongly favor the diagnosis; however occurs rarely	Absent	+++ (if present)

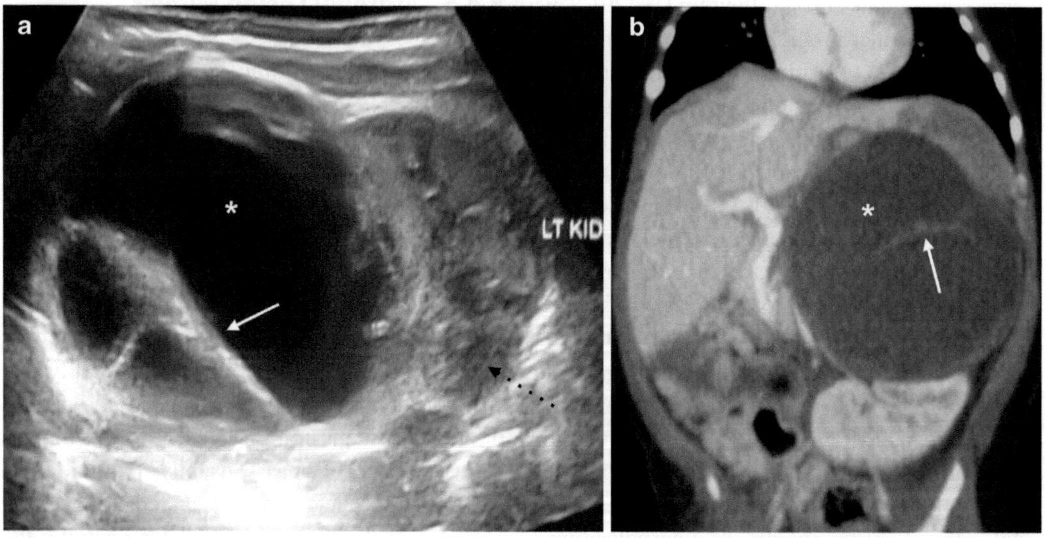

Fig. 8.11 Surgically proven case of left adrenal teratoma in a 2 month-old infant. (**a**) US image shows a large predominantly cystic left suprarenal lesion (asterisk) with a thick echogenic wall and internal septations (arrow), causing inferior displacement of the left kidney (dotted arrow). (**b**) Coronal contrast-enhanced CT abdomen image shows the lesion to be predominantly hypodense (asterisk) with enhancing internal septations (arrow). A large chronic adrenal hematoma remains a differential on imaging

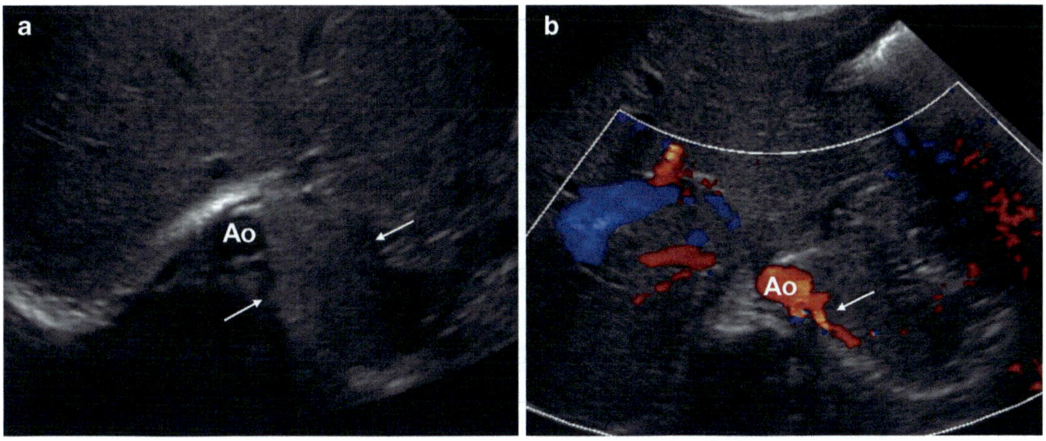

Fig. 8.12 Antenatally diagnosed infra-diaphragmatic extralobar sequestration. (**a**) The transverse US view shows an echogenic lesion (arrows) in the left paravertebral location. (**b**) Color Doppler image shows an anomalous artery (arrow) arising from the aorta feeding the left paravertebral sequestration. *Ao* Aorta

8.5 Neonatal Thromboembolism Involving Major Retroperitoneal Vessels

Neonatal vascular (venous or arterial) thromboses are uncommon pathology occurring in 0.2% of newborns admitted to the neonatal intensive care unit [33]. Neonatal thromboembolism (TE) shows remarkable variability, significantly influenced by the thrombus's size and location. Risk factors for neonatal TE encompass maternal diabetes or lupus, delayed rupture of membranes, polycythemia, dehydration, asphyxia, patent ductus arteriosus, and coagulation disorders [34]. The preferred diagnostic tool for neonatal arterial or venous thrombosis is Doppler ultrasound, which can identify the absence of flow in cases of complete occlusion and reduced flow in partial occlusion. Additionally, abnormal arterial waveforms can indicate partial or complete arterial blockages, even when the thrombus itself isn't visible, with echocardiography or abdominal ultrasound also being utilized to either confirm TE suspicion or screen for asymptomatic cases [33].

Inferior vena cava syndrome (IVCS): IVCS occurs when the IVC is blocked due to tumor growth, compression, or lumen thrombosis, leading to reduced blood flow back to the heart. This can present with tachycardia, peripheral edema, and renal failure. While thrombosis of the IVC is the primary cause of IVCS, not every instance of IVC thrombosis develops into full-blown IVCS [35]. In newborns, thrombosis is the leading cause of IVC obstruction occurring in 98% of the cases and the overall mortality rate is 23% [35]. Grayscale US is the method most commonly used for diagnosing and precisely evaluating IVC obstruction. It is important to note that newly formed clots may not be easily visible on US, whereas color Doppler imaging provides a clearer visualization of the clot's location, extent of blockage, and blood flow beyond the site of the clot (Fig. 8.13 a, b). However, this finding contrasts with results from various studies in both children and adults, which have definitively shown that US is not an effective technique for detecting IVC thrombosis [36].

Aortic thrombosis: Symptomatic aortic thrombosis in neonates is particularly severe and occurs at a rate of 0.1–1.1 in every 100,000 newborns [33]. The symptoms of aortic thrombosis in this age group can vary widely, from general irritability to severe complications like acute ischemia threatening limb viability, poor blood flow to the intestines, and kidney failure. Up to 80% of these cases are linked to the use of umbilical artery catheters

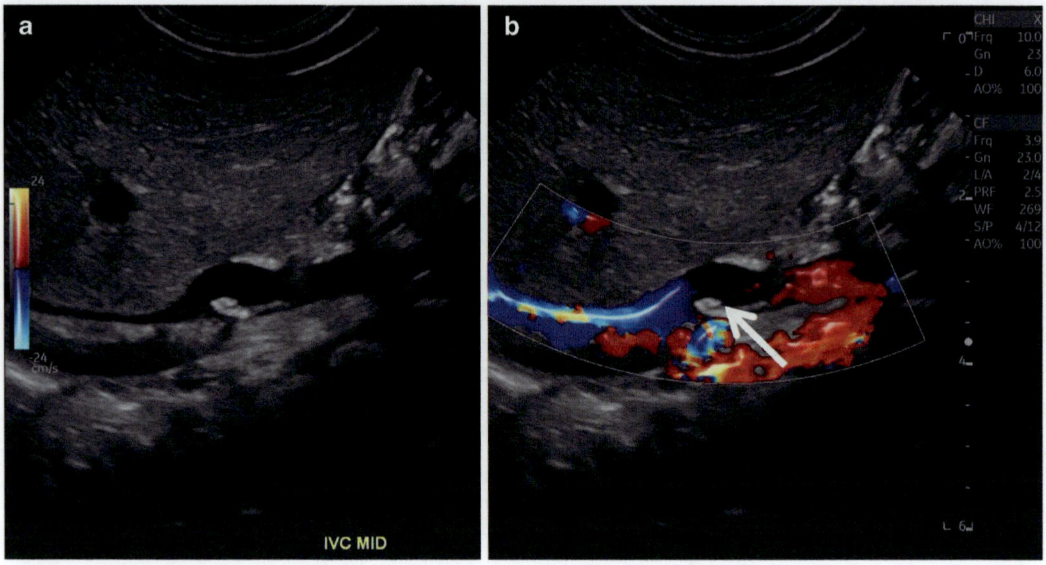

Fig. 8.13 Sagittal ultrasound of abdomen in a neonate with grayscale (**a**) and color Doppler image (**b**) showing a thrombus (white arrow) in the mid part of inferior vena cava (Image courtesy: Dr. Prakash M Masand, Texas Children's Hospital, Houston, Texas)

(UAC) although sepsis, being born extremely premature, and conditions that predispose to clot formation also pose significant risks [37, 38]. Previous research on the prevalence of aortic thrombus linked to UAC underscores the importance of US as a primary method for examining the neonatal abdominal aorta [33]. US enables a comprehensive and precise assessment of the aortic anatomy, aiding in the detection and diagnosis of thrombus and foreign objects. The US appearance of a thrombus can vary from being isoechoic as surrounding tissues to hypoechoic or more echogenic (Fig. 8.14), partially depending on whether the condition is acute or chronic.

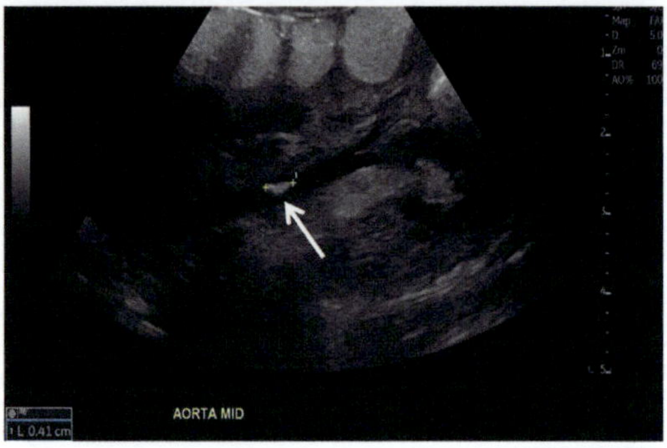

Fig. 8.14 Sagittal ultrasound of abdomen in a neonate with grayscale image showing an echogenic calcific thrombus (white arrow) in the mid part of abdominal aorta (Image courtesy: Dr. Prakash M Masand, Texas Children's Hospital, Houston, Texas)

8.6 Primary Retroperitoneal Masses

Retroperitoneal teratoma is an extremely rare tumor reported in neonates and infants. Both the indolent mature and rapidly enlarging immature teratomas have been seen in this location [39]. Typical radiological features of mature teratomas as in other locations of the body include the presence of cystic components along with calcifications, teeth, and fat within the mass (Fig. 8.15). Immature teratomas, on the other hand, show enhancing heterogeneous soft-tissue components and are difficult to differentiate from retroperitoneal neurogenic tumors and yolk sac tumors.

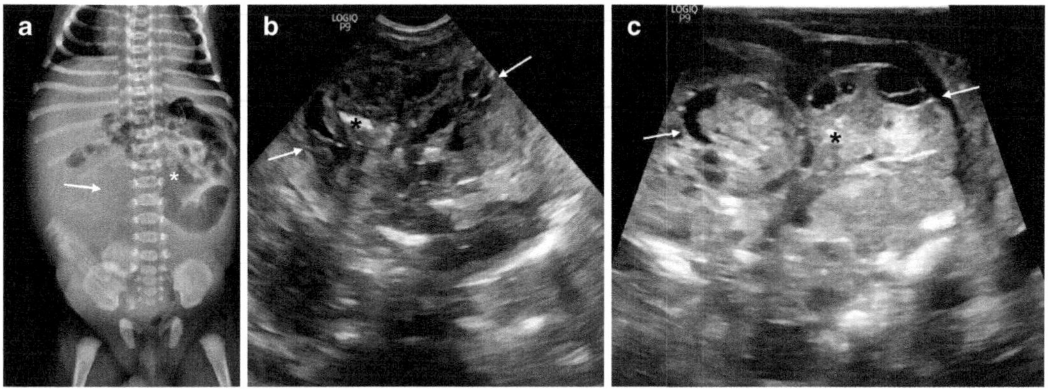

Fig. 8.15 Antenatally diagnosed retroperitoneal teratoma. (**a**) The abdominal radiograph shows bowel loops (asterisk) displaced to the left with the presence of calcific foci (arrow) on the right side of the abdomen. (**b**, **c**) US images show the presence of a heterogeneous mass (arrows) with both cystic and solid areas along with areas of calcifications (asterisks) (Image Courtesy: Dr Kanimozhi Vendhan, Kanchi Kamakoti CHILDS Trust Hospital, Chennai)

8.7 Conclusion

US is a useful modality for adrenal gland assessment in neonates and neonates presenting with a palpable abdominal mass. US can help in narrowing down the differential diagnoses of suprarenal neonatal masses; however, correlation with biochemical findings and other cross-sectional imaging is usually required to reach the correct diagnosis.

References

1. Aderotimi TS, Kraft JK. Ultrasound of the adrenal gland in children. Ultrasound Leeds Engl. 2021;29(1):48–56.
2. Sargar KM, Khanna G, Hulett Bowling R. Imaging of nonmalignant adrenal lesions in children. Radiogr Rev Publ Radiol Soc N Am Inc. 2017;37(6):1648–64.
3. Bittman ME, Lee EY, Restrepo R, Eisenberg RL. Focal adrenal lesions in pediatric patients. AJR Am J Roentgenol. 2013;200(6):W542–56.
4. Butler P. Applied radiological anatomy. Cambridge University Press; 1999. 458 p
5. van Vuuren SH, Damen-Elias HAM, Stigter RH, van der Doef R, Goldschmeding R, de Jong TPVM, et al. Size and volume charts of fetal kidney, renal pelvis and adrenal gland. Ultrasound Obstet Gynecol Off J Int Soc. 2012;40(6):659–64.
6. Barwick TD, Malhotra A, Webb JAW, Savage MO, Reznek RH. Embryology of the adrenal glands and its relevance to diagnostic imaging. Clin Radiol. 2005;60(9):953–9.
7. Ditkofsky N, Bradley N, Jeon P. Horseshoe adrenal gland: a rare congenital anomaly. Surg Radiol Anat. 2013;35(8):749–54.
8. Strouse PJ, Haller JO, Berdon WE, Rosovsky MA, Bellah RD, Barr M. Horseshoe adrenal gland in association with asplenia: presentation of six new cases and review of the literature. Pediatr Radiol. 2002;32(11):778–82.
9. Kawashima A, Sandler CM, Ernst RD, Takahashi N, Roubidoux MA, Goldman SM, et al. Imaging of nontraumatic hemorrhage of the adrenal gland. Radiogr Rev Publ Radiol Soc N Am Inc. 1999;19(4): 949–63.
10. Deeg KH, Bettendorf U, Hofmann V. Differential diagnosis of neonatal adrenal haemorrhage and congenital neuroblastoma by colour coded Doppler sonography and power Doppler sonography. Eur J Pediatr. 1998;157(4):294–7.
11. Paterson A. Adrenal pathology in childhood: a spectrum of disease. Eur Radiol. 2002;12(10):2491–508.
12. Elsayes KM, Emad-Eldin S, Morani AC, Jensen CT. Practical approach to adrenal imaging. Radiol Clin North Am. 2017;55(2):279–301.
13. Fulcher AS, Das Narla L, Hingsbergen EA. Pediatric case of the day. Wolman disease (primary familial xanthomatosis with involvement and classification of the adrenal glands). Radiogr Rev Publ Radiol Soc N Am Inc. 1998;18(2):533–5.
14. Chung EM, Biko DM, Schroeder JW, Cube R, Conran RM. From the radiologic pathology archives: precocious puberty: radiologic-pathologic correlation. Radiogr Rev Publ Radiol Soc N Am Inc. 2012;32(7):2071–99.
15. Lambert SM, Vilain EJN, Kolon TF. A practical approach to ambiguous genitalia in the newborn period. Urol Clin North Am. 2010;37(2):195–205.
16. Chavhan GB, Parra DA, Oudjhane K, Miller SF, Babyn PS, Pippi Salle FL. Imaging of ambiguous genitalia:

classification and diagnostic approach. Radiogr Rev Publ Radiol Soc N Am Inc. 2008;28(7):1891–904.
17. Hernanz-Schulman M, Brock JW, Russell W. Sonographic findings in infants with congenital adrenal hyperplasia. Pediatr Radiol. 2002;32(2):130–7.
18. Al-Alwan I, Navarro O, Daneman D, Daneman A. Clinical utility of adrenal ultrasonography in the diagnosis of congenital adrenal hyperplasia. J Pediatr. 1999;135(1):71–5.
19. Stikkelbroeck NMML, Suliman HM, Otten BJ, Hermus ARMM, Blickman JG, Jager GJ. Testicular adrenal rest tumours in postpubertal males with congenital adrenal hyperplasia: sonographic and MR features. Eur Radiol. 2003;13(7):1597–603.
20. Chen CP, Chen SH, Chuang CY, Lee HC, Hwu YM, Chang PY, et al. Clinical and perinatal sonographic features of congenital adrenal cystic neuroblastoma: a case report with review of the literature. Ultrasound Obstet Gynecol Off J Int Soc Ultrasound Obstet Gynecol. 1997;10(1):68–73.
21. Nuchtern JG. Perinatal neuroblastoma. Semin Pediatr Surg. 2006;15(1):10–6.
22. Isaacs H. Fetal and neonatal neuroblastoma: retrospective review of 271 cases. Fetal Pediatr Pathol. 2007;26(4):177–84.
23. Fisher JPH, Tweddle DA. Neonatal neuroblastoma. Semin Fetal Neonatal Med. 2012;17(4):207–15.
24. McCarville MB. New frontiers in pediatric oncologic imaging. Cancer Imaging Off Publ Int Cancer Imaging Soc. 2008;8(1):87–92.
25. Baun J, Garcia K. Prenatal diagnosis of neuroblastomacolor Doppler imaging may increase accuracy. J Diagn Med Sonogr. 2004;20:134–7.
26. Mehta SV, Lim-Dunham JE. Ultrasonographic appearance of pediatric abdominal neuroblastoma with inferior vena cava extension. J Ultrasound Med Off J Am Inst Ultrasound Med. 2003;22(10):1091–5.
27. Yamamoto K, Hanada R, Kikuchi A, Ichikawa M, Aihara T, Oguma E, et al. Spontaneous regression of localized neuroblastoma detected by mass screening. J Clin Oncol Off J Am Soc Clin Oncol. 1998;16(4):1265–9.
28. Hwang SM, Yoo SY, Kim JH, Jeon TY. Congenital adrenal neuroblastoma with and without cystic change: differentiating features with an emphasis on the of value of ultrasound. AJR Am J Roentgenol. 2016;207(5):1105–11.
29. Eo H, Kim JH, Jang KM, Yoo SY, Lim GY, Kim MJ, et al. Comparison of clinico-radiological features between congenital cystic neuroblastoma and neonatal adrenal hemorrhagic pseudocyst. Korean J Radiol. 2011;12(1):52–8.
30. Malhotra S, Waikar AR, Singh P, Guarini L, Jacobson-Dickman E, Motaghedi R, et al. Rare presentation of adrenocortical carcinoma in a 4-month-old boy. World J Oncol. 2017;8(3):81–5.
31. Corbett HJ, Humphrey GME. Pulmonary sequestration. Paediatr Respir Rev. 2004;5(1):59–68.
32. Pumberger W, Moroder W, Wiesbauer P. Intraabdominal extralobar pulmonary sequestration exhibiting cystic adenomatoid malformation: prenatal diagnosis and characterization of a left suprarenal mass in the newborn. Abdom Imaging. 2001;26(1):28–31.
33. Imad N, El Idrissi SN, Alaoui S, Zalle I, Boumzebra D, Bennaoui F, et al. Thrombosis of the abdominal aorta in newborn: about two cases. J Neonatal-Perinat Med. 2022;15(1):187–93.
34. Aslam M, Guglietti D, Hansen AR. Neonatal arterial thrombosis at birth: case report and literature review. Am J Perinatol. 2008;25(6):347–52.
35. Tieu P, Paes B, Ahmed A, Matino D, Chan A, Bhatt M. Inferior vena cava syndrome in neonates: an evidence-based systematic review of the literature. Pediatr Blood Cancer. 2020;67(4):e28114.
36. McAree BJ, O'Donnell ME, Fitzmaurice GJ, Reid JA, Spence RAJ, Lee B. Inferior vena cava thrombosis: a review of current practice. Vasc Med Lond Engl. 2013;18(1):32–43.
37. Langan M. Neonatal abdominal aortic thrombus: an associated risk of umbilical artery catheterization. J Diagn Med Sonogr. 2015;31(5):322–6. https://doi.org/10.1177/8756479315598864.
38. Nagel K, Tuckuviene R, Paes B, Chan AK. Neonatal aortic thrombosis: a comprehensive review. Klin Padiatr. 2010;222(3):134–9.
39. Kumar C, Sisodiya RS, Panda SS, Sarin YK. Retroperitoneal immature teratoma in a neonate. J Neonatal Surg. 2017;6(2):42.

Neonatal Urinary Tract

9

Joanna Kasznia-Brown, Kanimozhi Vendhan,
Tejas Kapadia, and Anmol Bhatia

9.1 Introduction

9.1.1 Ultrasound of the Renal Tract

Ultrasound is the main imaging modality in assessment of the urinary system in children and adults, including kidneys, ureters, urinary bladder, and urethra [1, 2].

Ultrasound is often performed on premature and low weight babies (LBW) as portable examination in the Neonatal Intensive Care Units, with lower quality machines and suboptimal scanning surroundings. Using an appropriate probes and appropriate machine settings is vital when performing neonatal ultrasound study. Optimisation of the paediatric pre-sets on the machines is necessary, especially in a general ultrasound department, where scanning equipment is shared with adult patients. Linear high frequency probe (9 MHz or higher) is recommended in neonates to achieve the best quality and results (Fig. 9.1). In older children, a 6 MHz curvilinear probe will be used for an initial assessment, when the linear probe being reserved for more focused views [3].

Urinary bladder should be examined first in the assessment of the neonatal urinary tract. Newborn may micturate after placement of the probe on the abdomen and important information could be lost. Several components of bladder assessments need to be remembered: thickness and appearance of the bladder wall, bladder volume and its contents, vesicoureteric junctions (VUJs), and distal part of ureters, as well as other structures located in the pelvis.

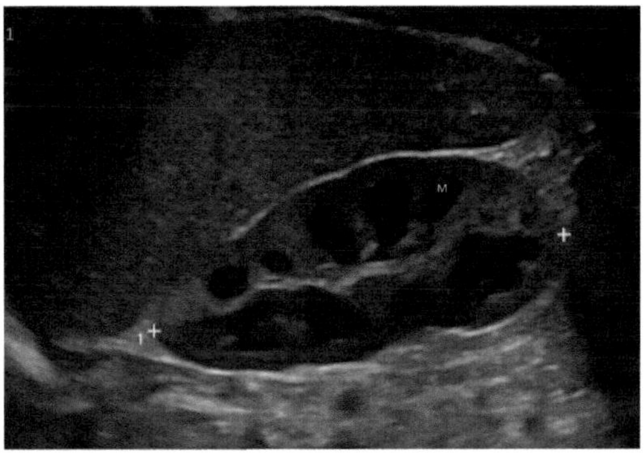

Fig. 9.1 Normal renal appearance in newborn : Coronal view of left kidney shows normal cortex and medulla (M)

J. Kasznia-Brown (✉)
Department of Radiology, Musgrove Park Hospital, University of Bristol, Bristol, UK
e-mail: joanna_kasznia-brown@rcr.ac.uk

K. Vendhan
Department of Paediatric Radiology, Kanchi Kamakoti CHILDS Trust Hospital, Chennai, Tamil Nadu, India

T. Kapadia
Royal Manchester Children's Hospital, Manchester University Hospitals NHS Foundation Trust, North West School of Radiology, Manchester, UK

A. Bhatia
Department of Radiodiagnosis and Imaging, Post Graduate Institute of Medical Education and Research, Chandigarh, India
e-mail: anmol_bhatia26@yahoo.co.in

K. S. Sodhi (ed.), *Neonatal Ultrasound*, https://doi.org/10.1007/978-981-97-8576-6_9

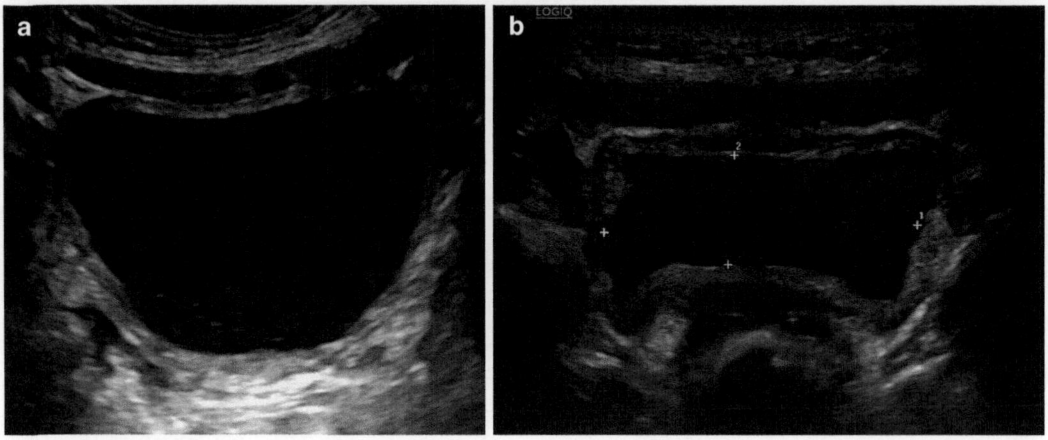

Fig. 9.2 Urinary bladder in neonate. Subtle internal echoes within the bladder lumen are commonly seen in newborns, secondary to dehydration. Various thickness of the bladder wall in relation to the bladder distention/volume. (**a**) Moderate bladder distention, with an impression of mild wall thickening and subtle internal echoes. (**b**) Diffuse bladder wall thickening due to poor bladder distention

Bladder wall thickness can only be accurately assessed, with a well-distended lumen (Fig. 9.2a, b). If bladder distension is suboptimal, obtained images and measurements need to be carefully evaluated to avoid a misinterpretation and false results. Often, an ultrasound study needs to be repeated to assure the right assessment, as there is a proven linear relationship between the bladder wall thickness and its distension [4]. The bladder wall thickness should be <3 mm in a well-filled bladder and <5 mm in an under-filled bladder. Wall thickness should be measured away from the trigone, as muscle layer increases the wall thickness in this region.

Normal urine should be anechoic in adult patients, but in neonates it can contain internal echoes. This feature is commonly seen in dehydrated babies and completely resolves with an adequate hydration. It is often related to transient dehydration after birth and corresponds to normal physiological finding (Fig. 9.2).

Kidneys can be scanned in the supine or prone position, depending on operator choice and general condition of the baby. Ultrasound should confirm normal anatomical position and structure of kidneys; assess the size, outline, corticomedullary differentiation, pelvicalyceal system, and renal vessels (Fig. 9.1)

9.1.2 Neonatal Kidneys - Anatomy

9.1.2.1 Renal Structure

1. The kidneys are formed in utero from several separate distinct lobules, which fuse during development. The fusion may not be complete and may result in the smooth indentations within the renal outline, visible between the medullary pyramids. Foetal lobulation of the kidneys can be very prominent in the infancy and could also persist into the teenage or adult age (Fig. 9.3) [5]. Focal lobulations shouldn't be confused with focal scarring, which is usually more irregular and triangular. An indentation within an outline due to focal scaring is usually located over the renal pyramids while an indentation due to foetal lobulation is visible between the medullary pyramids.
2. Renal cortex is thinner in newborns than in older children, with a ratio of cortex to medulla in neonates of 1.64:1 (compared to adults of 2.59:1). Therefore, renal pyramids often appear dilated and hypoechoic on ultrasound, which could be easily mistaken by inexperienced operator for hydronephrosis or cystic changes [6].

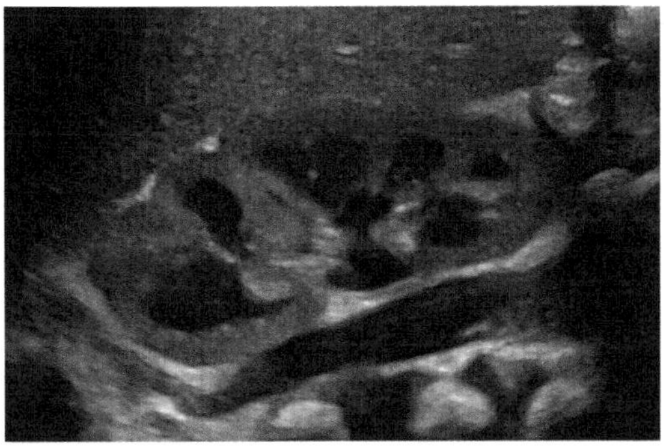

Fig. 9.3 Normal appearance of neonatal kidneys with persistent foetal lobulation. Renal outline is lobulated with small indentations over the pyramids

3. Structure of the renal cortex is also different in newborns. It contains the higher number and volume of glomeruli during the first 2 months of life (18% as compared with 8.6% in the adults) [7]. The neonatal renal cortex is similar or of increased echogenicity in comparison to hepatic parenchyma. This is a unique feature for newborns (renal parenchyma is of lower echogenicity than liver in older children and adults) and shouldn't be mistaken for pathology [8]. The kidneys become hypoechoic to the liver around 4 months of life. Increased echogenicity is usually more prominent in the preterm and low weight babies.
4. An increased cortical echogenicity and hypoechoic pyramids amplify the appearance of corticomedullary differentiation. Increased corticomedullary differentiation is often seen in older patients with hydronephrosis but remains a normal physiological finding in neonates [3, 9]. A hyperechoic focus at the tip of the papillae is also physiological in this group and helps to differentiate the medullary pyramids from dilated calyces.
5. An increased hyperechogenicity of renal medulla (Figs. 9.4 and 9.5) is commonly seen in neonates with severe perinatal renal injury, kidney malformations, nephrocalcinosis, and renal failure. However, this appearance has also been described as a transient finding in term and preterm babies without any abnormalities and with normal renal function. It is likely caused by stasis nephropathy (Tamm-Horsfall nephropathy) and needs to be interpreted as normal variation in this age group, possibly related to dehydration [10].
6. Lack of echogenicity within the renal sinus represents another anatomical difference. This reflects an absence of adipose tissue with the neonatal renal sinus [9]. Echogenicity of renal sinus becomes more prominent with age and increase in body fat deposition.

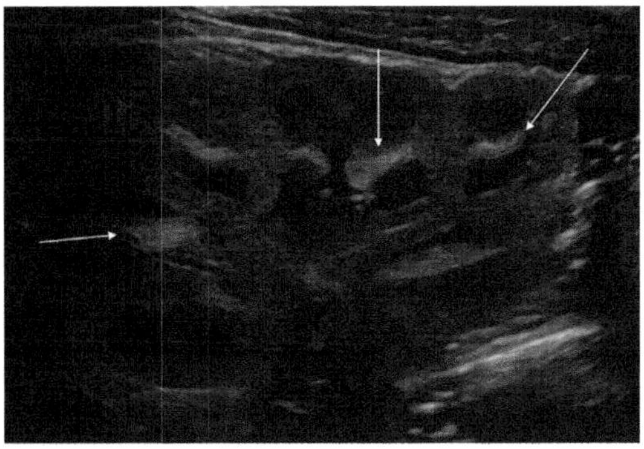

Fig. 9.4 Transient hyperechogenicty of the renal medulla. Ultrasound images show an increased echogenocity within medulla (arrows). This corresponds to a normal variant for patients age, often associated with dehydration

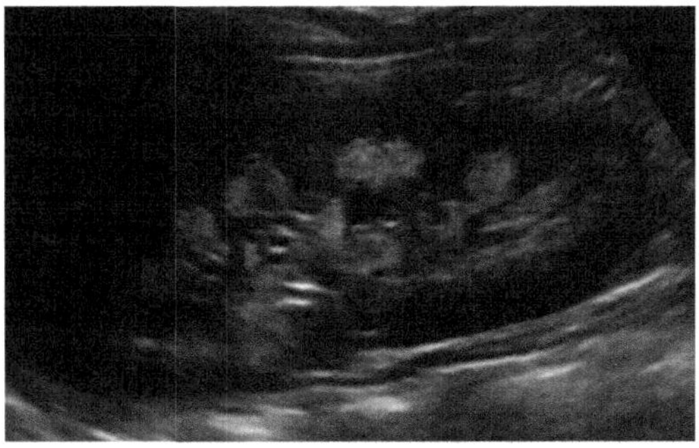

Fig. 9.5 Medullary nephrocalcinosis. Ultrasound showing an increased echogenicity within the medulla in a 4 week old newborn

Table 9.1 Renal length in neonates according to gestational age [12]

Gestational age	Right renal length in cm with 1 SD	Range of right renal length (Min–Max)	Left Renal length in cm with 1 SD	Range of left renal length (Min–Max)
Term (38–41 wk.)	4.13 (0.33)	3.0–5.0	4.10 (0.40)	2.6–5.2
36–37 wk.	4.09 (0.35)	3.0–4.9	4.02 (0.35)	3.0–4.65
32–35 wk.	3.67 (0.42)	2.9–4.6	3.59 (0.40)	2.50–4.2
24–31 wk.	3.30 (0.38)	2.5–4.0	3.27 (0.34)	2.5–4.0

9.1.2.2 Renal Size

A correct evaluation of kidney size is very important for clinical diagnosis and treatment, especially in neonates. Renal length and parenchymal thickness seem to be most useful parameters in evaluation of the renal growth in individual babies [6, 11]. Normal renal size at birth in a term neonate is 4.1 cm (±0.8 cm for 2 standard deviations) (Table 9.1) [12]. Ethnic differences have also been shown, which could be an important consideration when correlating and interpreting measurements against a known reference range [13].

Renal length and its growth are commonly monitored using growth charts which provide the range within two standard deviations. These growth curves are also available online.

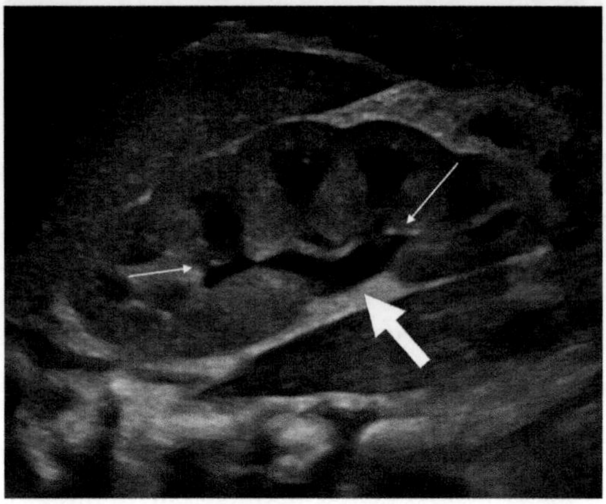

Fig. 9.6 Mild hydronephrosis of the right kidney. Mild dilatation of central aspect of renal pelvis (thick arrow), no calyceal dilatation (thin arrows)

9.2 Post-Natal Hydronephrosis

All newborns with diagnosis of prenatal hydronephrosis should have a postnatal ultrasound examination of the renal system [14]. It is recommended to delay the scan until fourth day after birth. The relative dehydration and decreased glomerular filtration rate, which are present after birth, may give the false-negative results or underestimate a degree of hydronephrosis [15]. However, an ultrasound should be performed earlier in cases of bilateral or severe hydronephrosis, in a solitary kidney or if posterior urethral valves are clinically suspected [15–17].

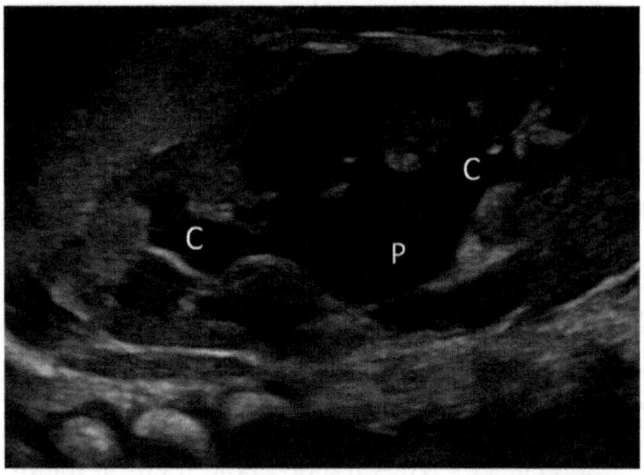

Fig. 9.7 Moderate hydronephrosis of the right kidney with dilated renal pelvis (P) and calyces (C)

All grades of persistent hydronephrosis (Figs. 9.6, 9.7, 9.8, 9.9, and 9.10) require a long-term follow-up, due to the risk of recurrence or possibility of worsening, and long-term impairment of renal function [18].

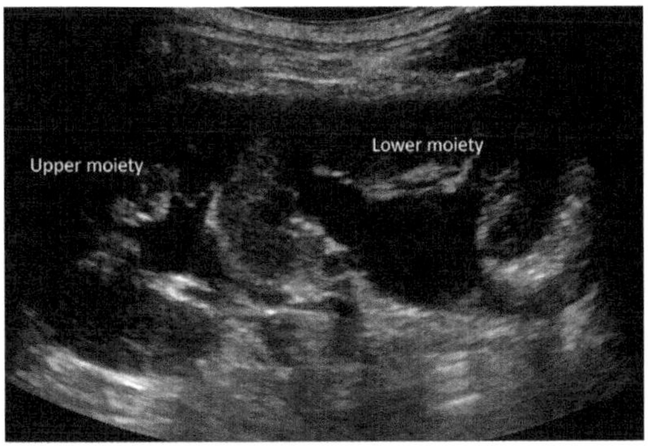

Fig. 9.8 Duplex kidney with moderate hydronephrosis. There is moderate dilatation of the renal pelvis, with mild-moderate dilatation of calyces. Shape of calyces and papillary projections are mostly preserved in upper moiety. Dilatation is more severe in the lower moiety

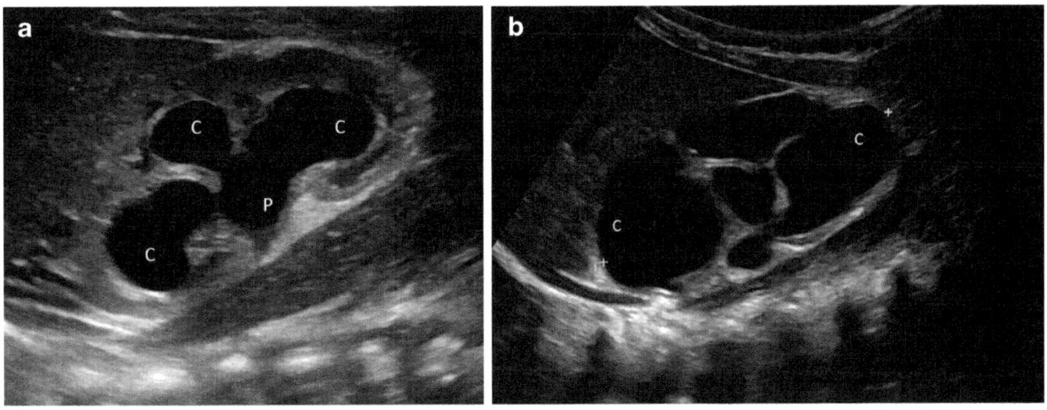

Fig. 9.9 (**a**) Severe hydronephrosis. Severe dilatation of renal pelvis (P) and all calyces (C). Blunting and flattening of calyces outline, with abnormal shape and stripe of increased echogenicity along their borders. Thinning of renal parenchyma. (**b**) Severe hydronephrosis. Kidney has been replaced by dilated calyces (C). Renal parenchyma is no longer visible

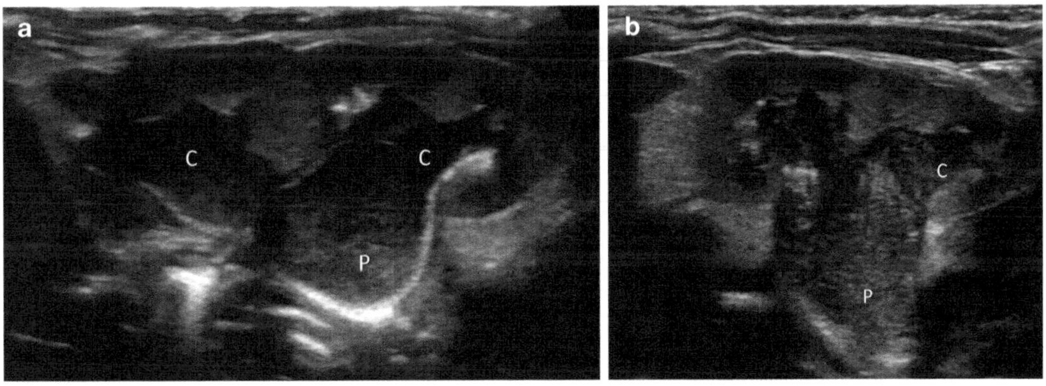

Fig. 9.10 Neonatal pyelonephritis, as complication of hydronephrosis and impaired flow of urine. (**a**) Heterogenous increase in echogenicity within the renal pelvis; calyces show normal appearance, with no features of infection. (**b**) Progression of infection, with thick and echogenic fluid within both the renal pelvis and calyces

9.3 Congenital Abnormalities

The urinary tract is most common site of congenital anomalies, which are seen in 3–4% of the general population and account for 15–20% of all prenatally detected congenital pathologies [19, 20].

Classification of the anomalies includes renal anomalies of the number, form and position, and anomalies in the development of the urinary collecting system.

9.3.1 Anomalies of Renal Number

Anomalies of renal number include a unilateral or bilateral renal agenesis, or supernumerary kidney.

9.3.1.1 Renal Agenesis

Renal agenesis is defined as a complete absence of one or both kidneys due to unsuccessful formation of the embryotic kidney [21, 22]. Bilateral agenesis is rare, and it is incompatible with life. It is often associated with pulmonary hypoplasia and typical facial features. Unilateral renal agenesis has an incidence 1:1000 births and can be sporadic or inherited as autosomal dominant trait. The left kidney is more commonly absent.

Unilateral agenesis is often asymptomatic and is normally diagnosed as incidental finding [21]. It is frequently associated with other anomalies which can be present in up to 50% of children. These include vesicoureteric reflux (28% of children), PUJ and VUJ obstruction (up to 20% of children) [23].

Supernumerary kidney is an additional accessory organ, which is commonly located inferior to the left kidney. Right-sided supernumerary kidney or bilateral accessory kidneys are very rare, with <100 cases published in the literature [24].

Supernumerary kidney is usually smaller than a native one and has a separate arterial supply originating from the aorta or the common iliac artery and separate venous drainage to the inferior vena cava. It is usually asymptomatic, but may present secondary to urinary complications as infection, renal calculi, or incontinence. It can be associated with other congenital abnormalities, as coarctation of aorta, vaginal atresia, or duplication of genitalia.

9.3.2 Anomalies of Renal Form

Anomalies of renal form can be divided into two groups: structural and fusion defects. Structural anomalies are anatomic variants related to the embryologic defects during the final stages of the renal development and include a persistent foetal lobulation, a hypertrophied column of Bertin and dromedary hump.

9.3.2.1 Persistent Foetal Lobulation

Persistent foetal lobulation is considered a normal physiological variant and is present in approximately 4–5% of the population [22]. It is characterised by small and smooth indentations of the renal outline between the pyramids, which corresponds to incomplete fusion of developing lobules (Fig. 9.3).

9.3.2.2 Hypertrophied Column of Bertin

Hypertrophied column of Bertin is a normal physiological variant and often presents as incidental finding during various radiological investigation. It is present up to 50% of the population, with 20% of the patients having hypertrophied columns in both kidneys [25, 26]. Hypertrophied column of Bertin represents a focal cortical hyperplasia and is characterised by extension of the cortical tissue into the renal sinus, which is

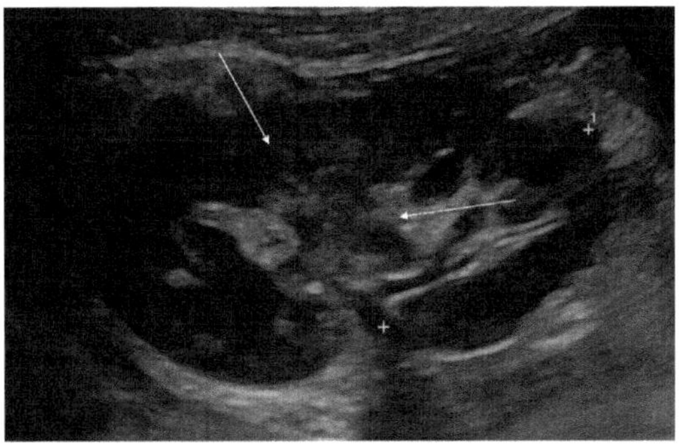

Fig. 9.11 Hypertrophied column of Bertin. Longitudinal image of the kidney shows a normal band of renal tissue (arrow) in the mid aspect of the kidney, visible between the pyramids in renal medulla

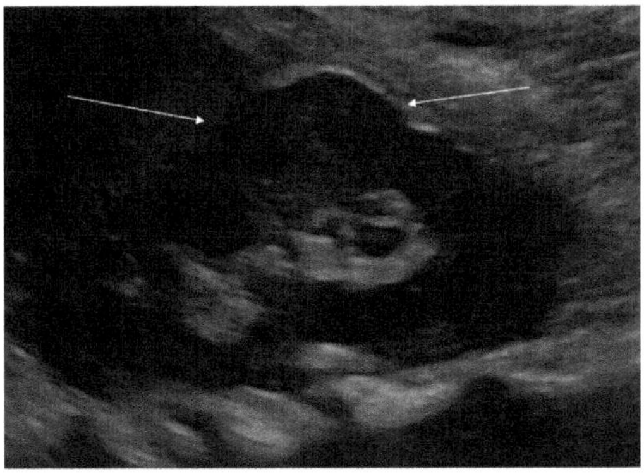

Fig. 9.12 Dromedary hump. Left kidney is abnormal in shape, with prominent renal tissue (arrow) in the mid aspect of renal cortex, causing a focal convex appearance. This corresponds to normal physiological variant and should not be mistaken as focal lesion

visible between the pyramids in the renal medulla. At ultrasound, it appears as a well-defined indentation in the renal sinus, which is in continuity and with similar echogenicity to the adjacent renal parenchyma [22, 25] (Fig. 9.11).

9.3.2.3 Dromedary Hump

Renal dromedary hump represents other anatomical variants of the kidney. It corresponds to a bulge or focal prominence in the lateral aspect of the kidney and is seen in approximately 0.5% of population. It is usually present in the lateral contour of the left kidney and caused by the splenic impression on the superior and lateral aspect of the kidney [27]. Similar to other renal variants, ultrasound examination is usually fully diagnostic, showing the features characteristic and identical to renal parenchyma, with a smooth and uninterrupted continuity of renal cortex and outline (Fig. 9.12).

9.3.3 Fusion Abnormalities

Fusion anomalies occur during the cranial migration of the kidneys from the pelvis to the lumbar region. The fusion can be partial (horseshoe kidney or crossed fused ectopia) or total (pancake kidney).

9.3.3.1 Horseshoe Kidney

Horseshoe kidney is the most common form of fusion anomalies, with an incidence of 1:400–800 babies. It is twice as common in females as in males (2:1) and represents approximately 90% of all renal congenital abnormalities [21, 22]. Horseshoe configuration results from two normally functioning kidneys positioned on either side of the midline, which are connected by a parenchymal or fibrotic bridge [22]. Most commonly the isthmus connects the lower poles of the kidneys (95%). Most patients are asymptomatic (90%) and horseshoe kidney is found incidentally [28, 29].

On the postnatal ultrasound, a horseshoe kidney is usually positioned lower than the normal kidneys with inferior poles projecting medially. Transverse images of the retroperitoneum often demonstrate a band of soft tissue, representing a renal isthmus crossing the midline anterior to the abdominal great vessels. The abnormally rotated and inferiorly located kidney usually results in poor visuali-

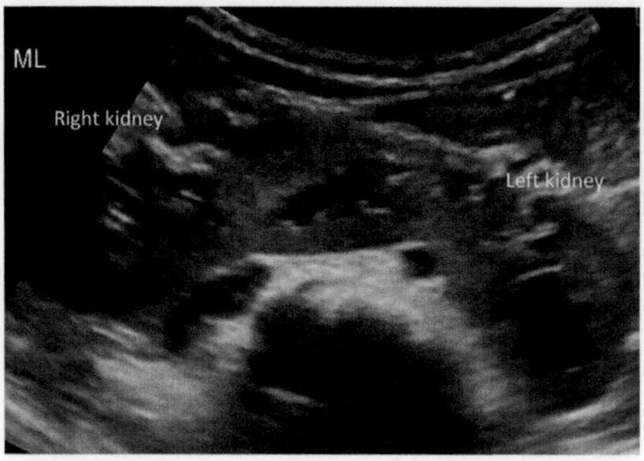

Fig. 9.13 Horseshoe kidney. Transverse image show connecting isthmus crossing the midline anterior to retroperitoneal vessels. Renal parenchyma extends and abuts the spine of each limb of horseshoe kidney

sation of the inferior pole and underestimation of the renal length (Fig. 9.13). Poor visualisation of the inferior part of the kidneys should always alert the clinician to a possibility of the horseshoe configuration. In this situation, it is necessary to perform ultrasound examination in the prone position for better visualisation of the retroperitoneum.

Known complications of the horseshoe configuration, hydronephrosis, and calculi within the collecting system are usually present at the later stages in older children and adults, and not be visible in the infancy.

9.3.3.2 Pancake Kidney

Pancake kidney is a rare abnormality of renal shape with an incidence of 1 in 65,000–2,37,500 and often presents with other genito-urinary and vertebral abnormalities. It is caused by a complete fusion of two kidneys in the pelvis with two separate collecting systems and ureters. Ureters are usually short, do not cross the midline and insert into bladder in the normal position [30].

9.3.4 Anomalies of Renal Position

Anomalies of the renal position correspond to abnormal orientation or location of the kidneys within the abdomen and pelvis [31] and include: renal malrotation, simple renal ectopia, and cross renal ectopia.

9.3.4.1 Renal Malrotation

Renal malrotation is defined as an abnormal position of the kidneys in relation to the hilum. It can be unilateral or bilateral and is present in 1:2000 patients. Renal malrotation includes spectrum of abnormalities: non-rotation, incomplete rotation, reverse rotation with dilatation, and sagittal rotation [22, 31]. Malrotation of kidneys is asymptomatic and usually found incidentally.

9.3.4.2 Renal Ectopia

Renal ectopia is characterised by the abnormal location of the kidneys within the abdomen, pelvis or thorax [22, 31]. Ectopic kidney can be simple (located at the same site of the ureter) or crossed (kidney is on the opposite side of ureteric orifice). It could be unilateral or bilateral. In the simple renal ectopia, kidney is most commonly located in the pelvis, follow by iliac region, abdomen, and chest [31]. The incidence of the pelvic kidney is 1:2000–3000 patients [32].

Pelvic kidneys are often small and abnormally rotated (Fig. 9.14a, b). The ureters are short with a poor drainage, which often results in dilatation of the collecting system, which may predispose to secondary infection and stone formation. Ectopic kidneys are also prone to traumatic injury, due to their abnormal location [32].

9.3.4.3 Crossed Renal Ectopia

Crossed renal ectopia is defined as a kidney located on the opposite side in relation to its embryologic position. Despite the ectopic position of the kidney, the ureter has normal insertion in the bladder. Left to right ectopia is more common, with a fusion reported in more than 90% of cases. Crossed fused ectopia is more commonly seen in males, with 3:2 predominance [31].

Depending on fusion site and final renal shape, different variants have been described (inferior/S-shaped/lump/disc/L-shaped/superior) [21, 22]:

In most cases, a crossed fused renal ectopia is found incidentally, with no associated symptoms. However, patients may present with clinical features related to complications such as hydrone-

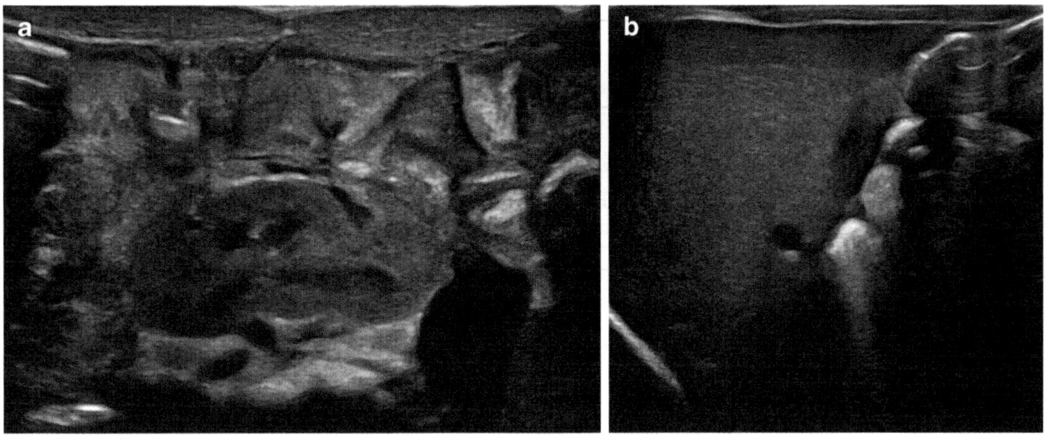

Fig. 9.14 Ectopic right kidney. (**a**) Small kidney located deep in the right iliac fossa. (**b**) Empty right renal fossa

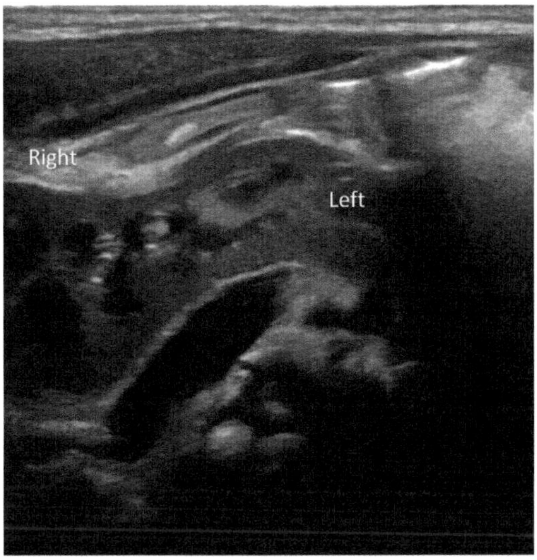

Fig. 9.15 Crossed fused renal ectopia. Left kidney is displaced to the right side of abdomen and fused with the right kidney. Fused kidneys demonstrate an abnormal shape and structure

phrosis, infections, VUR, or renal calculi [33]. Crossed fused ectopia may be associated with other congenital abnormalities, mainly skeletal, genital, anorectal, and cardiovascular [33].

Ultrasound is examination of choice. It will show both kidneys located on the same side of abdomen and typically fused with a characteristic anterior and posterior notch between the two fused kidneys (Fig. 9.15).

9.3.5 Anomalies Related to the Urinary Collecting System

9.3.5.1 Duplex Kidney

Duplex kidney is a common congenital abnormality, caused by duplication of the ureteric bud, which results in the formation of two collecting systems including two renal pelvises and two ureters (Figs. 9.8 and 9.16). It is often familial and occurs in 1% of population [21, 34].

Duplex system is more common in females (2:1 ratio) and is bilateral in 40% of cases [29]. It is often asymptomatic, it has been demonstrated in 10% of children with recurrent urinary tract infections [22, 34].

Duplex system can be classified as complete (two separate ureters) and incomplete (ureters fused together before the uretero-vesical junction).

In complete duplex kidney, the ureter from the lower pole follows a normal anatomic structure and insertion to the bladder. Ureter from the upper pole usually shows an ectopic orientation, being displaced medially and inferiorly. Distal end and insertion of the ectopic ureters varies between the girls and boys. In girls, an insertion could be above the external urethral sphincter (bladder) or below (urethra, upper vagina, uterus, or fallopian tubes). In boys, an ectopic insertion

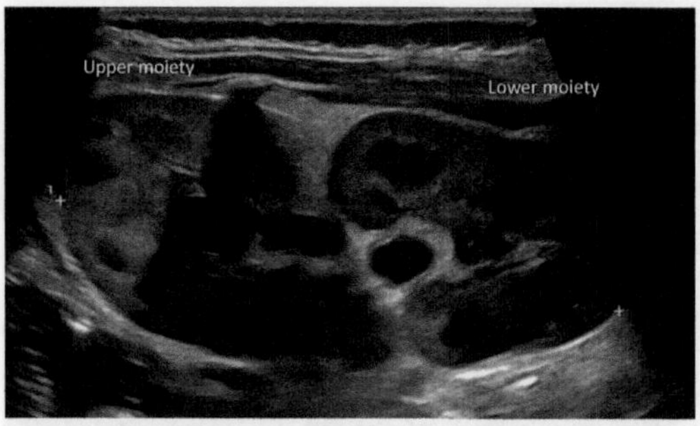

Fig. 9.16 Duplex left kidney with mild dilatation of the calyces. Complete separation of two moieties, with abnormal renal shape and fibrotic band in the central aspect

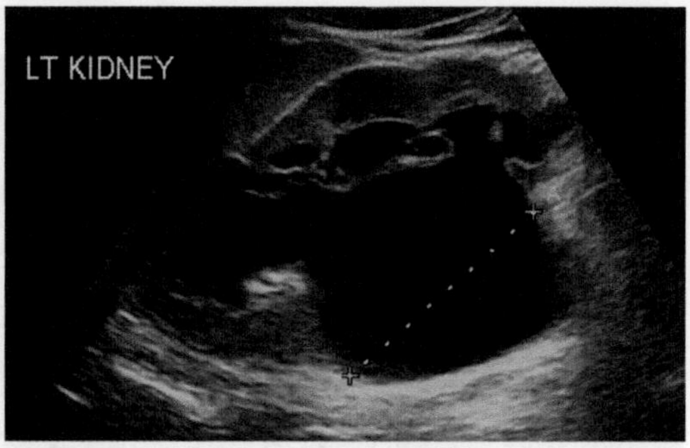

Fig. 9.17 Left pelvic-ureteric junction (PUJ) obstruction. Significant dilatation of left renal pelvis (calipers), with a large extrarenal component. Abrupt transition point at the PUJ, proximal ureter is collapsed

is always above the external sphincter (bladder, prostatic urethra, seminal vesicles, vas deferens, or ejaculatory ducts) [34–36].

The ureter draining the lower pole has more perpendicular course through the bladder wall, which makes it more prone to reflux. The ectopic ureter from the upper pole is usually prone to obstruction, causing a dilatation of the upper moiety. It is often associated with ureterocoele [21].

Most commonly, ultrasound findings include urinary tract dilation involving the upper pole system, with a normal appearance of the lower pole moiety. In case of long-standing dilatation, an atrophy of the renal parenchyma may occur [37, 38].

9.3.5.2 Pelvic-Ureteric Junction (PUJ) Obstruction

Dilatation of renal pelvis due to pelvic-ureteric junction obstruction is a common congenital abnormality, present in 1 per 1000–2000 newborns. It is estimated to represent approximately 50% of all urinary tract abnormalities in neonates [19, 20, 39]. It is more frequent in boys, with a 2:1 ratio; it could be bilateral in 10–30% of cases. Bilateral obstructions are associated with other non-urinary abnormalities, as oesophageal atresia, Hirschsprung disease or imperforate anus [39].

The left kidney is affected twice as often as the right kidney. PUJ obstruction is the most common cause of the postnatal hydronephrosis and second the most common cause of prenatal hydronephrosis (after transient or physiological hydronephrosis) [22].

Most cases of PUJ dilatation are diagnosed antenatally during the routine gestational scans. Characteristic features include a dilatation of the renal pelvis, with or without dilatation of renal calyces, and with an abrupt transition point at the ureteropelvic junction (Fig. 9.17).

Consequent parenchymal thinning, cystic changes and dysplasia depend on the degree and duration of obstruction [39]. The high-grade severe obstruction could be associated with developing perirenal urinomas and ascites.

9.3.5.3 Congenital Megacalyces and Megaureter

Megacalyces is a congenital malformation with an enlargement of the renal calyces, with normal non-dilated renal pelvis. Megacalyces are usually diagnosed as an incidental finding, but in older children could present with symptoms of recurrent infection, formation of calculi or haematuria. Ultrasound imaging shows enlarged calyces, with flattening of renal pyramids and normal renal pelvis. Imaging is helpful in differential diagnosis with obstructive and reflux related causes, and dynamic studies may be required to obtain a definite diagnosis.

Megaureter is a general term to describe dilatation of the ureter with or without dilatation of the colleting system within the kidneys. Mild transient dilatation (<5 mm) represents a normal physiological finding [40, 41]. Megaureter can be

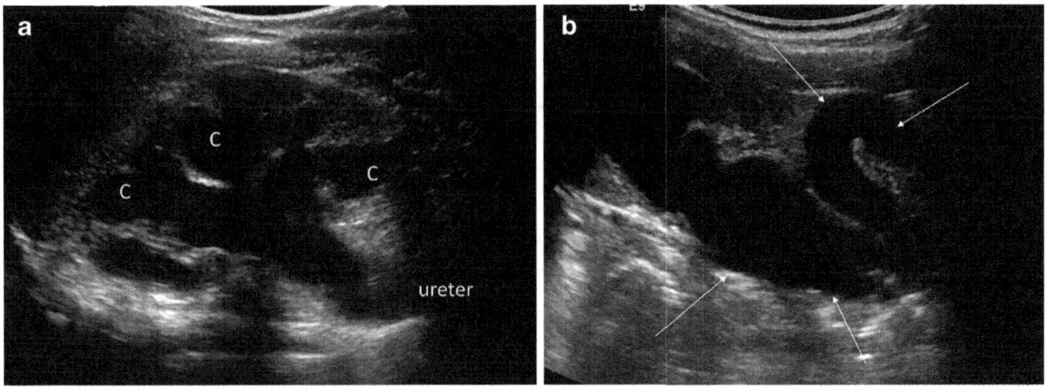

Fig. 9.18 Megaureter. (**a**) Coronal image of left kidney shows severe dilatation of left calyces, renal pelvis and upper part of left ureter, with an abnormal angulation and 'kink' in the upper part of ureter. (**b**) Longitudinal images through left side of abdomen shows a dilated and tortuous left ureter

classified as primary (idiopathic congenital abnormality) or secondary (due to other causes, as posterior urethral valves, neurogenic bladder, or calculi). Primary megaureter (known as congenital megaureter) is bilateral in 20% of cases, with contralateral genito-urinary abnormalities present in 5% of patients [41].

Characteristic ultrasound features include: a dilated, elongated and tortuous ureter, with a various degree of dilatation of renal pelvis and calyces (Fig. 9.18a, b). It is often demonstrated as tubular cystic structure, extending from the kidney to the urinary bladder [37, 38]. The role of imaging is to establish if ureteric dilatation is primary or secondary, and if it is associated with an obstruction and/or reflux. In case of obstructive pathology, there is usually dilation of the proximal and mid segment of ureter, with narrow and short segment inferiorly, near the vesicoureteric junction. This finding could be further evaluated with functional MRI urography or diuretic renography, as MAG3. Reflux within a dilated ureter could be confirmed by voiding cystourethrography or voiding ultrasound.

9.3.6 Vesicoureteral Reflux

Vesicoureteral reflux (VUR) represents an abnormal retrograde flow of urine from the urinary bladder into the ureters and kidneys due to abnormality of the vesicoureteral junction. In neonates, it's often caused by delayed maturation of the antireflux mechanisms [37, 42, 43].

VUR is seen in up to 40% of cases of urinary tract dilatation diagnosed prenatally [37]. It should be always suspected when renal dilatation is found in the pregnancy and warrants further postnatal evaluation. Early diagnosis of VUR is critical to prevent renal damage, due to an increased risk of the upper renal tract infection caused by ascending organisms, which could result in the parenchymal scarring and abnormal renal function.

In the clinical practice, a severity of the vesicoureteric reflux is described in grades [42]:

Grade 1—urine reflux into normal-size ureter.
Grade 2—reflux into the ureter and renal collecting system, without dilatation.
Grade 3—reflux with moderate dilatation of the ureter and collecting system, without blunting of calyces.
Grade 4—reflux, with dilated/tortuous ureter and dilated collecting system; blunting of the calyces and preservation of papillary impressions.
Grade 5—marked dilatation of ureter and collecting system, with blunting of calyces and papillary impressions.

Ultrasound reminds the first diagnostic test in evaluation of the VUR, and assessment of the renal system dilatation (Fig. 9.19 a–c). Ultrasound

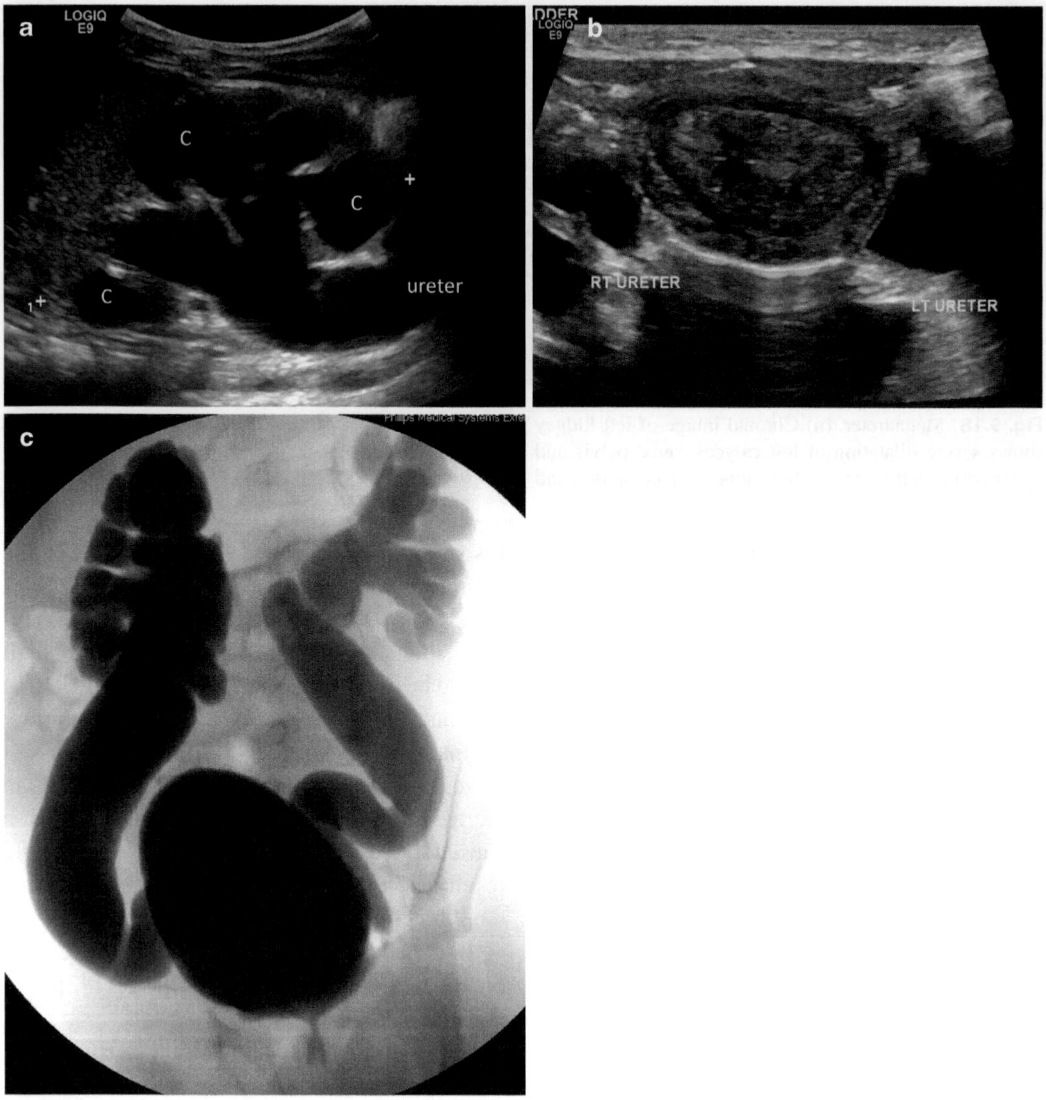

Fig. 9.19 Bilateral grade 5 vesico-ureteric reflux. Significant dilatation of the collecting systems in both kidneys, with blunting of the renal calyces and papillary projections. Dilated and tortuous ureters. (**a**) Coronal image of the left kidney. (**b**) Axial image through an empty urinary bladder and dilated both distal ureters. (**c**) Micturating cystoureterography (MCUG)

images demonstrate a tortuous and dilated ureter. Dilatation of renal pelvis and calyces depends on the degree of reflux. Size and shape of the calyces and papillary impressions are important ultrasound features, to determine a severity of reflux and guide treatment of follow-up. Historically, MCUG was required to confirm the presence of the refluxing urine. Currently, this examination has been slowly replaced by voiding ultrasonography, which has been proved in several studies to improve diagnostic accuracy and avoid an ionising radiation [1, 43].

9.3.7 Bladder and Urethral Anomalies

9.3.7.1 Ureterocoele

Ureterocoele is a cyst-like expansion of the terminal segment of the ureter that projects into the

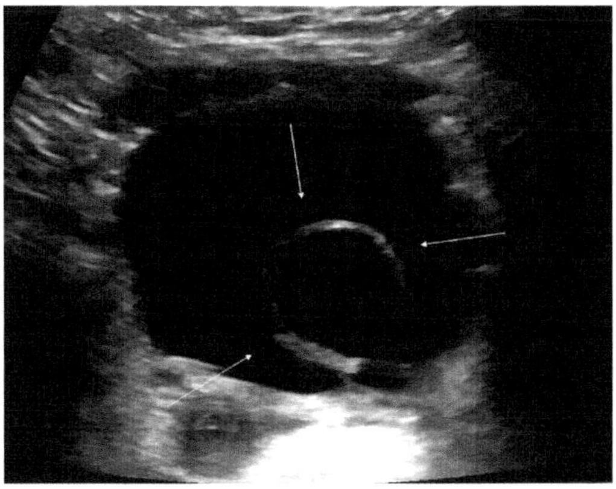

Fig. 9.20 Ultrasound image of the urinary bladder in a 5-week-old neonate shows cystic dilatation of the terminal portion of the left ureter (white arrows) confirming a ureterocele

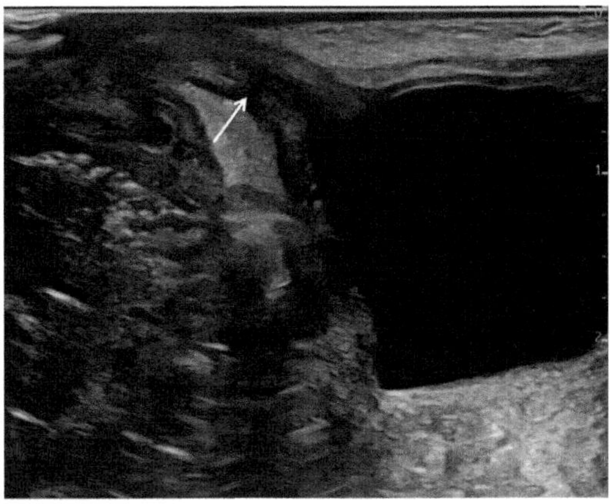

Fig. 9.21 5-day-old neonate with discharge from umbilicus. Grayscale ultrasound image shows a patent urachus (white arrow) extending cranially from the dome of the urinary bladder. Image courtesy: Dr. Adarsh Ghosh, Department of Radiology, Cincinnati Children's Hospital Medical Center, Ohio, USA

lumen of the urinary bladder at the site of its insertion (which may be orthotopic or ectopic). Most of the cases are diagnosed antenatally or in the neonatal period. The ectopic ureterocele is more commonly seen in children and is unilateral in 90% of cases [44].

Ureterocoele most often occurs in a duplicated system and is almost always connected with the ureter draining the upper pole. Intravesical ureterocoeles may be bilateral and, more commonly, seen in unduplicated collecting systems. In duplicated system, it may involve either the upper or the lower pole ureter of duplex kidney [44]. Occasionally, the ureterocoele herniates into the urethra, causing urethral obstruction. Ultrasound demonstrates an anechoic cystic lesion of variable size protruding into the bladder lumen (Fig. 9.20). A variable degree of upstream hydroureteronephrosis can be seen.

9.3.7.2 Urachal Anomalies

Urachus normally obliterates craniocaudally from the umbilicus towards the urinary bladder. Failure of this regression results in one of the following disorders [44, 45]: (1) patent urachus (50%), (2) urachal cyst (30%), (3) urachal sinus (15%), and (4) urachal diverticulum (3–5%). A patent urachus results in a vesicoumbilical fistula with urine coming out from the cutaneous opening (Fig. 9.21). Urachal cyst forms when the urachus gets obliterated at both ends but remains patent in its midpart. Urachal diverticulum results when the urachus is obliterated at the level of the umbilicus but communicates with the urinary bladder. Ultrasound readily demonstrates the urachal diverticulum at the dome of the urinary bladder.

9.3.7.3 Bladder Diverticula

Bladder diverticula can be primary, secondary, or iatrogenic (postoperative) [46, 47]. Primary diverticula are congenital and occur most frequently in the trigonal area, while the secondary bladder diverticula result due to chronically increased intravesical pressure and occur most frequently in the paraureteral area. Iatrogenic diverticula are seen most often in the wall of the bladder at the site of a previous surgery or intervention [47]. Ultrasound demonstrates urine-filled outpouching protruding beyond the bladder wall (Fig. 9.22).

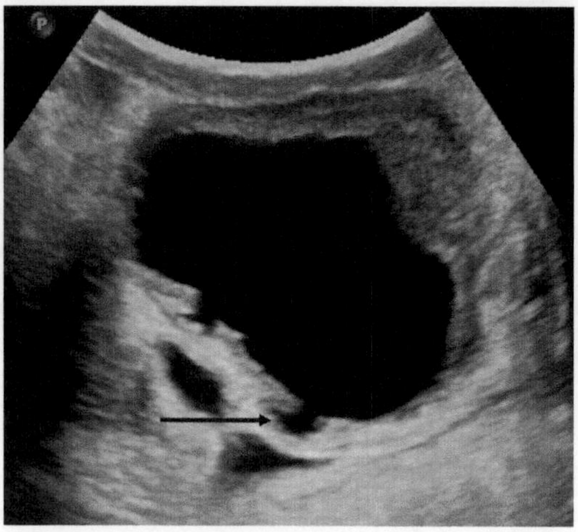

Fig. 9.22 3-week-old child with meningomyelocele. Gray scale ultrasound image shows an overdistended bladder with a small diverticulum arising from the right lateral wall of the urinary bladder

9.3.7.4 Posterior Urethral Valves

Posterior urethral valves (PUVs) are the most common cause of congenital bladder outlet obstruction [37, 48]. They are identified at the base of the verumontanum, causing narrowing of the urethra and impaired flow of urine. This leads to chronic bladder outlet obstruction and dilatation of the posterior urethra, proximal to the valves. They cause variable degrees of urethral obstruction, which depends on the size and shape of structural abnormality [37]. Ultrasound shows varying degrees of hydroureteronephrosis, thickened bladder wall, dysplastic kidneys with increased echogenicity, poor corticomedullary differentiation, and less commonly cortical cyst formation (Fig. 9.23).

Urinomas resulting in perinephric fluid collections may be seen, which occur due to forniceal rupture. The diagnosis of PUVs causing urinary

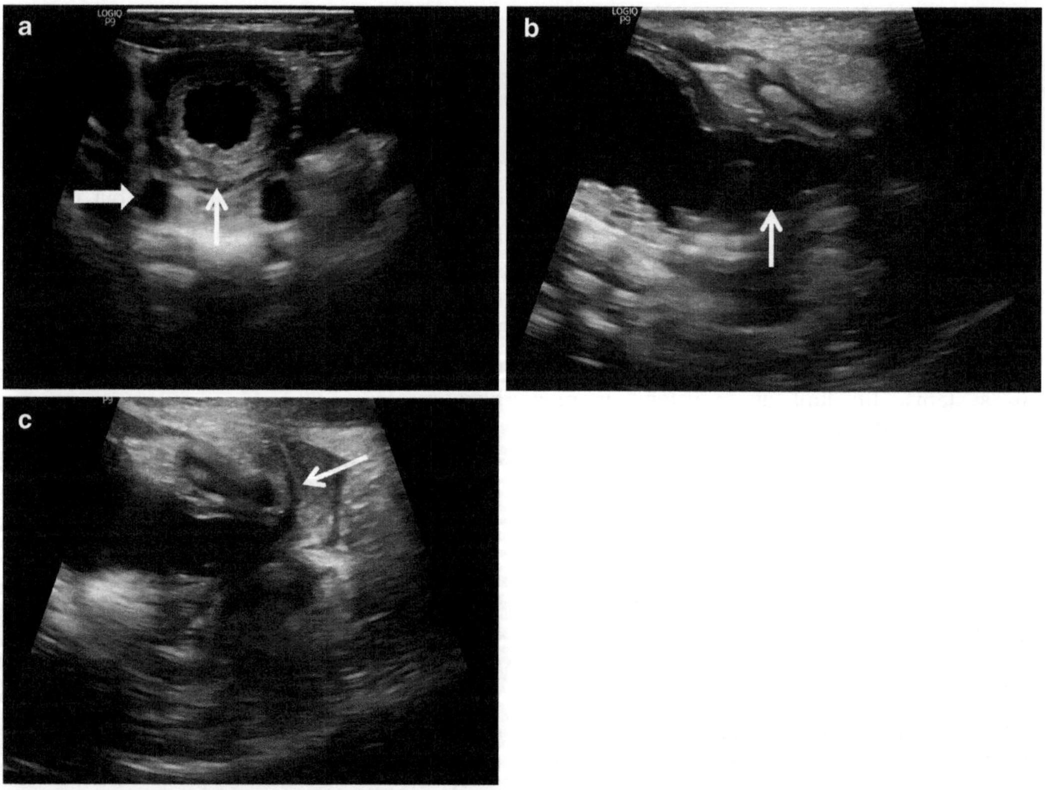

Fig. 9.23 Gray scale ultrasound images (**a**–**c**) show thickened irregular walls of the urinary bladder (solid white arrow in **a**) with dilated posterior urethra (white arrow in B) and thin caliber of the anterior urethra (white arrow in **c**) indicative of posterior urethral valves. In addition, dilated bilateral distal ureters are also seen (block white arrow in **a**). Image courtesy: Dr. CV Kanimozhi, Kanchi Kamakoti CHILDS Trust Hospital, Chennai, India

tract obstruction should be strongly considered in cases of unexplained ascites in a newborn male. In these cases, hydroureteronephrosis may not be present due to "pop off" mechanism as a result of the forniceal rupture and communication with the peritoneal cavity, which allows one or both kidneys to decompress [49].

9.4 Neonatal Medical Renal Disease

9.4.1 Neonatal Renal Cystic Disease

Renal cystic disease of the newborn may be grouped in several ways such as genetic and non-genetic in origin, or dysplasias and ciliopathies. As we gain a better understanding of the genotype-phenotype association and the pathology of these diseases, the classification of paediatric cystic kidney disease is constantly evolving.

Ultrasound is the imaging modality of choice to evaluate renal cystic disease. A renal evaluation must include the size of the kidney and the echogenicity of the cortex, as well as determination of corticomedullary differentiation (CMD), whether normal, absent, or reversed. A thorough evaluation of renal cysts, if present, should be made to assess the size, number and location (subcapsular, corticomedullary junction or medullary). Where available genetic testing may be offered to families, as the establishment of a genetic diagnosis is helpful for counselling regarding morbidity, disease progression and risk of recurrence in subsequent pregnancies.

9.4.1.1 Heritable Diseases

Ciliopathies

Ciliopathies are a genetically heterogeneous group of diseases that occur due to gene mutations in ciliary-associated proteins [50]. Renal cysts develop due to dysregulated cilia-dependent signalling. The common renal ciliopathies are autosomal recessive polycystic kidney disease, autosomal dominant polycystic kidney disease, nephronophthisis, and Bardet-Biedl syndrome.

Autosomal Recessive Polycystic Kidney Disease (ARPKD)

ARPKD is a hereditary hepatorenal cystic disease due to mutations in the PKHD1 gene and is the most common childhood ciliopathy. Pathologically there is dilatation of the renal collecting tubules that expand into multiple small cysts. Hepatobiliary disease occurs due ductal plate malformation and is present in varying degrees of severity in all patients. In neonates the renal involvement is more severe, and the hepatic disease is milder. The typical ultrasound findings in neonates are markedly enlarged kidneys (> + 4 standard deviations for age) that are hyperechoic with poor or absent CMD. The renal hyperechogenicity is the result of numerous acoustic interfaces produced by dilated tubules and microscopic cysts that are too small to be resolved on US. Often tiny echogenic foci with a 'comet-tail' artefact (Fig. 9.24) are seen which are caused by precipitation of crystalline material due to urine stagnation in dilated tubules [51]. High resolution sonogra-

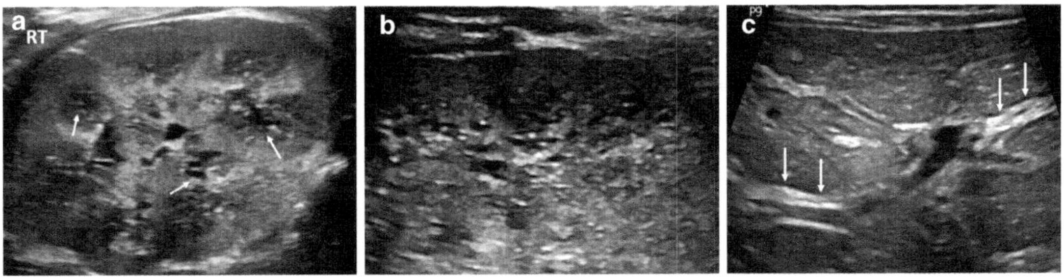

Fig. 9.24 Autosomal recessive polycystic kidney disease with hepatic fibrosis in an infant. (**a**) Coronal image of the right kidney shows multiple medullary microcysts and dilated tubules (arrows) with increased cortical echogenicity [similar findings were seen in the left kidney]. (**b**) High resolution image of the kidney shows innumerable small cysts radiating from the medulla to the cortex. The subcapsular cortex does not contain any cysts. (**c**) High resolution transverse of the liver in the same baby shows increased echogenicity surrounding the portal tracts (arrows) suggestive of periportal fibrosis

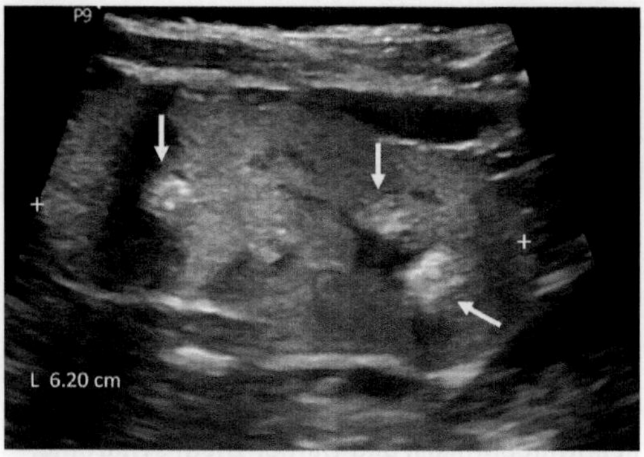

Fig. 9.25 Autosomal recessive polycystic kidney disease atypical pattern. Longitudinal image of the left kidney (in calipers) in a 4 wk. old neonate shows a moderately enlarged hyperechoic kidney with echogenic renal pyramids (arrows) leading to the appearance of reversed corticomedullary differentiation. Similar appearances were seen in the right kidney

phy can show cystic dilatations of the ducts radiating from the medulla to the cortex (Fig. 36). Discrete macrocysts (>10 mm) can be observed occasionally. The subcapsular cortex is unaffected (as it does not contain any tubules) and may be seen as a hypoechoic band in older children. An atypical sonographic appearance of ARPKD that is associated with a better clinical prognosis is characterised by moderately enlarged kidneys (around +2 to +4 SD) with reversed CMD (Fig. 9.25). This appearance is due to hyperechoic renal pyramids secondary to increased interfaces from dilated tubules in the medulla [52].

Autosomal Dominant Polycystic Kidney Disease (ADPKD)

ADPKD occurs usually in adulthood, but neonatal presentation of ADPKD can occur in a minority. Imaging findings in the neonatal period are characterised by markedly enlarged hyperechoic kidneys and as such, can be difficult to distinguish from ARPKD at this stage. Absence of renal macrocysts cannot be used as a criterion to rule out a diagnosis of ADPKD in infants and children. Extrarenal manifestations such as cysts in the liver, spleen and pancreas and cerebral aneurysms are rare in neonates.

Nephronophthisis (NPHP)

NPHP is group of autosomal recessive tubulointerstitial ciliopathy and can manifest in isolation but is more commonly seen as a component of several genetic syndromes. Cysts are not always evident on imaging, and their absence does not exclude a diagnosis of NPHP [53]. Ultrasound findings of infantile NPHP include enlarged hyperechoic kidneys with poor or absent CMD and cortical microcysts [54].

Other Renal Ciliopathies

Other ciliopathies than can present with multiple renal cysts are Bardet-Biedl syndrome, Meckel-Gruber syndrome, Joubert syndrome, Jeune syndrome, and Zellweger syndrome. A thorough clinical examination with further imaging is needed to detect multisystem involvement in these syndromes. Renal cysts can also be seen in Von Hippel-Lindau syndrome and tuberous sclerosis.

Hepatocyte Nuclear Factor 1β (HNF1β) Nephropathy

It is characterised by chronic tubulointerstitial nephritis [55]. Renal ultrasound findings in neonates include bilateral hyperechoic kidneys that are normal in size or slightly enlarged with unilateral or bilateral cysts (Fig. 9.26). Ultrasound appearances can be similar to that seen in ARPKD and its diagnosis requires genetic analysis.

9.4.1.2 Non-hereditary Diseases

Multicystic Dysplastic Kidney (MCDK)

MCDK is the most common form of cystic renal dysplasia. Abnormalities of the contralateral kidney, such as vesicoureteric reflux, pelviureteric junction (PUJ) obstruction and vesicoureteric

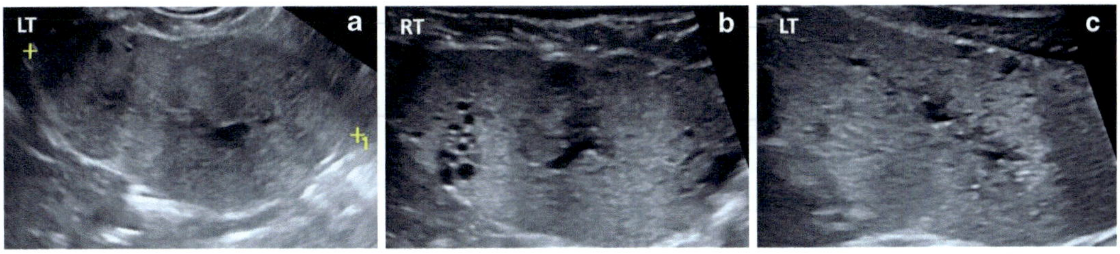

Fig. 9.26 HNF 1β nephropathy. 1 month old preterm neonate with h/o echogenic kidneys on the antenatal scan. (**a**) Longitudinal image of the left kidney shows a mildly enlarged kidney (left—5.70 cm, right—5.60 cm) with increased echogenicity and absent corticomedullary differentiation. (**b** and **c**) High resolution longitudinal images of the right and left kidneys show multiple small cysts in both kidneys. Cyst are located in the subcapsular cortex and medulla. Genetic testing revealed a 17q12 deletion

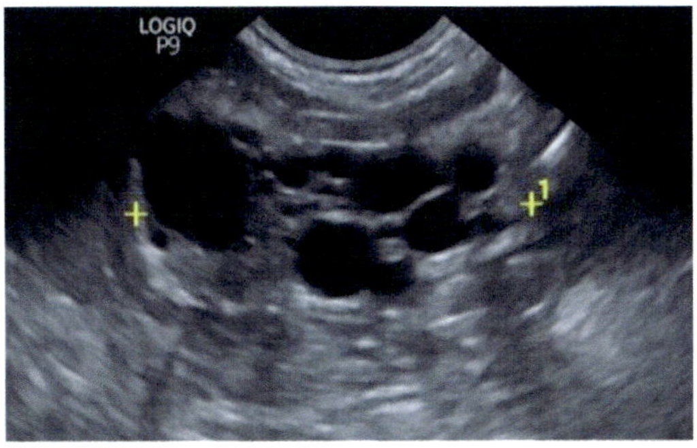

Fig. 9.27 Multicystic cystic dysplastic kidney (MCDK). A 6 week old female with antenatal diagnosis of MCDK. Longitudinal image of the left kidney (marked by calipers) shows multiple non-communicating cysts with intervening stromal tissue. Normal renal parenchyma is not seen

junction (VUJ) obstruction, are seen in 4–40% of patients [56, 57].

Ultrasound shows multiple non-communicating cysts of variable sizes with intervening echogenic stromal tissue. Normal renal parenchyma is not present, and the kidney does not have any function. Most commonly the entire kidney is involved, but the dysplasia can be segmental and can involve a moiety of a duplex kidney or affect an ectopic kidney (Fig. 9.27). An uncommon type of MCDK is the hydronephrotic variant, in which a renal pelvis can be seen on ultrasound. The natural course of MCDK is complete or partial involution and hence conservative management with periodic follow-up ultrasound studies is recommended.

Obstructive Cystic Dysplasia

Obstructive cystic dysplasia may be unilateral or bilateral and it occurs secondary to antenatal obstruction of the urinary tract which can occur due to PUJ obstruction, ureteric stenosis, VUJ obstruction or posterior urethral valves. On ultrasound the kidneys are of variable size. The renal cortex is hyperechoic with or without cysts and the CMD is usually absent. Often there is dilatation of the collecting system (Fig. 9.28).

Calyceal Diverticulum

A calyceal diverticulum is an outpouching of a calyx into the renal parenchyma and in children they are thought to be congenital in origin [58]. Calyceal diverticulae are of two types:- the more common type 1 cysts communicate with a minor calyx and are present in the upper pole; type 2 cysts are found in the central part of the kidney, are larger in size and communicate with the pelvis or a major calyx. On ultrasound a calyceal diverticulum appears as a simple thin-walled anechoic cyst. (Fig. 9.29).

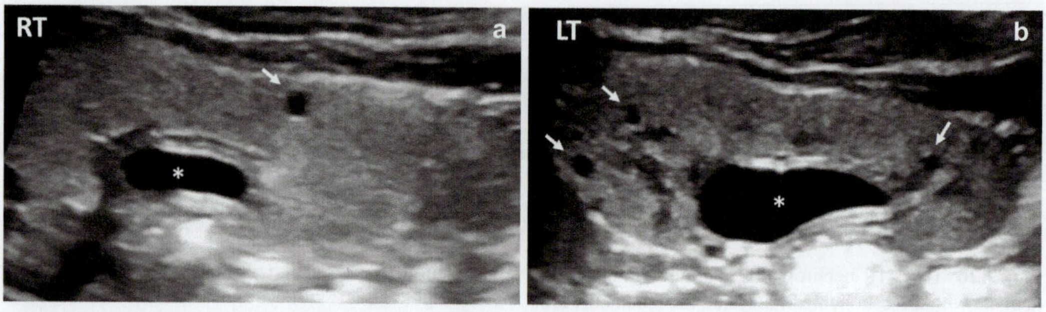

Fig. 9.28 Obstructive cystic dysplasia. (**a** and **b**) Longitudinal images of the kidneys in a 3 week old neonate show hyperechoic parenchyma in both kidneys with poor to absent corticomedullary differentiation. Small cysts (arrows) and a dilated renal pelvis (*) are seen in both kidneys

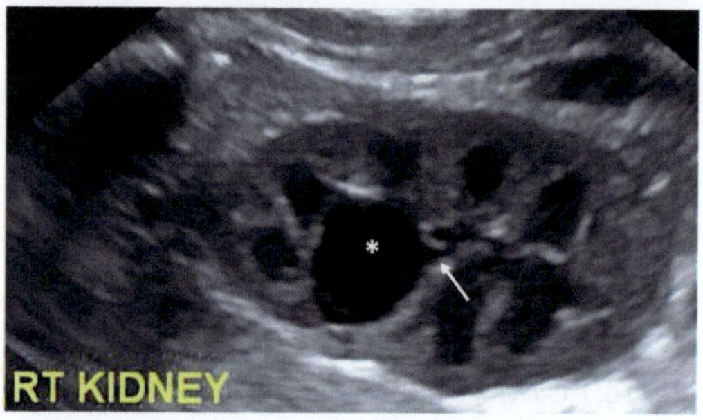

Fig. 9.29 Incidentally detected calyceal diverticulum in a neonate. Longitudinal image of the right kidney shows a well-defined thin-walled anechoic cyst (*) in the interpolar region with a thin tract (arrow) leading to the collecting system

9.4.2 Glomerulocystic Kidney Disease

Glomerulocystic kidney disease is not a single disease entity, but a descriptive term denoting the morphologic appearance of glomeruli on histopathology. Ultrasound shows bilateral enlarged hyperechoic kidneys with small subcapsular cortical cysts that correspond to dilated Bowman spaces. Glomerular cysts can be caused by a variety of underlying conditions including non-syndromic familial autosomal dominant tubulointerstitial disease, inheritable malformation syndromes (such as HNF1β nephropathy, tuberous sclerosis, Zellweger syndrome and Bardet-Biedel syndrome) and also as a component in acquired conditions such as obstructive renal dysplasia.

9.5 Renal Vascular Disease

9.5.1 Renal Vein Thrombosis (RVT)

RVT is the most frequent vascular condition of renal vessels in the neonate. The predisposing factors include coagulopathy, maternal diabetes mellitus, dehydration, sepsis, birth asphyxia, prematurity and prolonged femoral venous line.

Ultrasound findings in the early stages of obstruction include an enlarged oedematous kidney with increased cortical echogenicity and poor CMD. The thrombosis starts within the kidney in the interlobular veins and then extends proximally via the interlobar veins to the main renal vein and then to the IVC [59]. (Fig. 9.30). In about 40–50% of the cases, there is extension of the thrombus into the IVC. The venous outflow obstruction leads to secondary changes in flow pattern in the main renal artery seen as decreased or reversed end-diastolic flow and increased resistive index.

Ultrasound in the subacute phase shows a heterogeneous appearance of the renal parenchyma with hypo- and hyperechoic areas due to infarct, oedema, and haemorrhage. If collateral channels form early on and there is re-canalisation of the thrombosed renal veins, the kidney may recover favourably. However, if the renal perfusion is poor and haemorrhagic infarction occurs the final outcome is a small atrophic kidney.

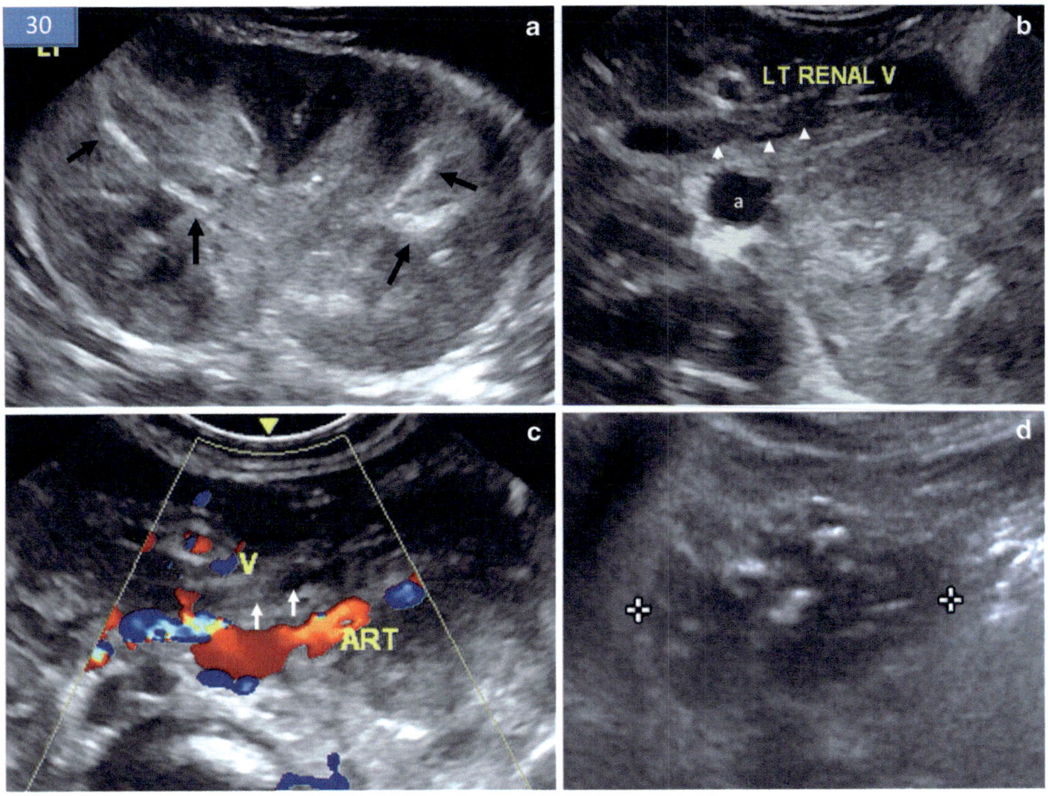

Fig. 9.30 Renal vein thrombosis. 4 day old neonate presenting with dehydration and decreased urine output. (**a**) Longitudinal image of the left kidney shows an enlarged kidney with increased echogenicity. Echogenic streaks (arrows) are seen in the parenchyma likely representing the thrombosed intra-renal veins. (**b**) Axial midline image of upper abdomen. Thrombus (arrowheads) is seen in the left main renal vein. [a—aorta]. (**c**) Axial color doppler image of upper abdomen shows absent flow (arrows) in the left main renal vein. Flow is seen in the left renal artery [ART]. (**d**) Longitudinal image of the left kidney at 2 month follow-up shows a contracted left kidney (measures 2.60 cm) with abnormal parenchymal echogenicity and multiple linear calcifications

9.5.2 Renal Artery Thrombosis (RAT)

RAT is a frequent cause of hypertension in neonates, but the incidence is far lower than that of RVT. Risk factors for RAT are indwelling umbilical artery catheter, femoral artery cannulation, sepsis, coagulopathy, shock, low birth weight, and congestive cardiac failure [60].

In the hyperacute phase of vascular obstruction the renal parenchyma can appear normal on ultrasound. With progression the affected kidney appears hyperechoic, due to oedema and haemorrhage, with loss of CMD. Intraluminal echogenic material, representing the thrombus, may be seen within the renal artery. However, fresh thrombus can appear isoechoic and may be missed on greyscale imaging. Colour Doppler imaging shows absent flow distal to the thrombus. There are often long-term sequelae, such as hypertension, renal atrophy and chronic kidney disease.

9.5.3 Congenital Renal Artery Stenosis

Congenital renal artery stenosis in the neonate is most commonly due to fibromuscular dysplasia (FMD) [61]. Other causes of renal artery stenosis in infants include mid-aortic syndrome, neurofibromatosis, Takayasu aortoarteritis, and Williams syndrome [62].

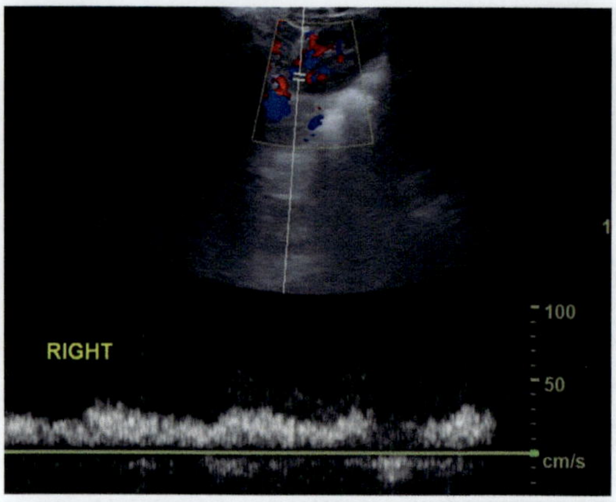

Fig. 9.31 Tardus-parvus pattern in a child with hypertension. Spectral doppler waveform of an intra-renal artery in the right kidney shows a slow systolic upstroke with rounding of the systolic peak and diminished amplitude typical of a tardus-parvus waveform. This pattern indicates a proximal stenosis. CT angiogram showed a high-grade stenosis of the mid-segment of the right main renal artery

Ultrasound is a useful baseline investigation that can be performed. A difference in renal length of >1.5 cm between the two kidneys is an indirect sign of renal artery stenosis. Spectral Doppler findings at the site of stenosis include elevated peak systolic velocity > 180–200 cm/s, renal artery-to-aorta flow velocity > 3 and a difference in resistive index >0.05 between the two kidneys [63]. The intra-renal vessels distal to the site of stenosis exhibit a tardus-parvus waveform characterised by a delayed systolic upsweep with a dampened systolic peak (Fig. 9.31). Ultrasound and Doppler studies have a poor sensitivity for detecting renal artery stenosis, particularly those in accessory renal arteries and in small intra-renal branches.

9.6 Neonatal Renal Tumours

Neonatal renal tumours account for 9% of solid abdominal tumours presenting antenatally or within the first year of life [64]. Neonatal renal masses are usually benign and have better prognosis in terms of overall survival.

9.6.1 Congenital Mesoblastic Nephroma (CMN)

CMN is the most common solid renal tumour of neonates, however they account for only 2–5% of all paediatric renal tumours [65]. CMN occur almost exclusively in the first year of life and over 15% cases are detected antenatally [65]. CMNs are of three histological subtypes, i.e., classic, cellular, and mixed type. Complete nephrectomy is the mainstay of treatment for CMN and chemotherapy is indicated for children >6 months of age [66]. Children with CMN show excellent outcomes with 5-year overall survival of 95% observed across different studies [65]. Poor prognosis is seen with cellular and mixed histological subtypes of CMN, which usually present at a later age (>3 months).

The perinatally common classic subtype presents as a solid tumour with intralesional vascularity and less commonly have necrotic/cystic changes (Fig. 9.32). The cellular and mixed subtypes present as large renal masses and frequently show heterogeneous appearances with numerous cystic/necrotic changes and intralesional haemorrhage (Fig. 9.33).

Age is one of the most important determinant factors to differentiate CMN from other possible but less common renal tumour in this age group, i.e. Wilms tumour. However, CMN lack a pseudo capsule, are well localised and lack venous invasion or renal vein/IVC tumour thrombus, features commonly seen in Wilms tumour [66].

9.6.2 Nephrogenic Rests

Nephrogenic rests (NR) are persistent embryonic metanephrogenic blastemal cells in foetal/neonatal kidney beyond 36 weeks of gestation. They are pre-neoplastic and are found in 30–40% cases of unilateral Wilms tumour and nearly 100% cases of bilateral Wilms tumour [67, 68]. The nephrogenic rests can be intralobar nephrogenic rests (ILNR) which are more central in location with ill-defined margins or can be perilobar neph-

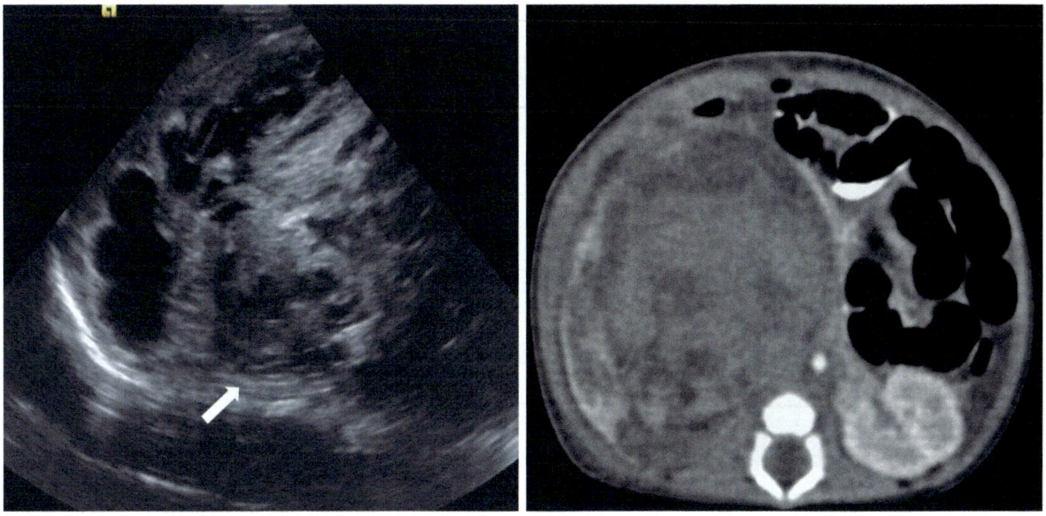

Fig. 9.32 Congenital mesoblastic nephroma (Classic). Newborn presented with bilious vomiting. Antenatal scans normal. US (Day 2 of life) showed a large right abdominal mass arising from the right kidney mid region and lower pole causing localised dilatation of the right renal upper pole calyces as seen on image a. The lesion (white arrow) is mostly solid appearing with peripheral cystic areas. CT scan (day 5 of life) confirms a right renal mass lesion showing predominantly solid enhancement with some cystic/necrotic components

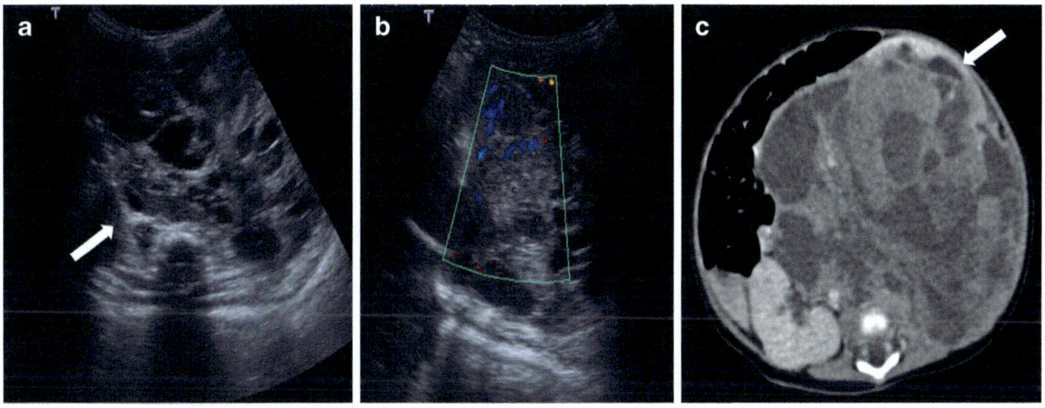

Fig. 9.33 Congenital mesoblastic nephroma (Cellular). 1 month old boy with a palpable abdominal lump. US abdomen (**a**). Left kidney was not identified on US imaging and the lesion (arrow) was mixed solid cystic and intralesional vascularity was noted in the solid component (**b**). CT abdomen (**c**) confirms the large left abdominal mass arising from the left kidney and the uninvolved left renal tissue seen more anteriorly (white arrow). The lesion displaces adjacent structures including the abdominal vessels. No renal vein or IVC invasion seen (not shown). Histopathology showed cellular variant of congenital mesoblastic nephroma

rogenic rests (PLNR), which are multiple peripherally located in renal cortex, can be exophytic and have well-defined margins. On US, nephrogenic rests appear as hypoechoic to isoechoic lesions, homogenous (perilobar), ovoid in shape and are localised to the kidney with no evidence of vascular or ureteric invasion (Fig. 9.34). Size is a feature used by many studies to differentiate NRs (<1.75 cm) from Wilms tumour [67], but few studies have reported otherwise [69].

A separate entity called nephroblastomatosis is often referred to multiple nephrogenic rests in both kidneys, but lately has been described as the diffuse hyperplastic variant of PLNR (DHPLNR)

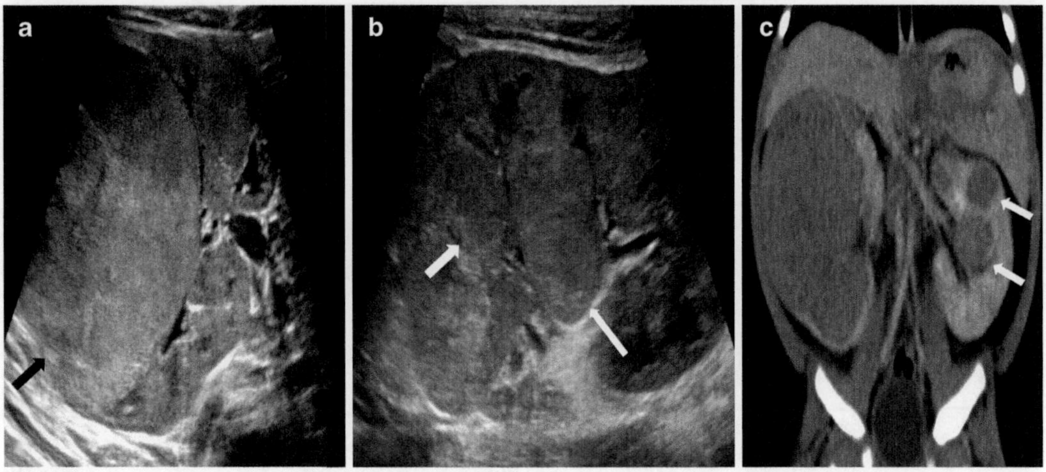

Fig. 9.34 Right Wilms tumour and bilateral nephroblastomatosis. 1 month old boy presented with right abdominal lump. US (**a**) shows a large partly exophytic multilobulated solid lesion arising from the upper pole and mid region of right kidney, showing well defined margins with a thin capsule around it (black arrow). No vascular or pelvicalyceal invasion. (**b**) Left kidney shows numerous small similar echogenicity lesions at the upper pole and mid region (white arrows). The US findings were confirmed on subsequently performed contrast CT abdomen (**c**) showing a large right renal tumour and multiple smaller rounded left renal lesions showing homogenous enhancement (white arrows). Right renal nephron sparing surgery with biopsy from smaller lesions was performed. Histopathology confirmed the large right renal lesion to be Wilms tumour and the smaller lesions in left kidney were nephrogenic rests

[69]. The DHPLNR are peripherally located as thick nephrogenic tissue causing enlargement of the kidney, and US characteristics similar to PLNR. Nephrogenic rests require regular follow-up imaging to look for occurrence of possible Wilms tumour in these lesions.

9.6.3 Less Common Neonatal Renal Tumours

9.6.3.1 Wilms Tumour

Wilms tumour (WT) is rare in the neonate accounting for <1% of renal tumours in the neonate. WT are commonly unilateral and bilateral WT always occur on a background of NR's in the kidneys. The most common age for presentation of WT is 2–5 years and more than 75% of cases occur before the age of 5. WT in neonatal period and infancy is commonly associated with various syndromes, Beckwith-Wiedemann syndrome, WAGR (WT, aniridia, genito-urinary abnormalities and range of developmental delays) [70, 71].

On US imaging, WT usually appear as large mass with heterogeneous appearance due to areas of necrosis and haemorrhage (Fig. 9.34). Renal vein and IVC invasion can be picked up on Doppler US in most of the cases except for very large lesions crossing midline. It is important to rule out lesion in the contralateral kidney to guide appropriate staging and management, and US is good at picking smaller lesions, especially with high resolution probe.

9.6.3.2 Other tumours

Malignant Rhabdoid Tumour of Kidney (MRTK) and Clear Cell Sarcoma of Kidney (CCSK) are less uncommon neonatal renal tumours with an incidence of 11% and 3%, respectively [72, 73]. The most common presenting symptom for both entities is a palpable abdominal mass and are associated with hydramnios and hydrops. Both are indistinguishable from WT on imaging, but have some other characteristics features.

MRTK is commonly seen around 1 year of age and show calcification in 70% of cases, can have synchronous brain tumour of rhabdoid type (Atypical teratoid rhabdoid tumour) [72, 73]. Lung, brain, and liver metastasis with a renal tumour in a neonate is quite diagnostic of MRTK.

CCSK is frequently associated with bone and lung metastasis at presentation and can be misdiagnosed as neuroblastoma if organ of origin is not clear on imaging. Local regional nodal spread is found in nearly 30% of cases which is more common compared to other neonatal renal tumours [70].

Metastases within the kidneys in neonates are rare, with neuroblastoma and lymphoma being the most common. Direct renal invasion from tumours arising adjacent to the kidneys can masquerade as a primary renal tumour.

References

1. Viteri B, Calle-Toro JS, Furth S, Darge K, Hartung EA, Otero H. State-of-the-art renal imaging in children. Pediatrics. 2020;145(2):e20190829. https://doi.org/10.1542/peds.2019-0829.
2. Dunnick R, Sandler C, Newhouse J. Anatomy and embryology. In: Textbook of uroradiology. 5th ed. Lippincott Williams & Wilkins; 2013. p. 1–12.
3. Paliwalla M, Park K. A practical guide to urinary tract ultrasound in a child: pearls and pitfalls. Ultrasound. 2014;22(4):213–22.
4. Jequier S, Rousseau O. Sonographic measurements of the normal bladder wall in children. Am J Roentgenol. 1987;149(3):563–6.
5. Nazim SM, Bangash M, Salam B. Persistent fetal lobulation of kidney mimicking renal tumour. BMJ Case Rep. 2017:bcr-2017-219856.
6. Brennan S, Kandasamy Y. Renal parenchymal thickness as a measure of renal growth in low-birth-weight infants versus normal-birth-weight infants. Ultrasound Med Biol. 2013;39(12):2315–20.
7. Caroli A, Remuzzi A, Lerman LO. Basic principles and new advances in kidney imaging. Kidney Int. 2021;100(5):1001–11.
8. Brennan S, Kandasamy Y. Ultrasound imaging of the renal parenchyma of premature neonates for the assessment of renal growth and glomerulomegaly. Ultrasound Med Biol. 2017;43(11):2546–9.
9. Riccabona M. Basics, principles, techniques and modern methods in paediatric ultrasonography. Eur J Radiol. 2014;83(9):1487–94.
10. Hemachandar R, Boopathy V. Transient renal medullary hyperechogenicity in a term neonate. BMJ Case Rep. 2015:bcr2015211285.
11. Kashaki M, Younesi L, Esmaeili M, Otoukesh H, Esmaeili M. Assessment of the kidney size in newborns. Rev Clin Med. 2017;4(4):160–4.
12. Soyupak SK, Narli N, Yapicioğlu H, Satar M, Aksungur EH. Sonographic measurements of the liver, spleen and kidney dimensions in the healthy term and preterm newborns. Eur J Radiol. 2002;43(1):73–8.
13. Bakker H, Kooijman M, van der Heijden A, et al. Kidney size and function in a multi-ethnic population-based cohort of school-age children. Pediatr Nephrol. 2014;29(9):1589–98.
14. Sinha A, Bagga A, Krishna A, Bajpai M, Srinivas M, Uppal R, et al. Revised guidelines on management of antenatal hydronephrosis. Indian J Nephrol. 2013;23(2):83.
15. Arnaud A, Laraqui Hossini S, Tunon de Lara S, Dobremez E, Chateil JF, Harper L. Managing children with hydronephrosis: common pitfall during ultrasound follow-up to remember. Arch Dis Child. 2020;105(6):610–1.
16. Choi YH, Cheon JE, Kim WS, Kim IO. Ultrasonography of hydronephrosis in the newborn: a practical review. Ultrasonography. 2016;35(3):198–211.
17. Sharma G. Postnatal management of antenatally detected hydronephrosis. World J Clin Urol. 2014;3(3):283.
18. Matsui F, Shimada K, Matsumoto F, Takano S. Late recurrence of symptomatic hydronephrosis in patients with prenatally detected Hydronephrosis and spontaneous improvement. J Urol. 2008;180(1):322–5.
19. Tyagi S, Chimurkar VK, Anjankar V. Congenital anomalies of kidney and urinary tract (CAKUT)-literature review. J Pharm Res Int. 2022:1–8.
20. Walker EYX, Winyard P, Marlais M. Congenital anomalies of the kidney and urinary tract: antenatal diagnosis, management and counselling of families. Pediatric Nephrol. 2024;39(4):1065–75. https://doi.org/10.1007/s00467-023-06137-z.
21. Patel NA, Suthar PP. Ultrasound appearance of congenital renal disease: pictorial review. Egypt J Radiol Nucl Med. 2014;45(4):1255–64.
22. Houat AP, Guimarães CTS, Takahashi MS, Rodi GP, Gasparetto TPD, Blasbalg R, et al. Congenital anomalies of the upper urinary tract: a comprehensive review. Radiographics. 2021;41(2):462–86.
23. Westland R, Schreuder MF, Ket JCF, van Wijk JAE. Unilateral renal agenesis: a systematic review on associated anomalies and renal injury. Nephrol Dial Transplant. 2013;28(7):1844–55.
24. Koureas AP, Panourgias EC, Gouliamos AD, Trakadas SJ, Vlahos LJ. Imaging of a supernumerary kidney. Eur Radiol. 2000;10(11):1722–3.
25. Algin O, Ozmen E, Gumus M. Hypertrophic columns of bertin: imaging findings. Eurasian J Med. 2014;46(1):61–3.
26. Ilounoh CE, Eteng RE, Leahy A. Renal mass mimicking prominent columns of Bertin: a case series. J Diagn Med Sonogr. 2023;39(5):533–8.
27. Koratala A, Bhattacharya D. Kidney hump, no need to jump! Clin Case Rep. 2018;6(8):1633–4.
28. Shah HU, Ojili V. Multimodality imaging spectrum of complications of horseshoe kidney. Indian J Radiol Imaging. 2017;27(02):133–40.

29. Schiappacasse G, Aguirre J, Soffia P, Silva CS, Zilleruelo N. CT findings of the main pathological conditions associated with horseshoe kidneys. Br J Radiol. 2015;88(1045):20140456.
30. Wong HYF, Lee KH. The pancake kidney. Abdom Radiol. 2019;44(1):381–2.
31. Benz-Bohm G. Anomalies of kidney rotation, position and fusion. In: Fotter R, editor. Pediatric uroradiology. Medical radiology. Berlin, Heidelberg: Springer; 2008. https://doi.org/10.1007/978-3-540-33005-9_4.
32. Bhoil R, Sood D, Singh YP, Nimkar K, Shukla A. An ectopic pelvic kidney. Pol J Radiol. 2015;80:425–7.
33. Solanki S, Bhatnagar V, Gupta A, Kumar R. Crossed fused renal ectopia: challenges in diagnosis and management. J Indian Assoc Pediatr Surg. 2013;18(1):7.
34. Didier RA, Chow JS, Kwatra NS, Retik AB, Lebowitz RL. The duplicated collecting system of the urinary tract: embryology, imaging appearances and clinical considerations. Pediatr Radiol. 2017;47(11):1526–38.
35. Lim R. Vesicoureteral reflux and urinary tract infection: evolving practices and current controversies in Pediatric imaging. Am J Roentgenol. 2009;192(5):1197–208.
36. Horgan JG, Rosenfield NS, Weiss RM, Rosenfield AT. Is renal ultrasound a reliable indicator of a non-obstructed duplication anomaly? Pediatr Radiol. 1984;14(6):388–91.
37. Berrocal T, López-Pereira P, Arjonilla A, Gutiérrez J. Anomalies of the distal ureter, bladder, and urethra in children: embryologic, radiologic, and pathologic features. Radiographics. 2002;22(5):1139–64.
38. Dickerson EC, Dillman JR, Smith EA, DiPietro MA, Lebowitz RL, Darge K. Pediatric MR urography: indications, techniques, and approach to review. Radiographics. 2015;35(4):1208–30.
39. Gopal M, Peycelon M, Caldamone A, Chrzan R, El-Ghoneimi A, Olsen H, et al. Management of ureteropelvic junction obstruction in children—a roundtable discussion. J Pediatr Urol. 2019;15(4):322–9.
40. Nguyen HT, Benson CB, Bromley B, Campbell JB, Chow J, Coleman B, et al. Multidisciplinary consensus on the classification of prenatal and postnatal urinary tract dilation (UTD classification system). J Pediatr Urol. 2014;10(6):982–98.
41. Shokeir AA, Nijman RJM. Primary megaureter: current trends in diagnosis and treatment. BJU Int. 2000;86(7):861–8.
42. Lebowitz RL, Olbing H, Parkkulainen KV, Smellie JM, Tamminen-Möbius TE. International system of radiographic grading of vesicoureteric reflux. Pediatr Radiol. 1985;15(2):105–9.
43. Duran C, Beltrán VP, González A, Gómez C, Riego JD. Contrast-enhanced voiding Urosonography for vesicoureteral reflux diagnosis in children. Radiographics. 2017;37(6):1854–69.
44. Yapo BR, Gerges B, Holland AJA. Investigation and management of suspected urachal anomalies in children. Pediatr Surg Int. 2008;24(5):589–92.
45. Buddha S, Menias CO, Katabathina VS. Imaging of urachal anomalies. Abdom Radiol. 2019;44(12):3978–89.
46. Boechat MI, Lebowitz RL. Diverticula of the bladder in children. Pediatr Radiol. 1978;7(1):22–8.
47. Alexander RE, Kum JB, Idrees M. Bladder diverticulum: clinicopathologic spectrum in pediatric patients. Pediatr Dev Pathol. 2012;15(4):281–5.
48. Hodges SJ, Patel B, McLorie G, Atala A. Posterior urethral valves. Sci World J. 2009;9:1119–26.
49. Feinstein K, Fernbach S. Septated urinomas in the neonate. Am J Roentgenol. 1987;149(5):997–1000.
50. McConnachie DJ, Stow JL, Mallett AJ. Ciliopathies and the kidney: a review. Am J Kidney Dis. 2021;77(3):410–9.
51. Lucaya J, Enriquez G, Nieto J, Callis L, Garcia Peña P, Dominguez C. Renal calcifications in patients with autosomal recessive polycystic kidney disease: prevalence and cause. Am J Roentgenol. 1993;160(2):359–62.
52. Avni FE, Garel L, Cassart M, Massez A, Eurin D, Didier F, et al. Perinatal assessment of hereditary cystic renal diseases: the contribution of sonography. Pediatr Radiol. 2006;36(5):405–14.
53. Omran H, Ermisch-Omran B. Nephronophthisis and medullary cystic kidney disease. In: Comprehensive Pediatric nephrology. Elsevier; 2008. p. 143–53.
54. Raina R, Chakraborty R, Sethi SK, Kumar D, Gibson K, Bergmann C. Diagnosis and management of renal cystic disease of the newborn: core curriculum 2021. Am J Kidney Dis. 2021;78(1):125–41.
55. Izzi C, Dordoni C, Econimo L, Delbarba E, Grati FR, Martin E, et al. Variable expressivity of HNF1B nephropathy, from renal cysts and diabetes to medullary sponge kidney through Tubulo-interstitial kidney disease. Kidney Int Rep. 2020;5(12):2341–50.
56. Verghese P, Miyashita Y. Neonatal polycystic kidney disease. Clin Perinatol. 2014;41(3):543–60.
57. Sharada S, Vijayakumar M, Nageswaran P, Ekambaram S, Udani A. Multicystic dysplastic kidney: a retrospective study. Indian Pediatr. 2014;51(8):641–3.
58. Waingankar N, Hayek S, Smith AD, Okeke Z. Calyceal diverticula: a comprehensive review. Rev Urol. 2014;16(1):29–43.
59. Cremin BJ, Davey H, Oleszczuk-Raszke K. Neonatal renal venous thrombosis: sequential ultrasonic appearances. Clin Radiol. 1991;44(1):52–5.
60. Adelman RD. Long-term follow-up of neonatal renovascular hypertension. Pediatr Nephrol. 1987;1(1):35–41.
61. Louis R, Levy-Erez D, Cahill AM, Meyers KE. Imaging studies in pediatric fibromuscular dysplasia (FMD): a single-center experience. Pediatr Nephrol. 2018;33(9):1593–9.
62. McLaren CA, Roebuck DJ. Interventional radiology for renovascular hypertension in children. Tech VascInterv Radiol. 2003;6(4):150–7.

63. Brun P, Kchouk H, Mouchet B, Baudouin V, Raynaud A, Loirat C, et al. Value of Doppler ultrasound for the diagnosis of renal artery stenosis in children. Pediatr Nephrol. 1997;11(1):27–30.
64. Chandrasekaran A. Neonatal solid tumors. Pediatr Neonatol. 2018;59(1):65–70.
65. Gooskens SL, Houwing ME, Vujanic GM, Dome JS, Diertens T, Coulomb-l'Herminé A, et al. Congenital mesoblastic nephroma 50 years after its recognition: a narrative review. Pediatr Blood Cancer. 2017;64(7):e26437.
66. van der Beek JN, Schenk JP, Morosi C, Watson TA, Coma A, Graf N, et al. Diagnostic magnetic resonance imaging characteristics of congenital mesoblastic nephroma: a retrospective multi-center International Society of Pediatric Oncology-Renal Tumor Study Group (SIOP-RTSG) radiology panel study. Pediatr Radiol. 2024;54(6):965–76.
67. Sandberg JK, Chi YY, Smith EA, Servaes S, Hoffer FA, Mullen EA, et al. Imaging characteristics of nephrogenic rests versus small Wilms tumors: a report from the Children's Oncology Group Study AREN03B2. Am J Roentgenol. 2020;214(5):987–94.
68. Rohrschneider WK, Weirich A, Rieden K, Darge K, Tröger J, Graf N. US, CT and MR imaging characteristics of nephroblastomatosis. Pediatr Radiol. 1998;28(6):435–43.
69. Fialkowski E, Sudour-Bonnange H, Vujanic GM, Shamberger RC, Chowdhury T, Aldrink JH, et al. The varied spectrum of nephroblastomatosis, nephrogenic rests, and Wilms tumors: review of current definitions and challenges of the field. Pediatr Blood Cancer. 2023;70(S2):e30162. https://doi.org/10.1002/pbc.30162.
70. Chung EM, Graeber AR, Conran RM. Renal Tumors of childhood: radiologic-pathologic correlation part 1. The 1st decade: from the radiologic pathology archives. Radiographics. 2016;36(2):499–522.
71. Isaacs H. Fetal and neonatal renal tumors. J Pediatr Surg. 2008;43(9):1587–95.
72. Li J, Zhang W, Hu H, Zhang Y, Wang Y, Gu H, et al. Case analysis of 14 children with malignant Rhabdoid tumor of the kidney. Cancer Manag Res. 2021;13:4865–72.
73. Tomlinson GE, Breslow NE, Dome J, Guthrie KA, Norkool P, Li S, et al. Rhabdoid tumor of the kidney in the National Wilms' tumor study: age at diagnosis as a prognostic factor. J Clin Oncol. 2005;23(30):7641–5.

Neonatal Genital Tract

10

Deeksha Bhalla and Ravikumar Hanumaiah

10.1 Introduction

Ultrasonography (US) forms the mainstay of imaging in neonates for most abdominal and pelvic pathology. It is particularly suitable for imaging of the reproductive organs for many reasons, the foremost being small and superficial organs that are easily identified on US. Further, there is also the possibility of dynamic evaluation, which is important in babies with conditions such as retractile testis and its differentiation from truly undescended testis. In addition, it also allows for Doppler evaluation, which is also valuable in suspected torsion and differentiation of mass lesions. The advent of transperineal sonography has allowed the evaluation of anomalies of the lower genitalia including the urethra and vagina, as well as fistulae and common channels in children with ambiguous genitalia. This chapter will discuss the technique of genital sonography in neonates, normal imaging appearance as well as common pathology that may be encountered in this age group.

10.2 Scanning Technique

Due to the small body size of neonates, linear high-resolution probes are ideal for evaluation. The frequency of the probe may range from 5 to 12 MHz, and in specialized systems may reach up to 17 or 20 MHz. A smaller footprint probe is preferred for ease of examination.

10.2.1 Transabdominal

The baby lies supine and US probe is placed cranial to the pubic symphysis. Scanning is performed in two planes, the transverse plane where the probe is placed perpendicular to the *Z* axis of the baby, and the longitudinal plane, where it is placed parallel to the *Z* axis.

In girls, the transabdominal plane is the mainstay, for identification of the uterus size and contour as well as the ovaries.

In boys, the transabdominal plane is used in babies with testis not palpable in the scrotum, to localize undescended or ectopic testis.

10.2.2 Transperineal

This technique refers to direct perineal visualization by US. The baby is made to lie in modified lithotomy position with knees flexed. Sequential scanning is performed in boys. First, the probe is placed over the scrotal sac and both testis and

D. Bhalla (✉)
Postgraduate Institute of Child Health, Noida, India

R. Hanumaiah
Pediatric Radiology, SUNY Upstate Medical University, Syracuse, NY, USA

K. S. Sodhi (ed.), *Neonatal Ultrasound*, https://doi.org/10.1007/978-981-97-8576-6_10

epididymal heads are identified. The spermatic cord is then followed retrograde till the inguinal region. Next, the probe is placed posterior to the scrotal sac for visualization of the posterior urethra and any fistulae in children with ambiguous genitalia.

In girls, the probe is placed overlying the labia. This allows identification of the urethra as well as the vagina and any abnormal communication between the two.

10.3 Normal Anatomy

10.3.1 Boys

Testicular length has been reported in several series and ranges from 1 to 1.8 cm on the right and from 1.3 to 1.7 cm on the left. The testicular breadth is ~1 cm (±0.15 cm) for both [1, 2]. No significant difference has been reported between the size of right and left testis.

The mean testicular volume is 0.6 ± 0.2 ml [3] (Fig. 10.1). Positive correlation of testicular dimensions is seen with baby length and weight.

On imaging of the perineum, the urethra is seen as a thin hypoechoic line posterior to the pubic symphysis and within the corpus spongiosum of the penis (Fig. 10.2).

10.3.2 Girls

The neonatal uterus is under influence of residual maternal hormones, and therefore is larger in size than the prepubertal uterus. The mean uterine length in studies is reported to be ~4.2 cm (±0.6 cm), and similar to the male genitalia, shows positive correlation with baby birth weight. The mean AP diameter of the fundus is ~1.5 cm (±0.2 cm). The length is between 0.5 and 1 cm longer than the prepubertal uterus, and the AP dimension is also approximately double that seen in older children [4]. The endometrium is identified as a central, thin echogenic line (Fig. 10.3). Hypoechoic myometrial halo may also be identified in some babies. The ratio between the cervical and fundal length is usually 1:1, but cervix may be longer and the ratio may reach 2:1.

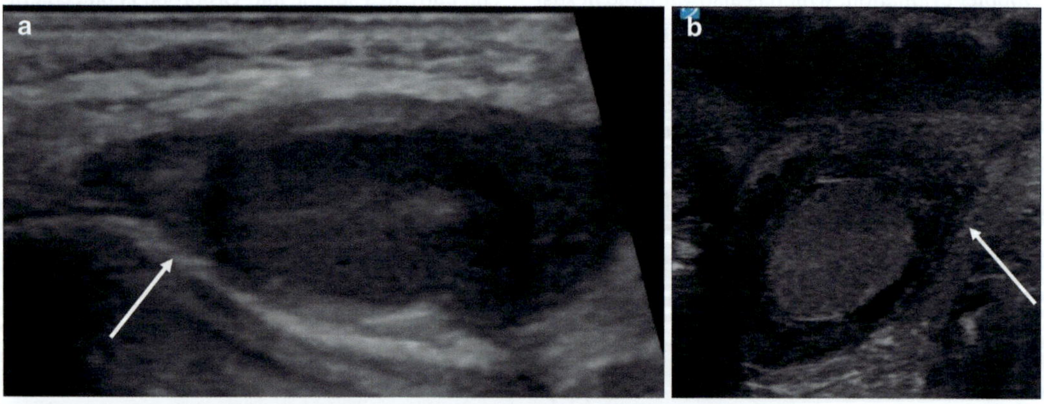

Fig. 10.1 Normal testicular appearance in a 20-day neonate. Longitudinal scan (**a**) and transverse scan (**b**). The epididymis (white arrow) is seen as a curved hypoechoic structure cranial to the testis

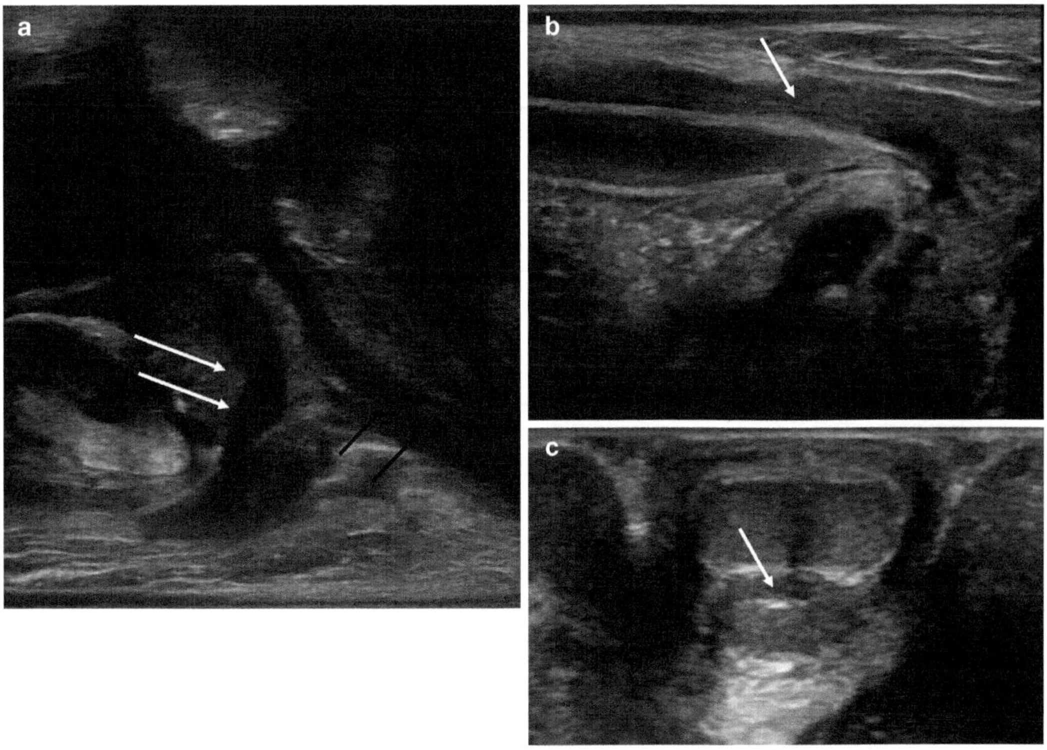

Fig. 10.2 Normal perineal anatomy in a boy. (**a**) Transperineal scan showing the bladder neck and urethra (white arrow) as well as hypoechoic muscular wall of the anal canal (black arrow). (**b**, **c**) Longitudinal (**b**) and transverse (**c**) scan of the penile shaft shows the superior corpora cavernosa and the inferior corpus spongiosum with the echogenic urethra (arrow)

Similar to the uterus, the ovaries are also larger in the first few months of life due to the high follicle-stimulating hormone levels in neonates. This leads to a multicystic appearance of the ovary with multiple follicles (Fig. 10.4). The mean ovarian volume has been reported ~0.8 cc; however, there is high variability due to the varying influence of gonadotropins. The 95% confidence interval is between 0.3 and 2.2 cc [5].

On transperineal sonography, the urethra and vagina are identified separately as thin hypoechoic lines posterior to the pubic symphysis with echogenic interface between them (Fig. 10.5). These have separate openings in the perineum.

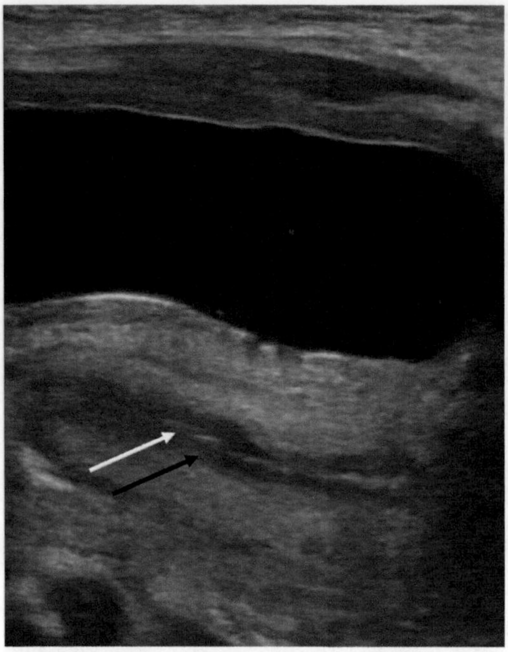

Fig. 10.3 Normal neonatal uterus. A well-defined echogenic endometrial stripe is seen (white arrow) along with a hypoechoic myometrial halo (arrow)

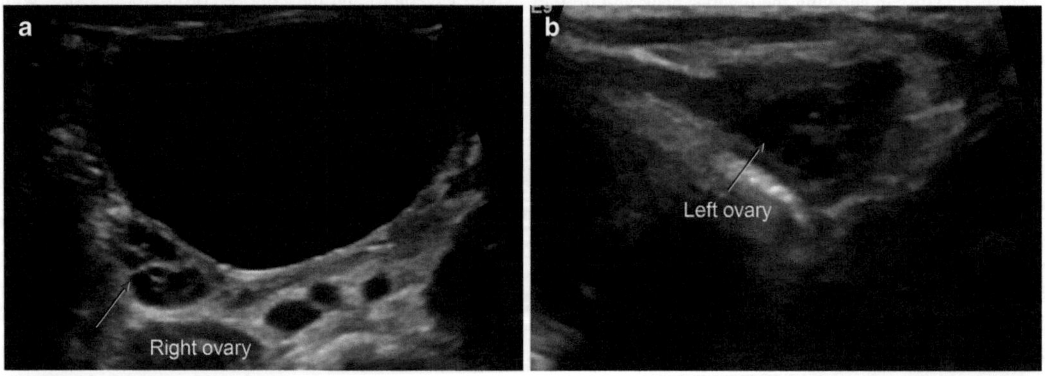

Fig. 10.4 Normal ovarian appearance in a 20-day neonate (**a**, **b**). There are multiple follicles in both ovaries (arrows)

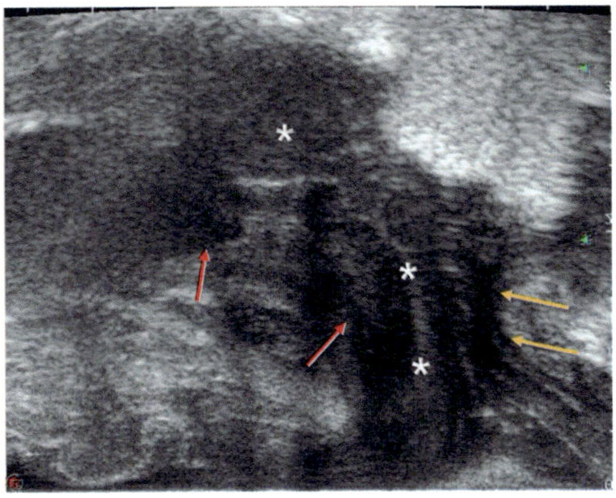

Fig. 10.5 Normal perineal anatomy in a girl. On the longitudinal scan, three tracts are seen, anteriorly is the bladder and urethra (red arrow), followed by the uterus and vagina (*) with an echogenic interface between them. The anal canal is most posterior, which is wide with a thick muscular wall (yellow arrow). All three have separate perineal openings

Table 10.1 Spectrum of congenital anomalies in boys

Organ of origin	Anomaly
Boys	
Testicular	Cryptorchidism Polyorchidism Torsion Microlithiasis Adrenal rests Neoplasms
Extratesticular	Scrotal hematoma Hydrocele Inguinal hernia
Ambiguous genitalia	Hypospadias, Mullerian remnants

10.4 Congenital Anomalies in Boys

There is a myriad of congenital anomalies that can be seen in the reproductive organs of boys, including the gonads as well as other structures such as the scrotal skin or inguinal canal. An organwise distribution is described in Table 10.1.

10.4.1 Congenital Anomalies in Boys: Testicular

10.4.1.1 Cryptorchidism

Cryptorchidism or undescended testis refers to abnormally located testes, which may be found anywhere along its path of descent from the upper scrotum to the lower pole of the kidney. The inguinal canal is the most common location for an undescended testis, seen in 80% of children. A related condition is ectopic testis, where the testis is located away from its path of usual descent. The common locations for an ectopic testis are in the femoral canal, at the superficial inguinal ring or in the perineum. Testes which are located outside of the scrotum are prone to several complications, the chief of these being decreased fertility due to high temperature for spermatogenesis. Other complications such as testicular torsion as well as malignancy are also higher in undescended testis. For localization of the testis, it is recommended to track the spermatic cord [6]. When it is identified in the inguinal region, it suggests an extra-abdominal testis. In case it is not identified, the common femoral vessels are traced up to the common iliac vessels to look for the testis along the course of the vessels. If still not identified, a thorough search of the pelvis and iliac region must be undertaken. In case the testis can be pulled down to the scrotum, orchidopexy is performed. In other, orchidectomy is performed due to risk of malignancy. A related condition is retractile testis, which occurs due to a hyperactive cremasteric reflex. These are normally descended testis, which move back and forth between scrotum and inguinal region, in response to stimuli such as touch (Fig. 10.6). These are not predisposed to complications like undescended testis and usually resolve by puberty.

10.4.1.2 Polyorchidism

Polyorchidism, or supernumerary testicle is labeled when more than two testes are present. The most common encountered form is one extra testicle, or triorchidism [7]. This is a rare anomaly and occurs due to defective embryogenesis causing the genital ridge to divide into two parts. The third testicle is most commonly left sided and usually smaller in size. Similar to the normal testis, the extra testicle may be orthotopic and ectopic and develop complications such as tor-

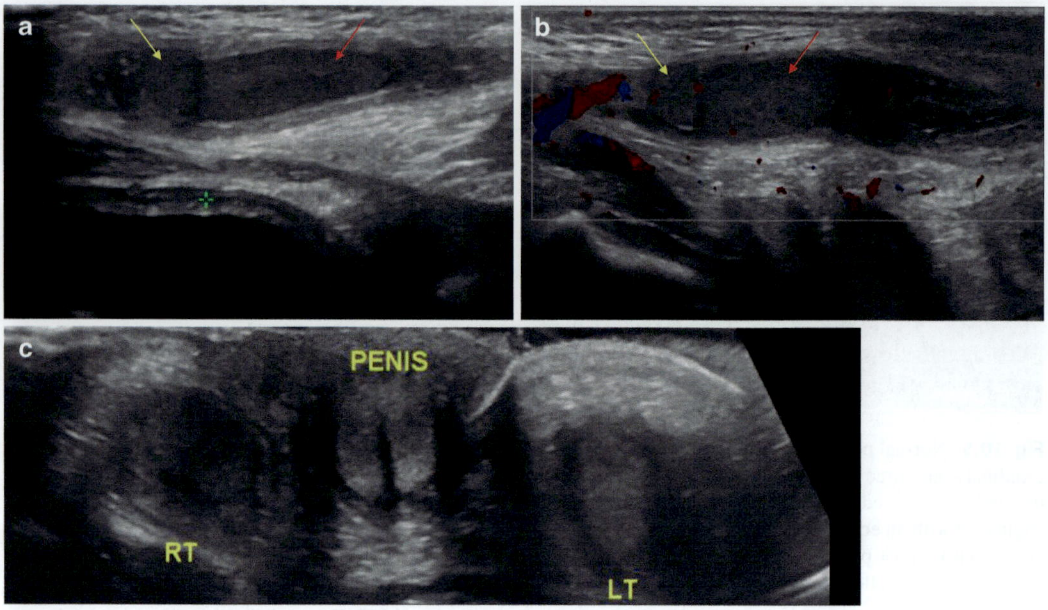

Fig. 10.6 Ultrasound images of the bilateral inguinal canals and scrotum in a 7-day neonate. Gray scale longitudinal ultrasound image of the left testis (**a**) and color Doppler image of the right testis (**b**) demonstrate the bilateral testicles (red arrows) in the inguinal canals. The epididymis appears normal bilaterally (yellow arrows). The testicles were seen to move into the scrotal sac (**c**) during the scan consistent with retractile testis. Undescended testis can have a similar appearance; however, the testis will never move into the scrotal sac

sion. In the absence of complications, prophylactic removal of orthotopic extra testicle is not indicated.

10.4.1.3 Testicular Torsion

The mechanism for testicular torsion varies among neonates and older children. In older children, an "intravaginal" torsion is seen due to abnormally high attachment of the tunica on to the spermatic cord, which allows rotation of the spermatic cord along with the testis within the tunica, compromising the blood supply.

In neonates on the other hand, the gubernaculum testis, which anchors the tunica to the scrotal wall is often underdeveloped [8]. This allows an "extravaginal" type of torsion. The tunica itself, along with its contents, twists around the spermatic cord axis (Fig. 10.7). This is rarely seen beyond 3 months of age.

The appearance of testicular torsion varies with age of the torsion. In the first few hours, the testicle appears swollen and shows reduced echogenicity due to venous edema. Absent flow on color Doppler is characteristic. As it progresses to infarction, the testis shrinks in size and becomes hyperechoic with peripheral calcification. In a chronic testicular infarct, the testis is atrophic.

10.4.1.4 Testicular Microlithiasis

Testicular microlithiasis (TM) refers to deposition of tiny calcific foci in the seminiferous tubules. Based on criteria by the European Society of Urogenital Radiology, a minimum of five microcalcifications must be seen in a single ultrasound field [9] (Fig. 10.8). There are multiple conditions associated with microlithiasis such as Klinefelter syndrome, Down's syndrome, Fragile X syndrome, and McCune Albright syndrome. It is also often associated with infertility and testicular atrophy. There has been a concern of malignancy risk in these patients and they are often kept under surveillance. Based on the ESUR guidelines, surveillance is not routinely recommended unless TM is associated with risk factors. The risk factors include an undescended or ectopic testis, testicular atrophy (testicular volume < 12 ml) and history of germ cell tumor in a

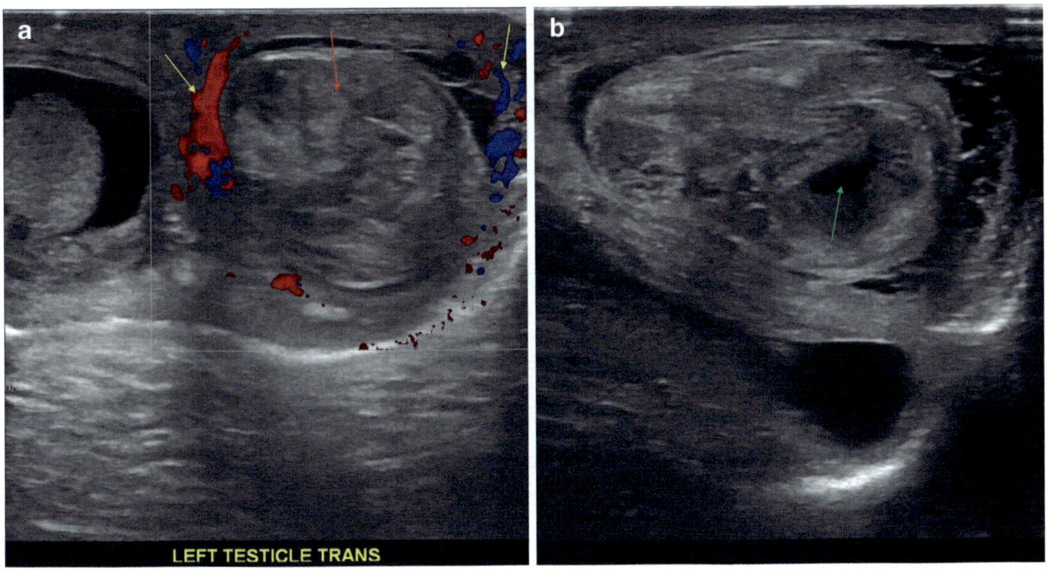

Fig. 10.7 Ultrasound images of the left scrotum in a 4-day neonate with left scrotal swelling since birth. Transverse color Doppler image (**a**) and gray scale ultrasound image of the left scrotum (**b**) demonstrate enlarged left testis with heterogeneous echotexture (red arrow) and lack of vascular flow consistent with testicular torsion. Reactive hyperemia is seen in the scrotal wall (yellow arrow). A hypoechoic area within the testis represents necrosis (green arrow). At surgery, extravaginal torsion was diagnosed; left orchiectomy and right orchiopexy were performed

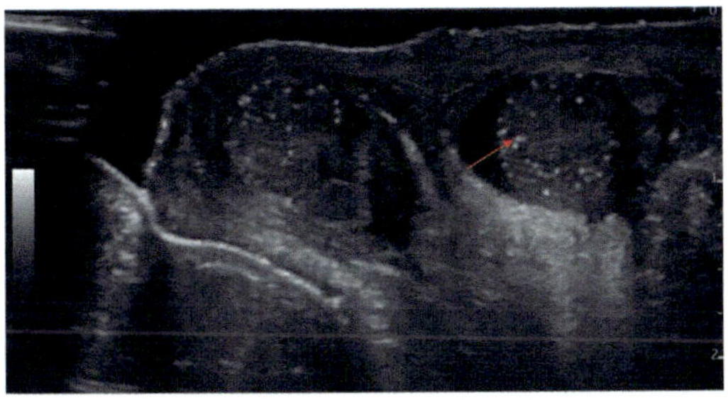

Fig. 10.8 Ultrasound images of the scrotum in a 38-day-old baby. Gray scale transverse ultrasound image of the scrotum demonstrate multiple tiny echogenic foci (red arrow) in the bilateral testicles suggestive of microlithiasis

first-degree relative. In these patients, annual surveillance by US must be performed. In children with Klinefelter syndrome, follow-up US must be performed at 6 months and 12 months for assessment of testicular nodules.

10.4.1.5 Adrenal Rests

Adrenal rests, or testicular adrenal rest tumors (TART) are seen in ~10% of neonates. These are benign, and usually asymptomatic, but can enlarge under adrenocorticotropic hormone to form masses. These occur secondary to trapped adrenal tissue in the testis during development. Adrenal rests are often associated with congenital adrenal hyperplasia and show bilateral involvement. Irregular hypoechoic areas are seen on sonography which are well vascularized on color Doppler [10]. The latter helps to differentiate them from segmental infarcts, which show lack of color flow.

10.4.1.6 Testicular Neoplasms

Testicular neoplasms are rare in the pediatric population, and even more so in neonates. These are of two histological types, germ cell tumors and sex cord stromal tumors. In the neonatal population, germ cell tumors are by far the more common. The most common among these are teratomas and yolk sac tumors though their usual age of presentation is in older infants (18–24 months old) [11]. Heterogeneous discrete masses in the testis are seen, which may occasionally replace the entire testis. In terato-

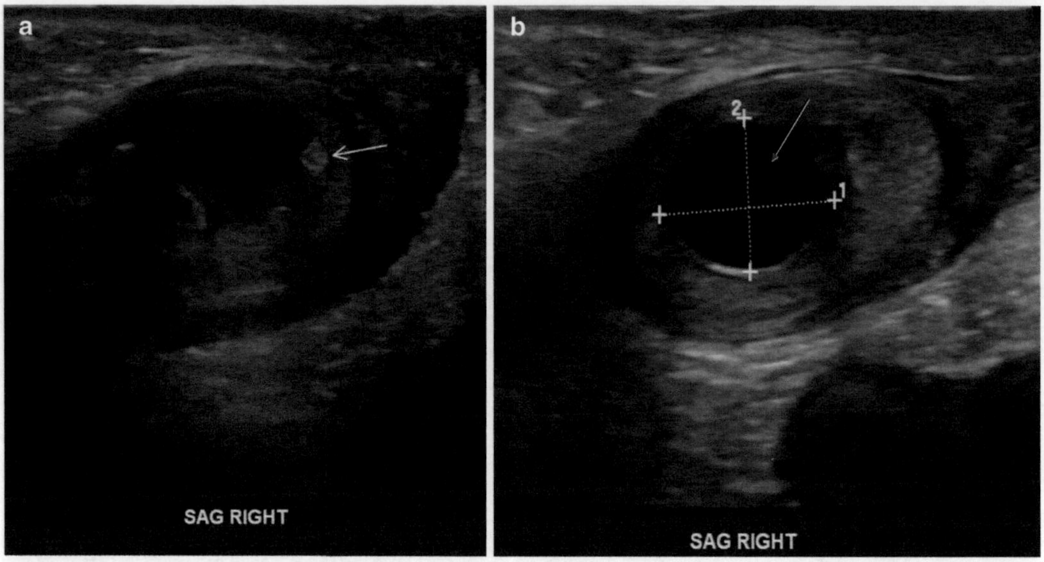

Fig. 10.9 Ultrasound images of the right scrotum in a 24-day neonate. Gray scale longitudinal ultrasound images of the right testis (**a**, **b**) demonstrate a complex cystic lesion (red arrow) with echogenic nodules at the periphery (green arrow). A partial orchiectomy was performed at 6 months, and the lesion was diagnosed as benign mature teratoma on histopathology

mas, fat and calcification are present which are seen as echogenic foci without and with posterior shadowing, respectively (Fig. 10.9). The solid component of the mass is usually hypervascular on color Doppler. Occasionally, they may be seen as cysts with septa, wherein the septa also show vascularity on color Doppler. This helps to differentiate it from other conditions such as cystic dysplasia of testis, which are avascular on Doppler.

10.4.2 Congenital Anomalies in Boys: Extratesticular

10.4.2.1 Scrotal Hydrocele

Hydrocele refers to fluid collection between the testis and the tunica vaginalis. It may be simple or complex. Simple refers to an uncomplicated, anechoic fluid collection (Fig. 10.10). Complex hydroceles are collections which have echogenic content due to either blood (hematocele) or pus (pyocele) (Fig. 10.11). These are seen secondary to scrotal trauma or infection. Hydroceles may be classified as communicating or noncommunicating (Fig. 10.12). Often in infants, hydroceles are seen due to failure of involution of the processus vaginalis, which is an outpouching from the peritoneum and descends along with the gubernaculum testis into the scrotum. This outpouching is sealed off and forms the tunica in its distal part. Varying manifestations are seen with failure of involution, which are summarized in Table 10.2 [12].

10.4.2.2 Inguinal Hernia

Similar to communicating hydroceles, inguinal hernias are seen in neonates with a patent processus vaginalis due to herniation of bowel loops into the sac. The incidence in boys is nearly ten times that of girls. Further, prematurity is another risk factor, inguinal hernia is seen in ~30% of babies below 1 kg birth weight. Since the left testicle descends earlier, hernias on the left side are infrequently seen (25%) compared to the right (75%). Bilateral hernia may be seen in up to 15% patients [13].

On US, herniation of bowel loops into the inguinal region and the scrotum is seen. Upright position may be used for scanning in case the abnormality is not visible in supine position.

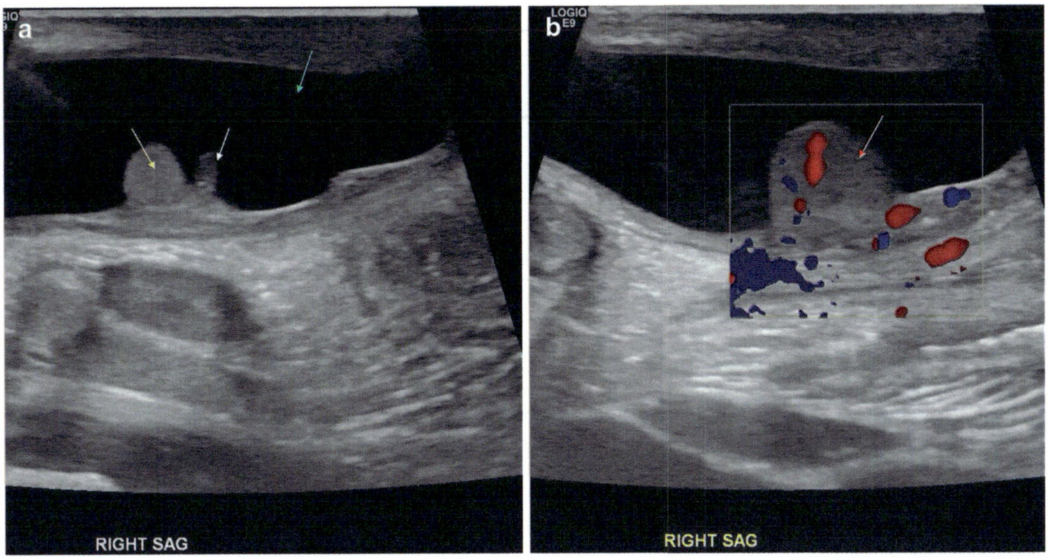

Fig. 10.10 Ultrasound images of the right scrotum in a 14-day neonate with right scrotal swelling. Gray scale ultrasound image of the right scrotum (**a**) and color Doppler image of the right scrotum (**b**) demonstrate fluid around the testis (red arrow) and the epididymis (yellow arrow) suggestive of hydrocele (green arrow). Appendix epididymis is noted (white arrow)

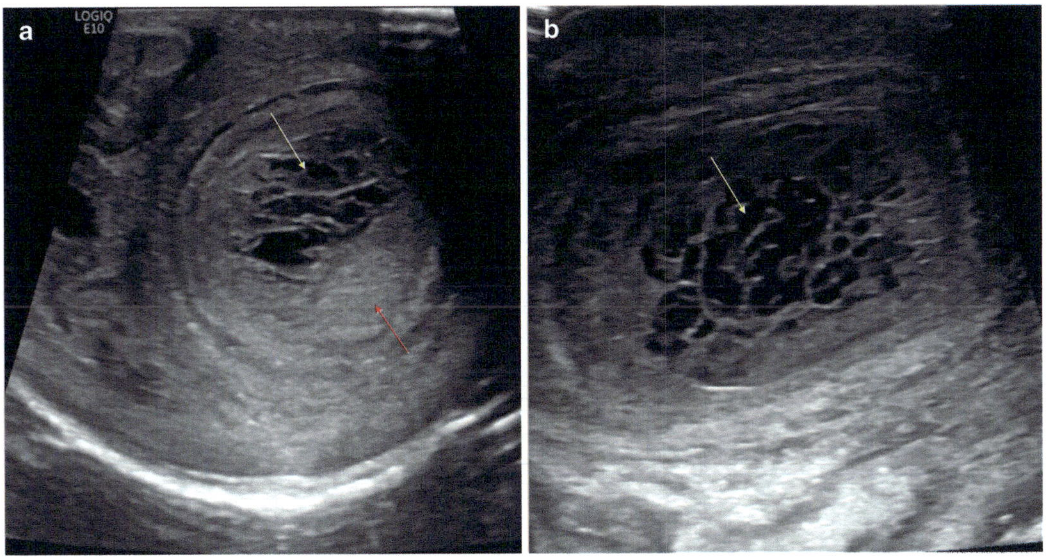

Fig. 10.11 Ultrasound images of the left scrotum in a 3-week-old neonate with left scrotal swelling and discoloration. Gray scale transverse ultrasound images (**a**, **b**) demonstrate a complex fluid collection with internal septations (yellow arrow) indicating complex hydrocele. The left testis is displaced posteriorly (red arrow). Bilateral scrotal exploration and drainage of complex left hydrocele and irrigation with antibiotic solution was performed

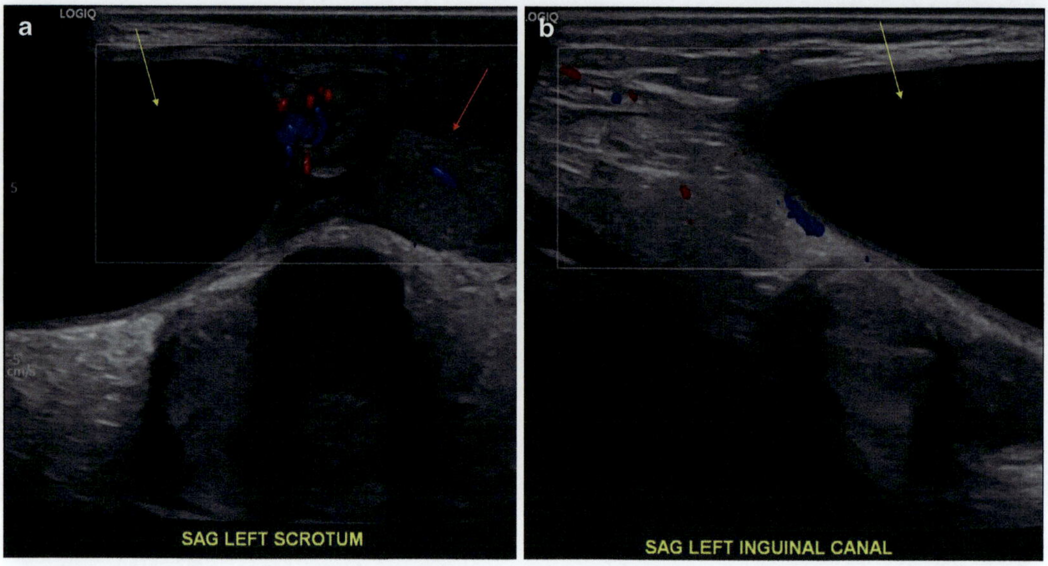

Fig. 10.12 Ultrasound images of the left scrotum in a 46-day-old baby with history of left inguinal hernia. Color Doppler longitudinal ultrasound image of the left scrotum (**a**) and inguinal canal (**b**) demonstrate a well-defined fluid collection (yellow arrow) in the left inguinal canal extending up to the superior aspect of left testis (red arrow), suggestive of encysted spermatic cord hydrocele

Table 10.2 Types of hydrocele based on embryological origin

	Communicating	Noncommunicating
Etiology	Entire processes vaginalis remains patent	Part of the processus vaginalis fails to involute Two types: Funicular: When proximal peritoneal communication remains patent Encysted: Middle part fails to involute, no peritoneal communication
Peritoneal communication	Present	Present in funicular, absent in encysted
Extension	From the peritoneal cavity till the scrotum	Funicular: Inguinal region, does not extend till scrotum Encysted: Between deep inguinal ring and scrotum along spermatic cord
Reducible	Yes	Funicular: yes Encysted: no
Treatment	Often resolve spontaneously	May resolve, surgery if persistent >12 months of age

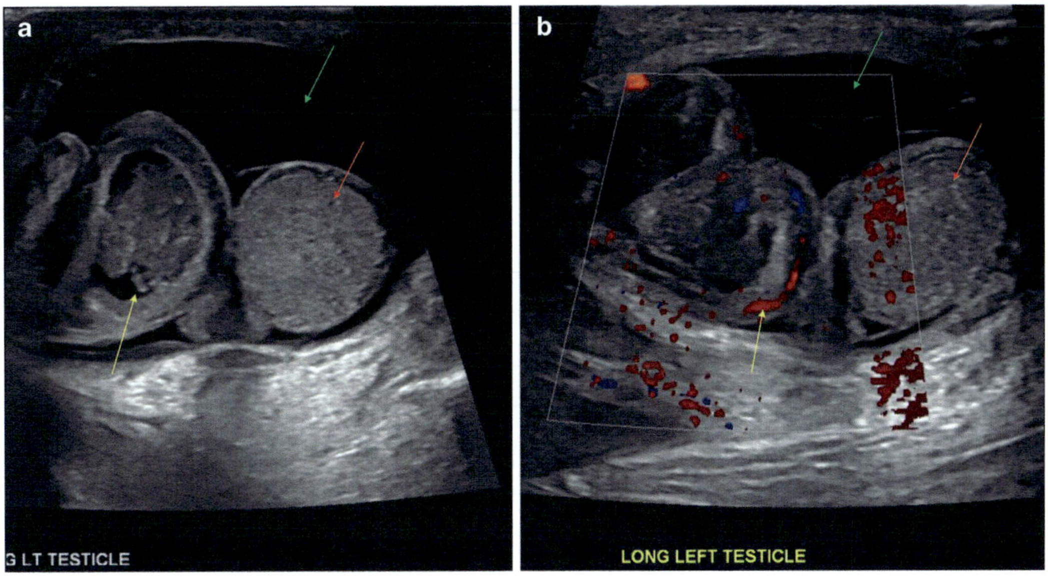

Fig. 10.13 Ultrasound images of the left scrotum in a 23-day neonate with history of left scrotal swelling. Gray scale longitudinal ultrasound image (**a**) and color Doppler longitudinal image (**b**) of the left scrotum demonstrate a bowel loop with intact vascular flow (yellow arrow) in the left scrotum extending up to the superior aspect of testis (red arrow), consistent with inguinal hernia. Fluid is also seen in the left scrotum (green arrow). At surgery, an incarcerated left indirect inguinal hernia was diagnosed, and hernia repair was performed

Elective repair may be performed in hernias that do not present with acute symptoms.

In infants however, there is a ~30% risk of incarceration, and thus timing of repair, immediate, or elective is controversial.

Complicated hernias may be incarcerated or strangulated (Fig. 10.13). These usually present with erythematous, tender swelling, and signs such as fever or leucocytosis. An incarcerated hernia means one that is not reducible; this may progress to a strangulated hernia, where the blood supply to the bowel loops is disrupted. Incarcerated bowel loops are thickened and edematous, peristalsis may be reduced with free fluid in the hernia sac. Color flow is typically preserved. In strangulated hernias on the other hand, an a-peristaltic, dilated loop is usually seen with absent flow on color Doppler [14]. Bowel obstruction, mural necrosis, and perforation are seen in complicated hernias, and therefore these warrant urgent repair.

10.4.2.3 Scrotal Hematoma

Scrotal hematomas may be seen in neonates in the setting of birth trauma, coagulopathy, or sepsis. Like hematomas elsewhere, it presents with thickening of the scrotal wall or extratesticular soft tissue showing raised echogenicity. There is evolution of the echogenicity with time, the hematoma becomes progressively hypoechoic. It may be associated with a hematocele, or even intrastesticular hematomas. Intratesticular hematomas appear as echogenic lesions within the testis and can be differentiated from tumors based on the absence of color flow [15].

10.4.3 Congenital Anomalies in Boys: Others

10.4.3.1 Ambiguous Genitalia

Ambiguous genitalia in boys include underdeveloped penile shaft, referred to as micropenis along with an ectopic urethral opening, hypospadias or epispadias. A detailed discussion of disorders of sex differentiation is beyond the scope of this chapter, but an effort must be made to scan the urethra and look for mullerian remnants including prostatic utricle or even a fully developed uterus in children with ambiguous genitalia [16, 17]. Mullerian remnants present as central midline projections from the urethra.

Table 10.3 Spectrum of congenital anomalies in girls

Organ of origin	Anomaly
Girls	
Uterine	Lateral fusion fault Vertical fusion fault
Ovarian	Cysts Torsion Neoplasms
Others	Urogenital sinus Cloacal malformation

10.5 Congenital Anomalies in Girls

The spectrum of congenital abnormalities in girls ranges from anomalies of uterine development, to ovarian lesions and defects in development of the urethra and vagina. These are listed in Table 10.3.

10.5.1 Congenital Anomalies in Girls: Uterine

10.5.1.1 Mullerian Anomalies

Mullerian anomalies occur secondary to developmental abnormality in the Mullers ducts, which form the fallopian tubes, uterus, and the upper two thirds of the vagina. While Mullerian anomalies often present around the pubertal period or even later in adult life with reproductive problems, few can present in the neonatal period due to vaginal or cervical obstruction and large hydrocolpos. These are of two types:

(a) Lateral fusion fault:

Common among these is uterus didelphys with obstructed hemivagina which occurs due to failure of lateral fusion of the two ducts (Fig. 10.14). Two separate uterine cavities are noted with a longitudinal vaginal septum. A large anechoic fluid-filled cavity may be seen in case of obstruction of one of the vaginal cavities.

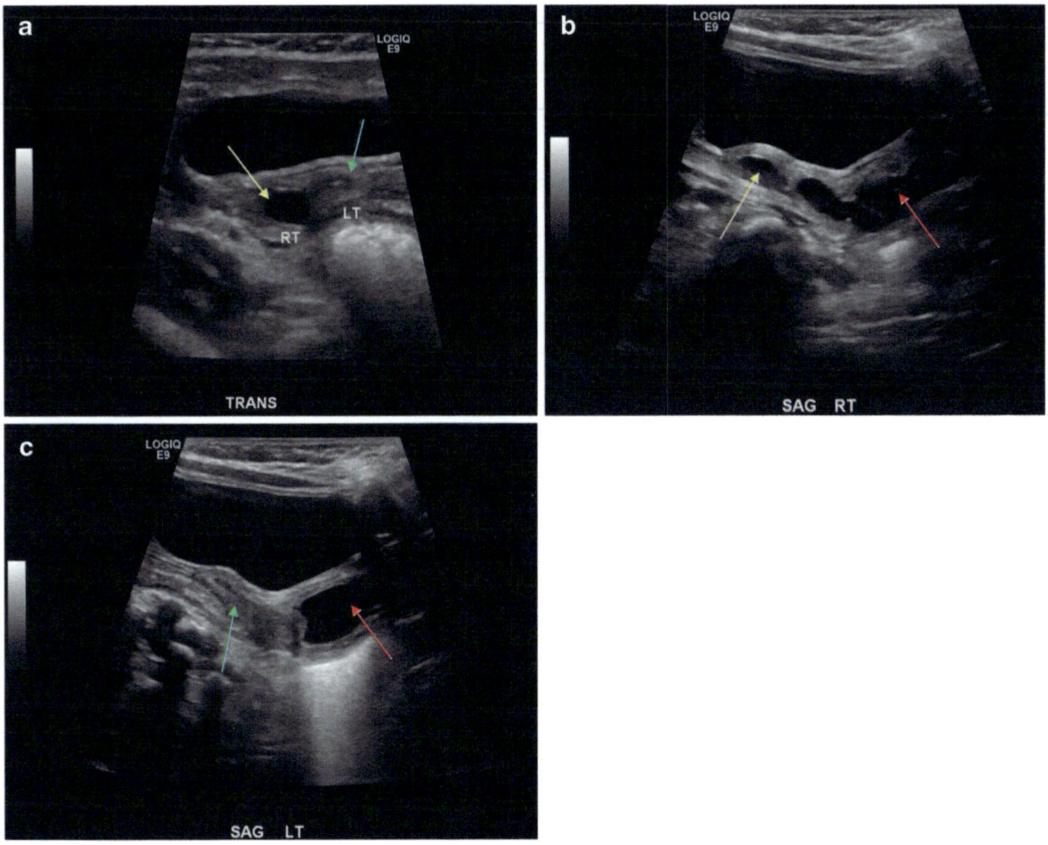

Fig. 10.14 Ultrasound images of the pelvis in a 43 days old baby. Gray scale transverse ultrasound image (**a**) demonstrates uterus didelphys with fluid in the right horn (yellow arrow). Longitudinal ultrasound image (**b**) shows fluid in the vagina (red arrow) and the endometrial cavity of right horn of uterus (yellow arrow). Longitudinal ultrasound image (**c**) demonstrates the left horn of uterus (green arrow) and fluid-filled vagina (red arrow). Findings are suggestive of vaginal septum with hydrometrocolpos of right mullerian structures. Resection of the vaginal septum was performed at 8 months

(b) Vertical fusion fault:

In cases with vertical fusion anomalies, such as distal vaginal atresia or vaginal septum, similar obstructive pathology may be seen. Single uterine cavity is seen with hydrometra as well as dilatation of the cervix and vagina with fluid or mucus.

10.5.2 Congenital Anomalies in Girls: Ovarian

10.5.2.1 Ovarian Cysts

Due to the influence of maternal hormones, many ovaries may develop cysts during the fetal period. These can be seen during the neonatal period, as simple thin-walled, anechoic cysts which are unilocular (Fig. 10.15). Since these represent functional cysts that have formed under hormonal influence, these undergo gradual regression after birth. However, some cysts, particularly those that are large in size (>5 cm) are prone to develop complications such as torsion and intracystic hemorrhage. Management of these cysts is controversial, while most may advocate a conservative, wait-and-watch approach, some advocate early surgery in large cysts due to risk of torsion, in order to preserve the ipsilateral ovary [18].

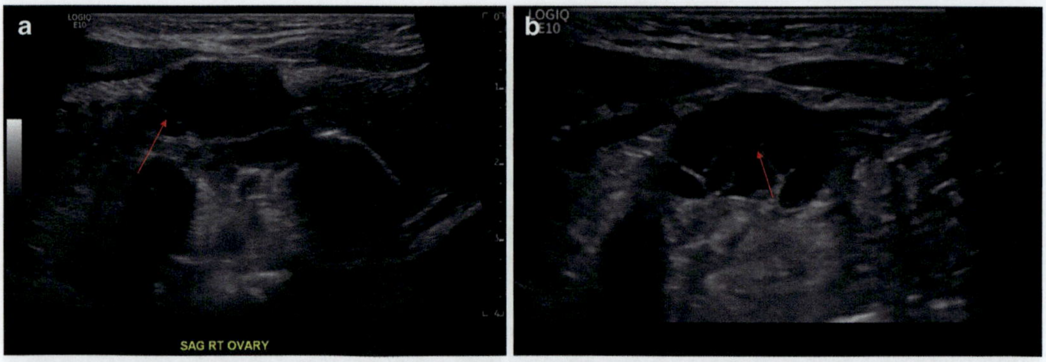

Fig. 10.15 Ultrasound images of the pelvis in a 20-day neonate. Gray scale longitudinal (**a**) and transverse (**b**) ultrasound images demonstrate the right ovary with multiple follicles and one cyst (red arrow)

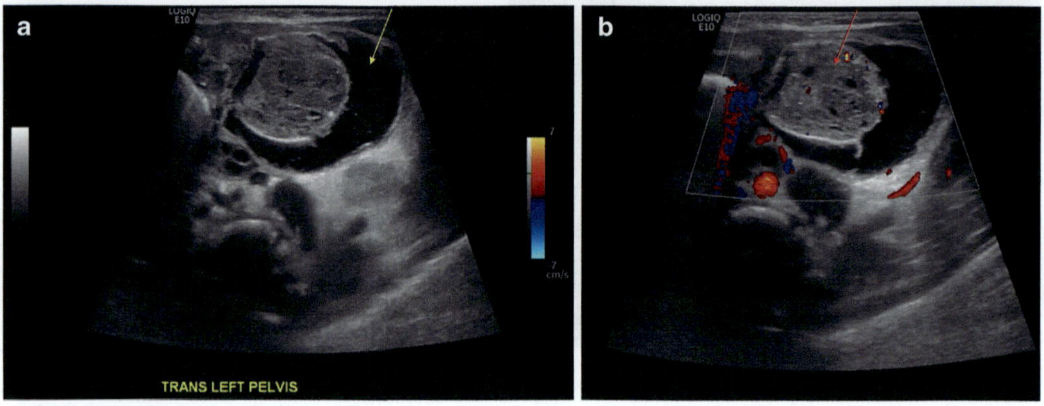

Fig. 10.16 Ultrasound images of the pelvis in a 3-week-old neonate with pelvic mass seen on antenatal scan. Gray scale transverse ultrasound image (**a**) and color Doppler image (**b**) of the pelvis demonstrates a complex mass with cystic (yellow arrow) and echogenic solid components (red arrow) without significant vascularity, suggestive of in utero ovarian torsion. The right ovary was not separately visualized. Surgery confirmed ovarian torsion

10.5.2.2 Ovarian Torsion

As described previously, ovarian torsion in neonates is most frequently seen in association with ovarian cysts. Rather, some patients may undergo in utero torsion that is detected on postnatal sonography (Fig. 10.16). Ovarian torsion should be suspected when there is change in character of the cysts from simple to complex, that is, new development of intracystic debris or septae within the cyst [19], which are mostly secondary to intracystic hemorrhage (Fig. 10.17). Not just development of complexity, but also a decrease in size of the cyst if associated with increased echogenicity or calcification indicates that torsion has occurred in the ovary. In many patients, auto-amputated ovaries are found in the peritoneal cavity since ovarian torsion in babies is not easily suspected or recognized, unlike in older children. Thus, a high index of suspicion should be kept in children with ovarian cysts, any complexity in the cyst, change in character, or change in position from previous examinations should raise the alarm for possibility of torsion. Color Doppler may sometimes be used as an adjunct for diagnosis of ovarian torsion though the classical signs seen in older children are often not seen in this age group [20]. Reduced venous flow is usually seen first, followed by compromise of arterial inflow as well, secondary to edema. In advanced cases, flow into the affected ovary will be absent. However, it has been reported that peripheral vascularity may be

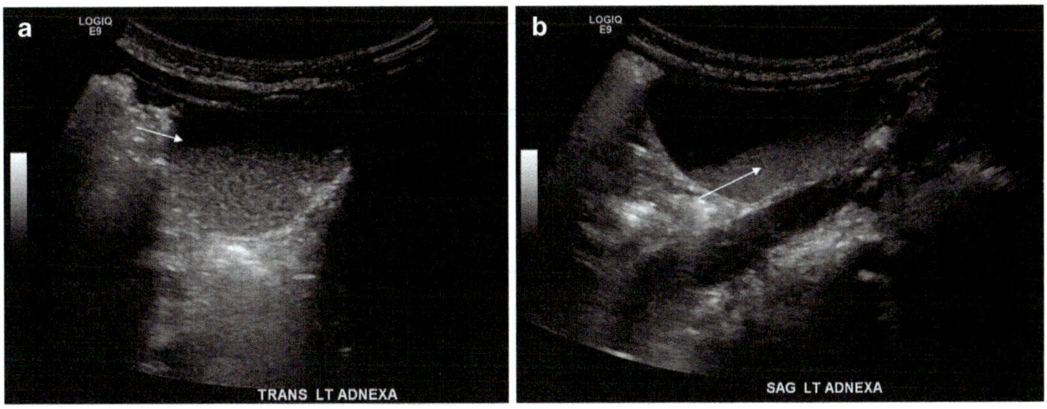

Fig. 10.17 Ultrasound images of the pelvis in a 27-day neonate. Gray scale transverse ultrasound image (**a**) and color Doppler image (**b**) of the pelvis demonstrates a complex cyst (arrow) with layering echogenic debris (arrow), representing left ovarian hemorrhagic cyst/infarcted ovary. The left ovary was not separately visualized. On the subsequent follow-up ultrasound after 3 months, this complex cyst disappeared, and the left ovary was not visualized. Findings consistent with in utero left ovarian torsion

seen in walls of cysts in neonates with chronic torsion due to neovascularization in the wall. Thus, the reliability of Doppler for diagnosis remains low.

10.5.2.3 Ovarian Neoplasms

Ovarian neoplasms are rare in the neonatal age group. In studies performed on pathological correlation of surgically resected ovarian cysts, no tumors were found [21]. In fact, contrary to testicular neoplasms, ovarian teratomas are also not found in the neonatal age group. Thus, the risk of malignancy is exceedingly rare and is generally not a consideration, even when dealing with complex cysts in this age group.

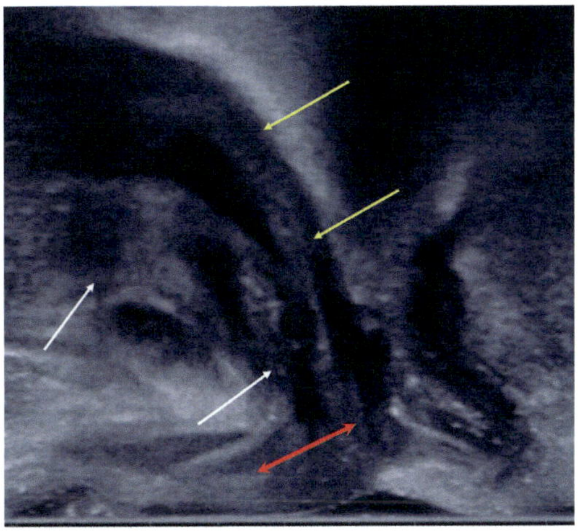

Fig. 10.18 Transperineal sonography in persistent urogenital sinus. The bladder neck and urethra seen anteriorly, and the vaginal canal seen posteriorly (white arrows) are seen opening into a short common channel (double arrow)

10.5.3 Congenital Anomalies in Girls: Others

10.5.3.1 Ambiguous Genitalia

Ambiguous genitalia may be in the form of clitoromegaly that resembles a small penile shaft, or labial fusion. In normal development of the distal genitourinary tract, the mullerian ducts join the urogenital sinus. Subsequently, the vaginal plate forms at the point of joining of mullerian ducts. The urogenital sinus then everts to form the vestibule, and vaginal plate canalizes to form the distal vagina, leading to separate urethral and vaginal canals [22]. Persistent urogenital sinus is seen in case of defects in this process. In case of early stage defects, there will be a short vagina, point of union will be close to the bladder neck and a long common channel is seen. In children with late defects, the point of union is distal and a short common channel is present (Fig. 10.18). On transperineal sonography, the length of the common channel must be measured and conveyed to surgeons for adequate surgical planning [23].

10.5.3.2 Common Cloaca

During the first 6 weeks of gestation, both the primitive hindgut and the primitive urogenital sinus enter into the cloaca. At around the seventh week of gestation, the urorectal membrane divides the cloaca into two parts, the ventral urogenital sinus and the dorsal anal canal. Defect in this cleavage leads to a common cloaca, which is considered the most complex anorectal malformation, and is seen exclusively in girls. There is a single perineal opening, which is the common tract for the gastrointestinal as well as urogenital system. Similar to a persistent urogenital sinus, the foremost role of the radiologist is to define the length of the common tract since that is an important determinant of prognosis [24]. Transperineal US is an important tool, which helps define the distal anal and urogenital tracts. In these patients, the anal canal musculature is often poorly developed and thus it resembles the genitourinary tract with thin walls, rather than the thick hypoechoic muscular wall that is usually identified [25].

10.6 Conclusion

Genital pathology in neonates is a unique spectrum which varies from that in older children. There is a myriad of congenital malformations, as well as their associated complications that are predominant in this age group. It is important for radiologists to be aware of anatomical differences from older children; and perform organ-based localization of pathology in order to provide accurate differential diagnosis and requisite information to treating clinicians.

References

1. Vasudevan G, Manivarmane, Bhat BV, Bhatia BD, Kumar S. Genital standards for south Indian male newborns. Indian J Pediatr. 1995;62(5):593–6. https://doi.org/10.1007/BF02761887.
2. Hagag AA, Erfan AA, Elrifaey SM, Gamal RM, Harakan AI. Penile and testicular measurements in male neonates and infants: Single Center Egyptian Study. Endocr Metab Immune Disord Drug Targets. 2017;17(4):309–16. https://doi.org/10.2174/1871530317666170912152351.
3. Mondal R, Ray S, Chatterjee K, et al. Penile length and testicular volume in newborns. Indian J Pediatr. 2016;83(12–13):1398–404. https://doi.org/10.1007/s12098-016-2163-6.
4. Kaplan SL, Edgar JC, Ford EG, Adgent MA, Schall JI, Kelly A, et al. Size of testes, ovaries, uterus and breast buds by ultrasound in healthy full-term neonates ages 0–3 days. Pediatr Radiol. 2016;46(13):1837–47. https://doi.org/10.1007/s00247-016-3681-0.
5. Orbak Z, Kantarci M, Yildirim ZK, Karaca L, Doneray H. Ovarian volume and uterine length in neonatal girls. J Pediatr Endocrinol Metab. 2007;20(3):397–403. https://doi.org/10.1515/jpem.2007.20.3.397.
6. Vijayaraghavan SB. Sonographic localization of nonpalpable testis: tracking the cord technique. Indian J Radiol Imaging. 2011;21(2):134–41. https://doi.org/10.4103/0971-3026.82298.
7. Khedis M, Nohra J, Dierickx L, et al. Polyorchidism: presentation of 2 cases, review of the literature and a new management strategy. Urol Int. 2008;80(1):98–101. https://doi.org/10.1159/000111738.
8. Basta AM, Courtier J, Phelps A, Copp HL, MacKenzie JD. Scrotal swelling in the neonate. J Ultrasound Med. 2015;34(3):495–505. https://doi.org/10.7863/ultra.34.3.495.
9. Richenberg J, Belfield J, Ramchandani P, et al. Testicular microlithiasis imaging and follow-up: guidelines of the ESUR scrotal imaging subcommittee. Eur Radiol. 2015;25(2):323–30. https://doi.org/10.1007/s00330-014-3437-x.
10. Sung EK, Setty BN, Castro-Aragon I. Sonography of the pediatric scrotum: emphasis on the Ts—torsion, trauma, and tumors. AJR Am J Roentgenol. 2012;198(5):996–1003. https://doi.org/10.2214/AJR.11.8034.
11. Wu D, Shen N, Lin X, Chen X. Prepubertal testicular tumors in China: a 10-year experience with 67 cases. Pediatr Surg Int. 2018;34(12):1339–43. https://doi.org/10.1007/s00383-018-4366-6.
12. Brainwood M, Beirne G, Fenech M. Persistence of the processus vaginalis and its related disorders. Australas J Ultrasound Med. 2020;23(1):22–9. https://doi.org/10.1002/ajum.12195.
13. Lao OB, Fitzgibbons RJ, Cusick RA. Pediatric inguinal hernias, hydroceles, and undescended testicles. Surg Clin North Am. 2012;92(3):487–504, vii. https://doi.org/10.1016/j.suc.2012.03.017.
14. Meena D, Jhuria R, Saxena S, Saini U. Inguinoscrotal hernia in infants: three case reports in ultrasound diagnosis. Indian J Radiol Imaging. 2017;27(1):78–81. https://doi.org/10.4103/0971-3026.202951.
15. Rao MS, Arjun K. Sonography of scrotal trauma. Indian J Radiol Imaging. 2012;22(4):293–7. https://doi.org/10.4103/0971-3026.111482.
16. Rangarajan K, Jana M, Wadgera N, Gupta AK, Bajpai M, Kandasamy D. Role of transperineal ultrasound (TPUS) in children with ambiguous genitalia. Indian

J Radiol Imaging. 2021;31(1):49–56. https://doi.org/10.1055/s-0041-1729123.
17. Schoellnast H, Lindbichler F, Riccabona M. Sonographic diagnosis of urethral anomalies in infants: value of perineal sonography. J Ultrasound Med. 2004;23(6):769–76. https://doi.org/10.7863/jum.2004.23.6.769.
18. Ozcan HN, Balci S, Ekinci S, et al. Imaging findings of Fetal-neonatal ovarian cysts complicated with ovarian torsion and autoamputation. AJR Am J Roentgenol. 2015;205(1):185–9. https://doi.org/10.2214/AJR.14.13426.
19. Kim HS, Yoo SY, Cha MJ, Kim JH, Jeon TY, Kim WK. Diagnosis of neonatal ovarian torsion: emphasis on prenatal and postnatal sonographic findings. J Clin Ultrasound. 2016;44(5):290–7. https://doi.org/10.1002/jcu.22327.
20. Sintim-Damoa A, Majmudar AS, Cohen HL, Parvey LS. Pediatric ovarian torsion: spectrum of imaging findings. Radiographics. 2017;37(6):1892–908. https://doi.org/10.1148/rg.2017170026.
21. Fiegel HC, Gfroerer S, Theilen TM, Friedmacher F, Rolle U. Ovarian lesions and tumors in infants and older children. Innov Surg Sci. 2021;6(4):173–9. https://doi.org/10.1515/iss-2021-0006.
22. Valentini AL, Giuliani M, Gui B, et al. Persistent urogenital sinus: diagnostic imaging for clinical management. What does the radiologist need to know? Am J Perinatol. 2016;33(5):425–32. https://doi.org/10.1055/s-0035-1565996.
23. Lindert J, Hiort O, Tüshaus L, Tafazzoli-Lari K, Wünsch L. Perineal ultrasound offers useful information in girls with congenital adrenal hyperplasia. J Pediatr Urol. 2016;12(6):427.e1–6. https://doi.org/10.1016/j.jpurol.2016.08.010.
24. Stafrace S, Lobo L, Augdal TA, Avni FE, Bruno C, Damasio MB, et al. Imaging of anorectal malformations: where are we now? Abdominal imaging task force of the European Society of Paediatric Radiology. Pediatr Radiol. 2022;52(9):1802–9. https://doi.org/10.1007/s00247-022-05395-7.
25. Alamo L, Meyrat BJ, Meuwly JY, Meuli RA, Gudinchet F. Anorectal malformations: finding the pathway out of the labyrinth. Radiographics. 2013;33(2):491–512. https://doi.org/10.1148/rg.332125046.

11 Neonatal Spine

Noah Seymore, Krystle Barhaghi, and Maja Herco

11.1 Introduction

Sonography is one of the first-line methods of imaging used in evaluating the neonatal spine, being well established for infants [1]. It is best performed before 3 months of age when the posterior elements begin to ossify and narrow the acoustic window [2]. Sonographic imaging of the spine beyond this time frame is of limited utility, except in specific cases with increased acoustic windows due to congenital defects or surgical laminectomies. Examinations are also predominantly of the lumbosacral spine, with few specific indications to examine the cervical and thoracic spine sonographically.

11.2 Clinical Indications

By far the most common reason for ultrasound of the lumbar spine is the presence of a cutaneous lesion on the lower back, including skin dimples, skin tags/tails, hairy patches, sinus tracts, hyperpigmented plaques, and hemangiomas [3, 4]. Although 5% of infants with normal spines will have these lesions [5], there is a strong association with spinal dysraphism (defective closure of the neural tube during development), which in turn is associated with tethering of the spinal cord and potential cord injury [1, 2]. Skin dimples in particular are a common reason, though only present an increased risk (and thus indication for imaging) if they are large (>5 mm in diameter) or in a paramedian or superior (>2.5 cm from anus) location [6].

Other indications concerning for potential spinal dysraphism are cloacal anomalies, imperforate anus, or vertebral/sacral anomalies (e.g., incidentally identified on other imaging) [4]. While symptoms of a tethered spinal cord (detailed below) may also be indications for imaging evaluation in older children, only lower extremity weakness can be identified in the neonate. Ultrasound may also be used in the setting of performing or evaluating for complications of lumbar punctures or aspiration of spinal fluid collections [7]. Sonographic evaluation of spinal tumors, post-traumatic lesions (e.g., cord transection/laceration or cord hematoma), or for intraoperative guidance may be done but is not routine and generally is best performed on a case-by-case basis. In general, an abnormal sonogram will be further evaluated with magnetic resonance imaging (MRI) of the region or lesion of interest.

The original version of the chapter has been revised. A correction to this chapter can be found at https://doi.org/10.1007/978-981-97-8576-6_13

N. Seymore (✉) · K. Barhaghi
Mallinckrodt Institute of Radiology, Washington University of St. Louis, St. Louis, MO, USA
e-mail: noahs@wustl.edu

M. Herco
Brody School of Medicine, East Carolina University, Greenville, NC, USA

K. S. Sodhi (ed.), *Neonatal Ultrasound*, https://doi.org/10.1007/978-981-97-8576-6_11

11.3 A Normal Study

11.3.1 Sonographic Technique

The patient should be positioned prone on a pillow or with legs flexed in order to widen the spaces between the spinous processes and increase the acoustic window [8]. A high frequency (7–18 MHz) linear or curved transducer should be selected, as the structures are superficial and a high level of detail is needed [1, 2, 8]. While spinal ultrasound is generally not recommended for patients older than 3 months, it can be performed in patients up to 6 months of age, with decreasing efficacy as the posterior elements progressively ossify during this time frame. A probe with a smaller surface area may be required as patients approach 6 months of life and the acoustic window concordantly decreases in size. If the patient cannot be placed prone due to anatomy or support devices, the study may be performed in left lateral decubitus position, though this is more technically challenging and may lead to pseudomass appearance of nerve roots (detailed below). Upright positioning may also be considered to allow CSF to pool in the thecal sac in the setting of attempted lumbar puncture [8].

Longitudinal and transverse still and real-time images should be performed at multiple levels of the lumbosacral spine to capture the anatomy and document normal cord and nerve root motion. M-mode may also be used to document motion though less commonly done as it is usually not needed [9].

11.3.2 Normal and Variant Sonographic Appearance and Anatomy

The deepest (most anterior) structures visible will be the echogenic, ossified block-shaped *vertebral bodies,* which will cause posterior shadowing and prevent imaging of deeper structures. *Intervertebral disks* will be seen as hypoechoic spaces between the vertebral bodies (Fig. 11.1a, b). As the imaging moves caudally, the coccygeal bones will be visible at the tip of the spine as hypoechoic, unossified cartilage just below the S5 vertebrae. The *coccyx* is almost always unossified in the newborn, but rarely (in older infants) a round echogenic ossification center can be seen, with shape being helpful to distinguish from the S5 vertebral body [1, 2, 8]. If it is difficult to tell, vertebral bodies can instead be counted from superior to inferior, starting with the most inferior rib-bearing T12 vertebrae. Longitudinal panoramic or extended field-of-view images are highly useful to count vertebral levels and identify the position of the tip of the *conus medullaris,* which should be documented on every study (Fig. 11.2) [10]. It should normally be at or above the level of the L2-L3 inter-

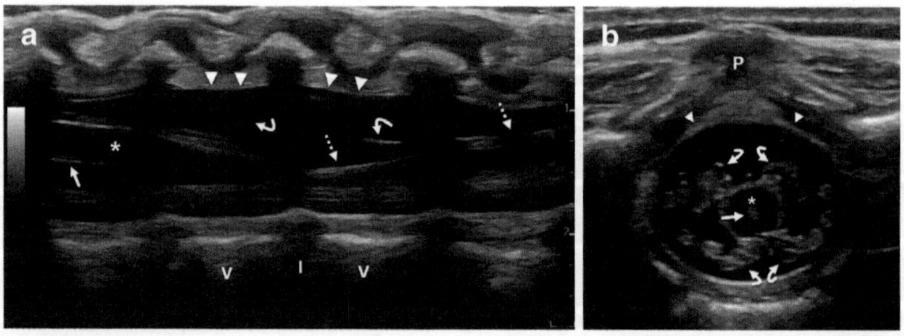

Fig. 11.1 Normal spinal ultrasound. Longitudinal (**a**) and transverse (**b**) grayscale views of normal neonatal spine. At the deepest visible region, the echogenic, shadowing vertebral bodies (V) and hypoechoic intervertebral disks (I) are seen. The spinal canal contains the hypoechoic tubular spinal cord (*) with a central echogenic complex representing the central canal (solid arrow). The cord terminates as the conus medullaris which is attached to the fibrous echogenic filum terminale (dotted arrow). Parasagittal to the conus and filum are echogenic tubular nerve roots composing the cauda equina (curved arrows). Lining the dorsal spinal canal is the echogenic linear dura mater (arrowheads), over which lie the hypoechoic posterior spinal elements (P) and superficial soft tissues

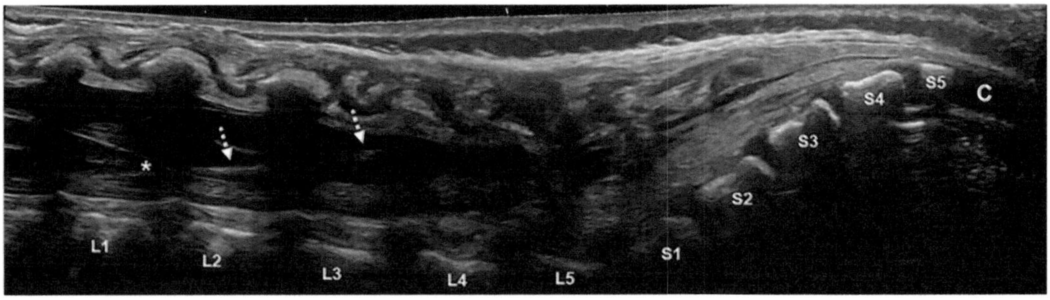

Fig. 11.2 Longitudinal extended field-of-view (FOV). Extended FOV imaging demonstrating normal location of the tip of the conus medullaris (*) as it connects with the filum terminale (dotted arrow). Counting of the lumbosacral vertebral elements (labeled L1–S5) from caudal-to-cranial typically begins with the echogenic, shadowing block-shaped most inferior ossified S5 vertebral body, directly adjacent to the non-ossified coccyx (C). When ossified, the coccyx is typically rounder in morphology

Table 11.1 Spinal cord sagittal diameters of healthy infants

Spinal cord level	Newborn [12] Mean ± SD (mm)	1–3mo [13] Mean ± SD (mm)
Cervical	4.1 ± 0.5	5.3 ± 0.28
Thoracic	3.3 ± 0.3	4.4 ± 0.42
Lumbar	4.4 ± 0.6	5.8 ± 0.66

vertebral space (most commonly L1–L2) [11]. In cases of anomalous anatomy resulting in difficulty counting vertebral levels, MRI or CT is usually performed, though an external radiopaque marker may be placed on the skin at the level of the conus (as identified by ultrasound) and radiographs may be done to aid localization [1, 2, 8].

The *conus medullaris* appears as a conical tapering which expands superiorly into the tubular hypoechoic *spinal cord* (Table 11.1) (Figs. 11.1 and 11.2) [1, 2, 8, 12, 13]. A normal variant that may be present at birth is the *ventriculus terminalis* or "fifth ventricle," a thin cystic remnant at the junction of the conus and filum terminale, approximately 8–10 mm long by 2–4 mm in diameter, that typically regresses as the patient ages (Fig. 11.3) [8, 14]. The cord and conus are surrounded by the anechoic CSF-filled *subarachnoid space*, which is most prominent anterior and posterior to the cord. Within the cord is the echogenic *central echo complex* which rep-

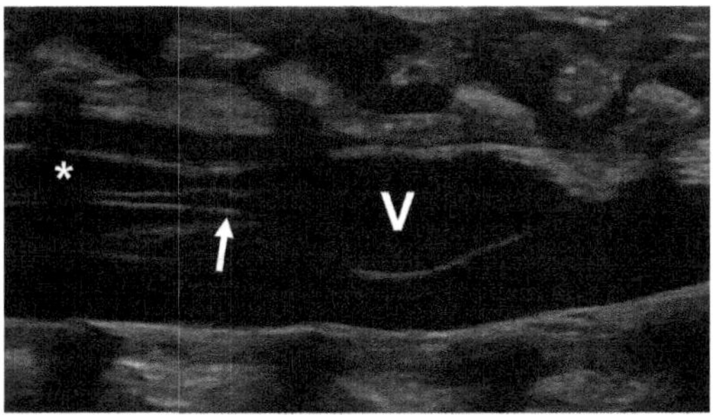

Fig. 11.3 Ventriculus terminalis. Grayscale longitudinal ultrasound images of a normal variant ventriculus terminalis (V), also known as the "fifth ventricle," which appears as a hypoechoic thin-walled cystic remnant in continuity with the central canal (arrow) at the tip of the conus medullaris (*)

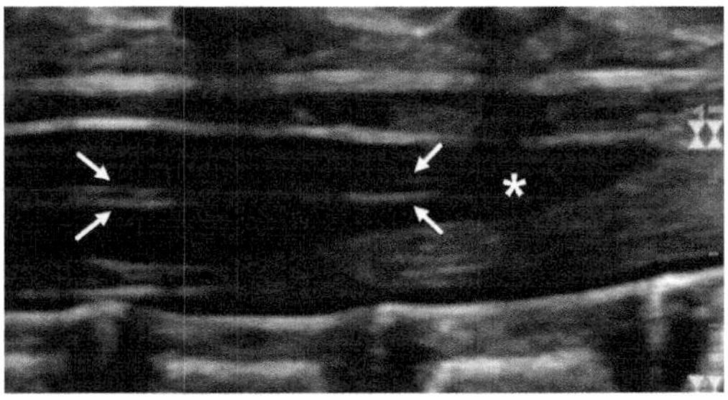

Fig. 11.4 Transient central canal dilation. Longitudinal (**a**) grayscale views demonstrating transient central canal dilatation in a 1-day-old infant. The central canal normally appears as a single linear echogenic line but resolves into parallel ventral and dorsal borders (solid arrows) with central anechoic fluid-filled canal when dilated

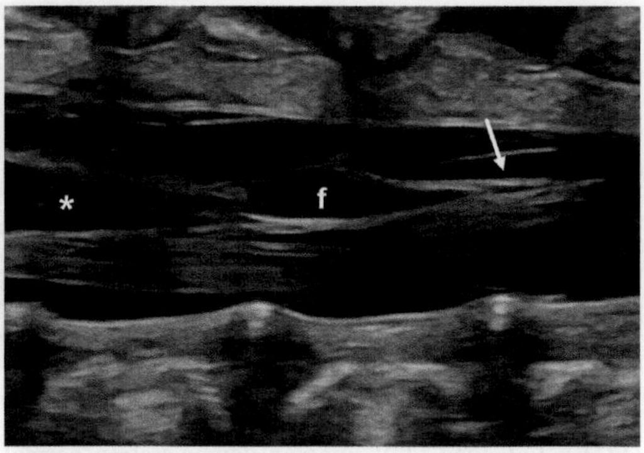

Fig. 11.5 **Filar cyst.** Longitudinal grayscale image of a normal variant filar cyst (f), an anechoic cystic structure in the cranial aspect of the filum terminale (solid arrow). It is distinguished from a ventriculus terminalis (Fig. 11.3a) by its separation from the adjacent conus medullaris (*) and lack of continuity with the central canal

resents the central canal, which appears linear longitudinally, and dot-like on transverse views (Fig. 11.1a, b) [1, 8]. Occasionally, a healthy, normal newborn may have mild but benign and transient *central canal dilation*, which should resolve soon after birth (Fig. 11.4) [2, 15].

Extending inferiorly from the tip of the conus medullaris is the *filum terminale*, an echogenic fibrous cord that measures <2 mm in thickness that crosses the subarachnoid space to attach to the dorsal aspect of S1 (Fig. 11.1a). *Filar cysts* are small, benign normal variant structures located within the filum (separate from the conus medullaris) (Fig. 11.5) [16]. The filumis surrounded by echogenic *nerve roots* (the *cauda equina*), which on transverse view can be separated into dorsal and ventral, right and left roots (Fig. 11.1a, b). Clumping of these nerves may occur when patient is imaged in decubitus positioning, forming a *pseudomass* (*positional nerve root clumping*), but this returns to a normal appearance in prone positioning and so is easily identified (Fig. 11.6a, b) [17].

At the posterior border of the spinal canal is the echogenic lining representing the *dura mater*, posterior/superficial to this are the hypoechoic, unossified cartilaginous *posterior spinal elements* appearing roughly triangular to rectangular on longitudinal imaging, which are in turn deep to the isoechoic paraspinal musculature and echogenic subcutaneous fat (Fig. 11.1a, b) [1, 2, 8]. The echogenic cutaneous structures are often difficult to see without a stand-off (gel) pad [2].

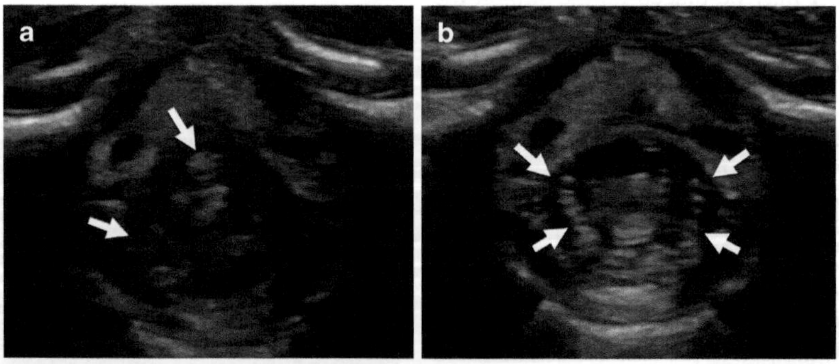

Fig. 11.6 **Positional nerve root clumping ("pseudomass").** Transverse grayscale views in decubitus (**a**) positioning demonstrating positional nerve root clumping forming a "pseudomass" (arrows). In prone positioning (**b**), there is resolution of the "pseudomass" with normal appearance of the nerve roots (arrows)

11.4 Spinal Dysraphism

Spinal dysraphism occurs when there is absent or incomplete fusion of the posterior midline structures during development, with complete, partial, or premature failure of separation of the developing spine from overlying cutaneous structures, resulting in an open defect, a skin-covered defect, or a skin-covered defect with an associated mass, respectively. Despite these variations, these pathologies share the common feature of spinal cord tethering, where lesions or anatomy limits natural movement of the cord. As the growing vertebral column elongates, this limited movement causes increasing mechanical traction and stretching of the cord, impairing the microcirculation, and resulting in ischemia and neural dysfunction [4]. Sonographically, this is demonstrated with a low-lying conus medullaris (below L2–L3), posteriorly located cord in the sac/canal, and decreased or absent cord and nerve root motion. The resulting clinical findings referred to as *tethered cord syndrome* include bladder and bowel incontinence, bladder retention, back pain and scoliosis, lower extremity motor and sensory deficits, and foot deformities (pes cavus and cavovarus) [1]. With the exception of lower extremity weakness, these findings are only detectable in older children.

Knowledge of certain fundamental word parts (also known as root words) can help with identification and description of the types of spinal dysraphism, as they correspond with the type of tissues contained in the lesion. These include the roots "*myel-*" (of the spinal cord)," "*mening-*" (of the meninges), "*lip-*" (fat), "*-cele*" (hernia or mass, i.e., a protrusion), and "*-cyst-*" (pouch or bladder). Thus, overt spinal dysraphism (non-skin covered lesions) such as *myelocele* (spinal cord + hernia) and *myelomeningocele* (spinal cord + meninges + hernia) can be understood as posterior spinal defects, through which herniates the spinal cord (which forms a reddish mass in the midline back, the *neural placode*), in addition to a fluid-filled space lined by meningeal tissue in the case of myelomeningocele. When a fluid-filled, meningeal tissue-lined space is present ventral to the neural placode, it elevates the neural placode from the skin and causes it to protrude dorsally; without the "meninges," the neural placode is flush with the skin surface. These pathologies typically have the clear clinical finding of the reddish, mass-like neural placode in the spinal midline, and are repaired as soon as possible following birth, therefore generally not requiring preoperative ultrasound (though MRI may be performed to look for associated pathologies such as Chiari II) [1, 4].

In contrast, closed spinal dysraphism (skin-covered lesions) may not be clinically obvious, and so imaging is needed. These may be associated with an echogenic fatty mass (lipoma) merging with the neural placode, such as in *a lipomyelocele* (fat + spinal cord + hernia) or *lipomyelomeningocele* (fat + spinal cord + meninges + hernia), or a cyst-like herniation of meninges forming a mass such as *meningocele* (meninges + hernia). Analogous to myelocele/myelomeningocele, ultrasound will show the echogenic lipoma/neural placode mass in the spinal midline between the splayed posterior elements. For a lipomyelocele, the lipoma/neural placode interface will be flush with the dorsal spinal canal (Fig. 11.7), while

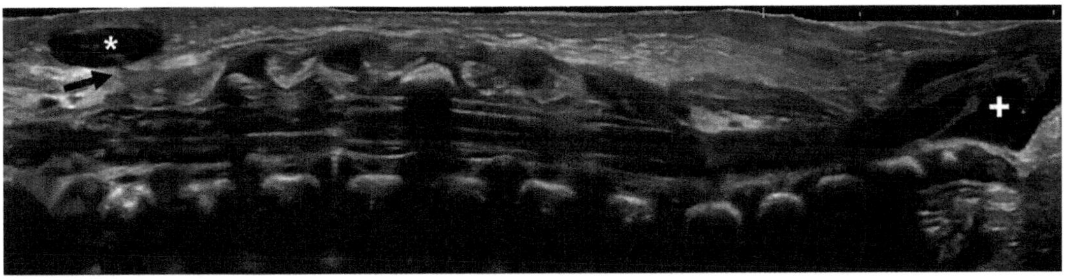

Fig. 11.7 Posterior meningocele and Lipomyelomeningocele. Longitudinal extended FOV grayscale ultrasound image demonstrates the anechoic ovoid fluid-filled posterior meningocele (*) at the mid-thoracic spine with a thin hypoechoic tract (solid arrow) extending to the spinal canal. The hypoechoic lipomyelomeningocele (+) protrudes from the posterior spinal canal defect with a poorly defined but certainly low-lying conus medullaris

a *lipomyelo meningocele* will have a ventral, anechoic fluid-filled space that displaces the lipoma/neural placode interface dorsally relative to the canal (Figs. 11.8 and 11.9). In both instances, findings of tethered spinal cord with low-lying conus medullaris will be seen [1, 4]. A meningocele will have no spinal elements/neural placode or lipoma, instead consisting solely of a fluid-filled anechoic space lined by meninges protruding through a spinal defect (Figs. 11.8 and 11.10). While a nerve root may occasionally drift into the space, these patients are usually neurologically intact and do not have tethering of the cord. Meningoceles are predominantly posteriorly located and may occur anywhere along the spine but with increased incidence caudally. Anterior and transverse meningoceles can occur, but almost always in older patients with associated conditions (e.g., neurofibromatosis type 1). Regardless, these are not well assessed by ultrasound and other imaging modalities predominate in their evaluation [1, 4]. Rarely, a meningocele with posterior spinal defect will also be associated with a dilated central canal of the spinal cord that terminates in a cystic structure, which is in continuity with both the central canal and the subarachnoid space of the spinal canal, called a terminal myelocystocele. If a lipoma is associated with this, it will be termed a terminal lipomyelocystocele (Fig. 11.11) [1, 4].

11.4.1 Caudal Regression Syndrome

Caudal Regression Syndrome is a sporadically occurring spectrum of anomalies involving the lower gastrointestinal tract, genitourinary tract, and spine (though they may rarely be familial). On clinical exam, there is lower extremity weakness and deformities, sometimes with sirenomelia ("mermaid deformity") in which the

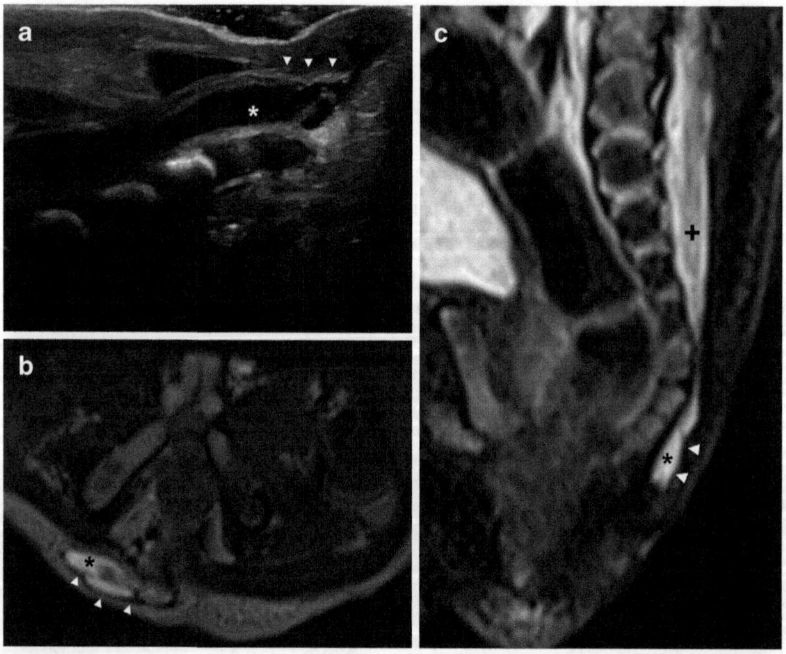

Fig. 11.8 Lipomyelomeningocele (*same patient as* Fig. 11.8). Longitudinal ultrasound (**a**), axial T2-weighted (**b**) and sagittal T2 fat-suppressed (**c**) imaging of the sacrococcygeal region demonstrates posterior spinal defect with intraspinal fluid collection (*) ("*meningo-*") elevating the neural placode-lipoma interface (arrowheads). The spinal cord (+) is clearly low-lying though the conus is difficult to distinguish

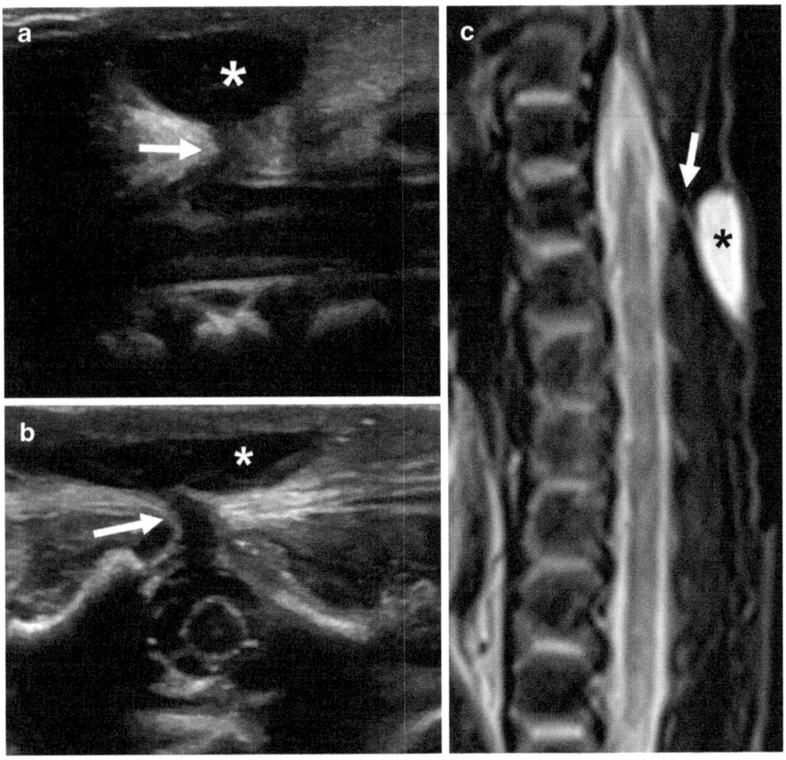

Fig. 11.9 **Posterior meningocele** (*same patient as* Fig. 11.8). Longitudinal (**a**) and transverse (**b**) ultrasound and sagittal T2 fat-suppressed (**c**) imaging of the mid-thoracic spine demonstrates the hypoechoic, T2-hyperintense fluid collection (*) with a similarly hypoechoic/T2-hyperintense tract (arrow) extending to the spinal canal

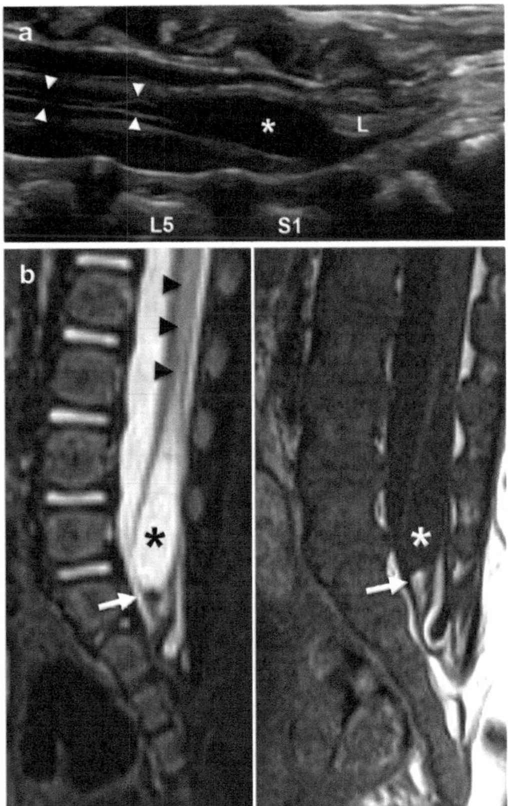

Fig. 11.10 **Terminal lipomyelocystocele.** Longitudinal ultrasound image (**a**) demonstrates a dilated central canal (arrowheads) terminating in an anechoic cystic structure (*). At the inferior aspect of this structure is an echogenic mass consistent with lipoma (L). While the tip of the spinal cord is difficult to delineate due to the terminal lipomyelocystocele, the cord is definitely low-lying, extending to at least L5, consistent with tethering. MR (**b**) sagittal T2 fat-suppressed (left image) and T1-weighted (right image) images shows the dilated central canal (arrowheads) with terminal cystic structure (*) and small associated lipoma (solid arrows)

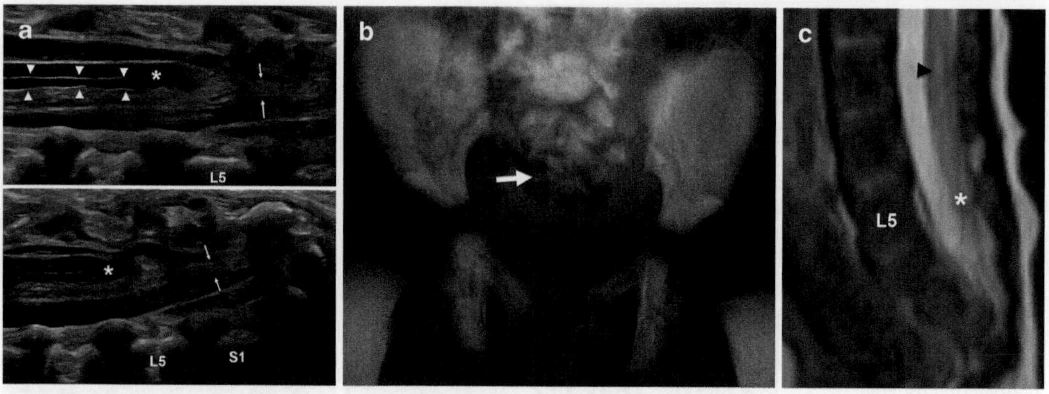

Fig. 11.11 **Caudal regression syndrome.** Two longitudinal ultrasound images (**a**) demonstrate a low-lying, blunted conus medullaris (*) at the level of L5 with a thickened filum terminale (arrows) consistent with cord tethering. Dilation of the central canal consistent with a syrinx is present (arrowheads, upper image). Dysplasia of the sacrum is seen (lower image), with vertebral bodies caudal to S1 not being clearly visible. Radiograph (**b**) confirms sacral dysplasia (arrow) and sagittal T2-weighted MR (**c**) confirms the low-lying, blunted cord (*) at L5 with the more proximal syrinx and poorly defined sacrum

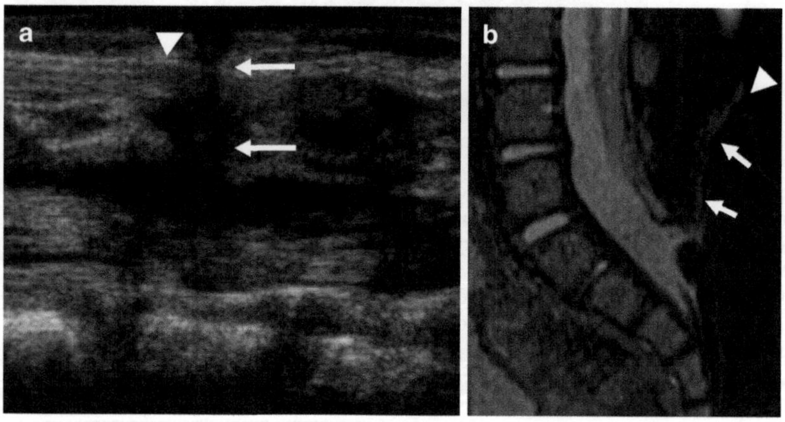

Fig. 11.12 **Dorsal dermal sinus.** Longitudinal grayscale ultrasound (**a**) demonstrates a hypoechoic tract (arrows) extending from a skin dimple (arrowhead) to the spinal canal. Sagittal T2-weighted MR images in a different patient show the T2 hyperintense tract (arrows) from the skin dimple (arrowhead) to the spinal canal, with defect and tenting of the dura

lower extremities are fused. Anal atresia/imperforate anus, renal aplasia, bladder exstrophy, and myelomeningoceles are also associated findings. Spinal anomalies range from lumbosacral agenesis to sacral hypoplasia [1, 4]. On ultrasound imaging, the spinal cord is hypoplastic. The conus is typically blunted or wedge-shaped, and located at or above the L1 level. If it appears elongated and extends below L1, this indicates tethering, usually with a thickened filum terminale (>2 mm) or intraspinal lipoma (Fig. 11.12) [15].

11.5 Superficial Soft Tissue Lesions

11.5.1 Dorsal Dermal Sinus

A *dorsal dermal sinus* is a fistula extending from the skin surface to the spine and is most commonly located at the lumbosacral level though it may be anywhere along the spine or occipital region. Clinically, they present with a midline dimple with fluid (CSF) discharge and may be associated with other cutaneous or intraspinal lesions or defects, including cord tethering [1, 4]. Sonographically, they appear linear and are hypoechoic relative to the subcutaneous tissues as they extend from the dimple/skin surface and appear echogenic as they pass through the hypoechoic/anechoic spinal canal and subarachnoid space (Fig. 11.13) [18]. A low/tethered cord is essentially confirmation that the fistula communicates with the spinal canal and is therefore at risk of meningitis or abscess formation.

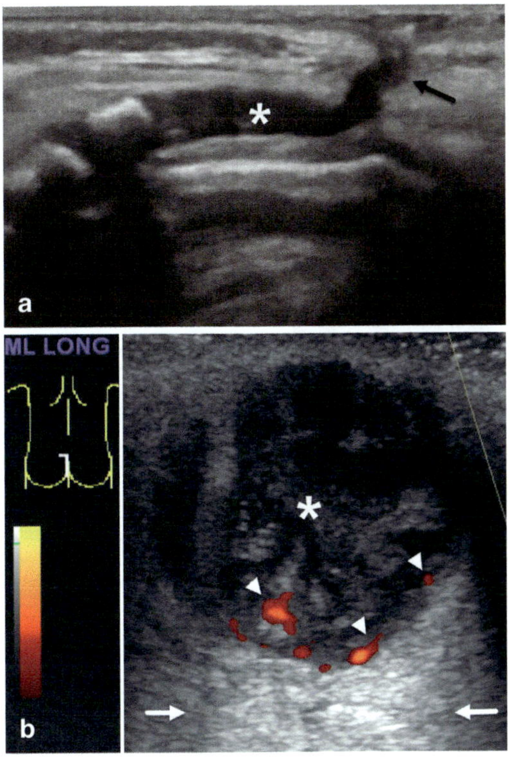

Fig. 11.13 Pilonidal sinus (pseudosinus) and Pilonidal cyst/abscess. Sonographic images of a pilonidal sinus (pseudosinus) tract (**a**) and pilonidal cyst/abscess (**b**). (**a**) Linear hypoechoic tract (solid arrow) extends from the skin surface to the inferior tip of the coccyx (*) consistent with a pilonidal sinus; a pseudosinus results when a pilonidal sinus completely closes and obliterates any potential spaces. (**b**) At the superior gluteal cleft a hypoechoic, well-defined spherical collection (*) containing echogenic debris and showing posterior acoustic enhancement (between solid arrows) is seen, consistent with pilonidal cyst. Hyperemia (arrowheads) along the periphery is suggestive of superimposed infection, and surgical drainage demonstrated purulent material consistent with pilonidal abscess

11.5.2 Pilonidal Sinus or Simple Sacral Dimple

The *pilonidal sinus* can sonographically appear similar to a dorsal dermal sinus, but does not extend into the spinal canal and therefore does not carry an increased risk of meningitis or tethered spinal cord. The etiology is different than dorsal dermal sinus though whether the origin is congenital or acquired is debated [19]. Clinically, they have distinguishing features such as small size (<5 mm), midline and caudal positioning <25 mm from the anus, and no other cutaneous lesions, which indicate a low risk of associated spinal cord tethering (Table 11.2). Sonographically, they are distinguishable as hypoechoic subcutaneous tracts that extend to the tip of the coccyx, where it termi-

Table 11.2 High risk features of skin dimples/pits

Size >5 mm
Paramedian location
>25 mm superior to anus

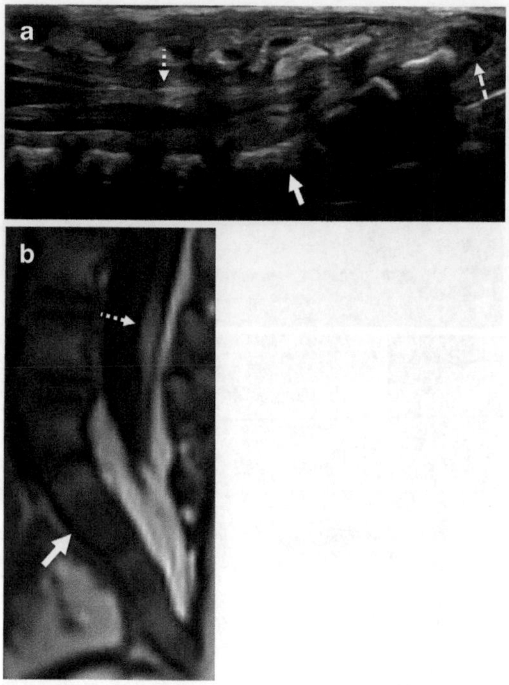

Fig. 11.14 **Filum lipoma.** Longitudinal grayscale ultrasound (**a**) demonstrates a thickened, echogenic filum terminale (dotted arrow). Counting of the vertebral bodies is complicated by apparent fusion of at least two sacral bodies (solid arrow) and truncated appearance of the coccyx (dashed arrow). Sagittal T1-weighted MR (**b**) again shows this along with T1-hyperintensity of the filum terminale (dotted arrow), confirming filum lipoma

nates. These tracts may close completely to form a thin hypoechoic fibrous remnant (*pseudosinus tract*) without a potential space (Fig. 11.14a) or may only partially close to form a potential space. These potential spaces may become dilated to form cysts, which may become superinfected to form pilonidal abscesses, appearing complex and cystic with surrounding hyperemia on ultrasound (Fig. 11.14b) [2, 20].

11.6 Filar Lesions

11.6.1 Tight Filum Terminale Syndrome

Tight Filum Terminale Syndrome is a form of spinal cord tethering due to an abnormally thickened and non-compliant filum terminale. The filum will measure >2 mm in thickness, and decreased or absent motion will be seen in the cord and nerve roots. Sonographically, it is indistinguishable from a tethered cord with associated filum lipoma (described below), and MRI is usually performed. The conus is usually low lying, but can be normally located, emphasizing the importance of examining the filum on every study [4]. A concurrent filum lipoma may be present.

11.6.2 Filum Lipoma

Small filum lipomas are common, occurring in up to 5% of asymptomatic adults [21]. They may be difficult to distinguish from a tight filum terminale syndrome, as the echogenicity of the lipoma matches the echogenic filum, and may make it appear thickened. They may also be present concurrently in a tethered and thickened filum. In these cases, MRI is often necessary to confirm the finding (Fig. 11.15). Larger filum lipomas may be associated with tethering. These may be difficult to distinguish from intradural lipomas (which are most commonly subpial, along the spinal cord) if they are at or near the conus, and MRI again may be needed to distinguish (Fig. 11.16) [4, 21].

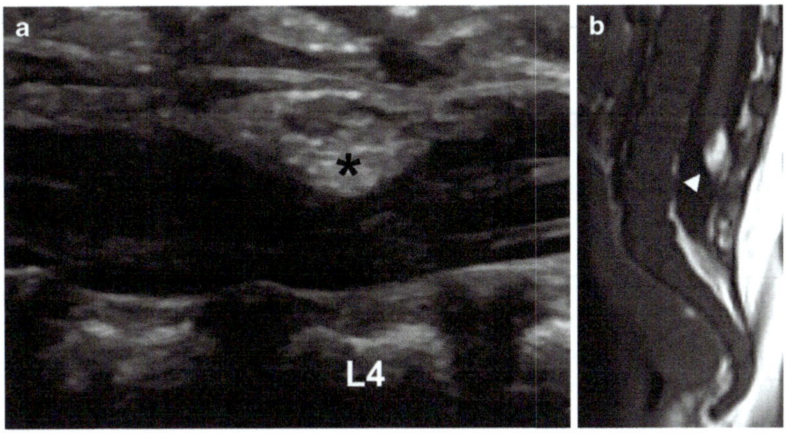

Fig. 11.15 Intradural lipoma. Ultrasound (**a**) and MR (**b**) images of a tethered spinal cord with intradural lipoma. (**a**) Longitudinal ultrasound images demonstrate an echogenic mass (*) along the posterior spinal canal consistent with intradural lipoma. The mass abuts but is not within the tip of the conus medullaris, which is low-lying at the level of the L4 vertebrae. (**b**) Sagittal T1-weighted image demonstrated a low-lying conus medullaris at the level of L4 with associated mass demonstrating fat-intensity signal (white arrowhead)

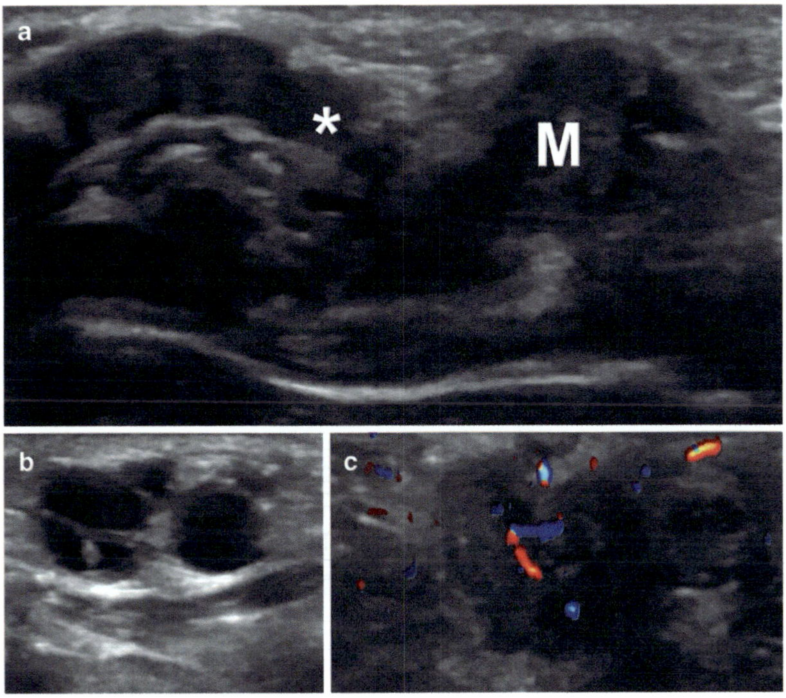

Fig. 11.16 Sacrococcygeal teratoma. Longitudinal grayscale ultrasound (**a**) of the coccyx (*) demonstrates an ill-defined heterogeneous hypoechoic mass (M), which is difficult to separate from the coccyx. Transverse grayscale (**b**) and color Doppler (**c**) images of the mass demonstrate anechoic cystic components with increased posterior acoustic transmission and solid components with internal vascular flow, respectively

11.7 Sacrococcygeal Teratoma

Teratomas are germ cell tumors containing elements from all three embryological layers, seen on imaging as fluid, fat, and soft tissue, often with calcifications. The sacrococcygeal teratoma is the most common site of germ cell tumor in prepubertal children and is typically centered at the coccyx [22]. In the most common sporadic form, there is no association with bony defects (other than coccygeal involvement) or spinal cord/canal involvement, but there is a risk of malignant degeneration and so surgical resection is performed even in asymptomatic cases. Sacrococcygeal teratomas are classified into types I–IV based on relative intra-pelvic versus external location of the majority of the mass. Type I is when the mass is almost entirely external with only a small presacral component, and is the most common type, with decreasing prevalence as the tumor is progressively more intrapelvic. In type II, the external component is larger than internal component. In type III, the internal component is larger than external component. In type IV, the lesion is essentially entirely presacral [23].

Most cases (being types I or II) are clinically obvious, with an easily identified skin-covered mass on exam that often extends into gluteal musculature. Type IV (internal) tumors may present later with mass effect causing constipation, buttock pain, and urinary retention, which may be identified on imaging as hydronephrosis [23].

Sonographically, their multi-tissue anatomy is reflected in their appearance, with hypoechoic, vascular soft tissue, anechoic fluid, and echogenic fatty components, possibly with echogenic shadowing calcifications (Fig. 11.17). Often ultrasound is not obtained when the lesion is clinically obvious or is prenatally diagnosed, and the patient goes directly to MRI to evaluate the extent of tumor and effects of the mass (Fig. 11.18).

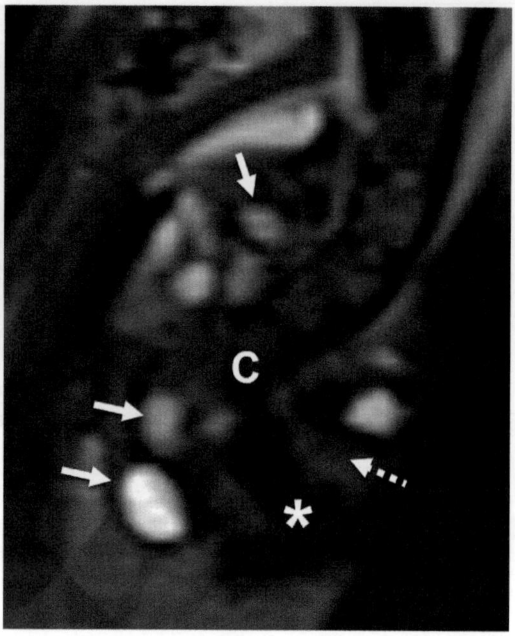

Fig. 11.17 **Sacrococcygeal teratoma** (*same patient as* Fig. 11.17). Sagittal MR images with T2-weighting without fat suppression demonstrates the irregular mass centered at the coccyx (C). Multiple tissue types are present including non-enhancing T2-bright fluid-filled cysts (solid arrows), T2-dark solid tissue (*) which enhanced on post-contrast images (not shown), and T2-intermediate fat-suppressing fat tissue (dotted arrow), consistent with a teratoma. The mass of the teratoma is split evenly between the pre- and post-sacral regions, consistent with Type II sacrococcygeal teratoma

Only in cases of uncertainty whether there is a mass (e.g., a small, deeper lesion) is an ultrasound usually performed [24]. In these cases, a variety of lesions may be included in the differential due to the variable cystic and solid nature, including rhabdomyosarcoma, neuroblastoma, sacral meningocele, and enteric (tailgut or presacral) duplication cyst (Fig. 11.18). Benign (mature) teratoma cannot definitively be distinguished from malignant teratoma by imaging, but is often predominantly cystic with small soft tissue component, while malignant is more often predominantly solid.

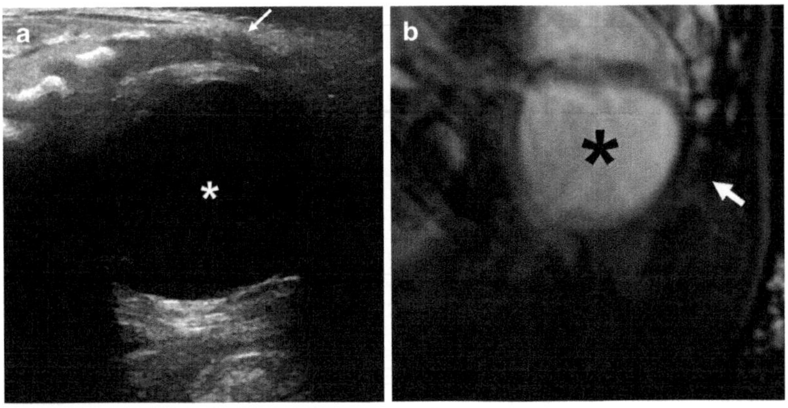

Fig. 11.18 **Presacral cystic mass.** A large cystic lesion (*) initially seen on spinal ultrasound, located in the pelvic presacral space near the coccyx (arrow). On ultrasound (**a**), the lesion could not be completely imaged and was difficult to separate from the coccyx, raising concern for cystic sacrococcygeal teratoma among other differential considerations. Sagittal T2 fat-suppressed MR (**b**) images showed the lesion was entirely cystic without solid component and was separated from the coccyx. Pathology after resection was consistent with enteric duplication cyst

11.8 Other Findings

Other tumors only rarely involve the neonatal spine, with spinal tumors making up only 1–10% of pediatric CNS tumors in total. While tumor features and location as intramedullary and extramedullary can be detected and described sonographically if incidentally found, MRI is necessary in all cases for characterization and determination of tumor extent, and so ultrasound is rarely performed [25]. Intramedullary tumors (arising within the spinal cord) enlarge the cord and have well-defined margins, and include teratomas, dermoids, epidermoids, hamartomas, lipomas, and enterogenous cysts [1]. Extramedullary tumors (arising external to the spinal cord) obliterate the CSF space surrounding the cord and displace or compress it. These tumors include neuroblastoma, rhabdomyosarcoma, lymphoma, and hemangioma [1]. Both intramedullary and extramedullary masses may be solid, cystic, or mixed, with fatty or vascular components depending on the underlying tumor.

Epidural collections may be identified on ultrasound in the lumbosacral region. These most commonly represent epidural hematoma secondary to lumbar puncture (Fig. 11.19), or less commonly due to birth trauma. It will appear on ultrasound as a heterogeneous echogenic collection along the posterior spinal canal within the epidural space. Epidural abscess would be a less common differential consideration that could appear similarly. Ultrasound may be helpful in these scenarios for procedural guidance to sample either the CSF or epidural collection for diagnostic purposes, as indicated clinically [26].

Post-traumatic spinal injuries including transection and laceration or intra-cord pathologies such as syringohydromyelia (syrinx) or hematomyelia can be identified and evaluated on ultrasound [4, 27]. Hemorrhage will appear echogenic acutely, gradually evolving into an anechoic collection. Thus, acute hematomyelia will appear as an echogenic focus within the cord parenchyma on ultrasound, and a laceration will appear as somewhat linear echogenicity extending from the surface of the cord into the deeper parenchyma.

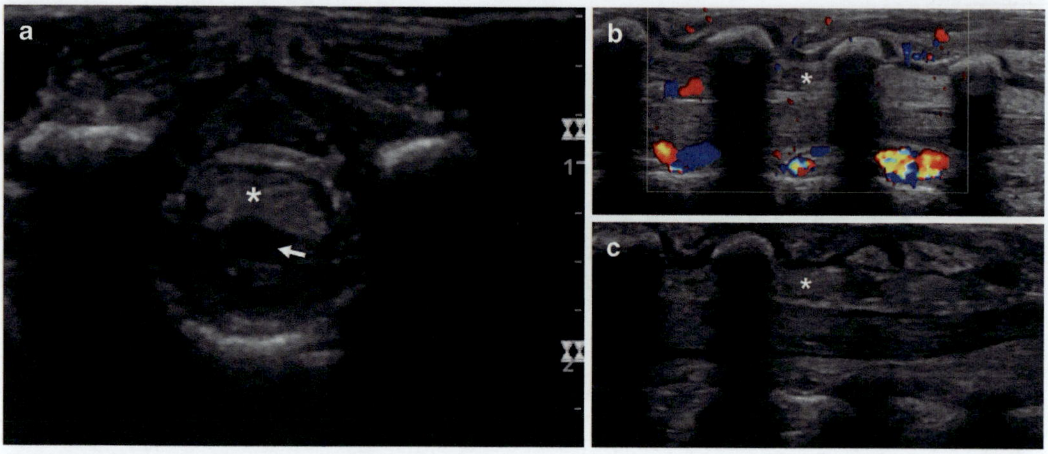

Fig. 11.19 **Epidural hematoma.** Transverse grayscale (**a**) and longitudinal Doppler (**b**) and grayscale (**c**) images of the lumbar spine in a patient following an unsuccessful lumbar puncture demonstrate an isoechoic to mildly hyperechoic collection without internal vascularity (*) in the epidural space, dorsal to the conus medullaris (arrow), consistent with epidural hematoma

In contrast, transection of the cord or nerve roots will show clear separation of the component parts, likely with anechoic CSF intervening (though possibly with echogenic debris). Syringohydromyelia (syrinx) will appear as a dilated central canal (though may be off-center) with central tubular anechoic region and echogenic lining.

References

1. Siegel MJ. Spinal ultrasonography. In: Pediatric sonography. 5th ed. Wolters Kluwer; 2019. p. 653–76.
2. Inarejos E, Irujo M, Navarro O, Flores B, Cacheiro P, Ladera E. Ultrasound of the spine in neonates and infants: a practical guide (digital presentation). Radiographics. 2021; https://doi.org/10.1148/rg.220136.pres. RSNA Annual Meeting, 2023
3. Schenk J-P, Herweh C, Günther P, Rohrschneider W, Zieger B, Tröger J. Imaging of congenital anomalies and variations of the caudal spine and back in neonates and small infants. Eur J Radiol. 2006;58(1):3–14. https://doi.org/10.1016/j.ejrad.2005.12.004.
4. Schwartz ES, Barkovich AJ. Congenital anomalies of the spine. In: Pediatric neuroimaging. 6th ed. Philadelphia, PA: Wolters Kluwer; 2019. p. 1043–71.
5. Kriss VM, Desai NS. Occult spinal dysraphism in neonates: assessment of high-risk cutaneous stigmata on sonography. Am J Roentgenol. 1998;171(6):1687–92. https://doi.org/10.2214/ajr.171.6.9843314.
6. Kucera JN, Coley I, O'Hara S, Kosnik EJ, Coley BD. The simple sacral dimple: diagnostic yield of ultrasound in neonates. Pediatr Radiol. 2014;45(2):211–6. https://doi.org/10.1007/s00247-014-3110-1.
7. Coley BD, Shiels WE II, Hogan MJ. Diagnostic and interventional ultrasonography in neonatal and infant lumbar puncture. Pediatr Radiol. 2001;31(6):399–402. https://doi.org/10.1007/s002470100453.
8. Rees MA, Squires JH, Coley BD, Hoehne B, Ho M-L. Ultrasound of congenital spine anomalies. Pediatr Radiol. 2021;51(13):2442–57. https://doi.org/10.1007/s00247-021-05178-6.
9. Schumacher R, Richter D. One-dimensional Fourier transformation of M-mode sonograms for frequency analysis of moving structures with application to spinal cord motion. Pediatr Radiol. 2004;34(10):793–7. https://doi.org/10.1007/s00247-004-1243-3.
10. Patterson S. Sonographic assessment of the neonatal spine and the potential for new technologies to aid in diagnoses. J Diagn Med Sonogr. 2009;25(1):4–22. https://doi.org/10.1177/8756479308327063.
11. Thakur NH, Lowe LH. Borderline low conus medullaris on infant lumbar sonography: what is the clinical outcome and the role of neuroimaging follow-up? Pediatr Radiol. 2010;41(4):483–7. https://doi.org/10.1007/s00247-010-1889-y.
12. Singh G, True AJ, Lui CC, Prasanna P, Orleans G, Partyka L, et al. Normal anterior-posterior diameters of the spinal cord and spinal canal in healthy term newborns on sonography. Pediatr Radiol. 2020;51(4):622–7. https://doi.org/10.1007/s00247-020-04879-8.
13. Lam WWM, Ai V, Wong V, Lui W, Chan F, Leong L. Ultrasound measurement of lumbosacral spine in

children. Pediatr Neurol. 2004;30(2):115–21. https://doi.org/10.1016/j.pediatrneurol.2003.07.002.
14. Sigal R, Denys A, Halimi P, Shapiro L, Doyon D, Boudghene F. Ventriculus terminalis of the conus medullaris: MR imaging in four patients with congenital dilatation. Am J Neuroradiol. 1991;12:733–7.
15. Unsinn KM, Geley T, Freund MC, Gassner I. US of the spinal cord in newborns: spectrum of normal findings, variants, congenital anomalies, and acquired diseases. Radiographics. 2000;20(4):923–38. https://doi.org/10.1148/radiographics.20.4.g00jl06923.
16. Irani N, Goud AR, Lowe LH. Isolated filar cyst on lumbar spine sonography in infants: a case-control study. Pediatr Radiol. 2006;36(12):1283–8. https://doi.org/10.1007/s00247-006-0317-9.
17. Nair N, Sreenivas M, Gupta AK, Kandasamy D, Jana M. Neonatal and infantile spinal sonography: a useful investigation often underutilized. Indian J Radiol Imaging. 2016;26(04):493–501. https://doi.org/10.4103/0971-3026.195788.
18. Kanat BH. Disease that should be remembered: Sacrococcygeal pilonidal sinus disease and short history. World J Clin Cases. 2015;3(10):876. https://doi.org/10.12998/wjcc.v3.i10.876.
19. Lin K-L, Wang H-S, Chou M-L, Lui T-N. Sonography for detection of spinal dermal sinus tracts. J Ultrasound Med. 2002;21(8):903–7. https://doi.org/10.7863/jum.2002.21.8.903.
20. Winningham P, Hutchinson L. Part 5: Vertebral column and spinal cord; chapter 40: embryology, anatomy, and Normal findings. In: Caffey's pediatric diagnostic imaging. 13th ed. Philadelphia: Elsevier; 2019. p. 395.
21. Rossi A, Biancheri R, Cama A, Piatelli G, Ravegnani M, Tortori-Donati P. Imaging in spine and spinal cord malformations. Eur J Radiol. 2004;50(2):177–200. https://doi.org/10.1016/j.ejrad.2003.10.015.
22. Pizzo PA, Poplack DG, Adamson PC, Blaney SM, Helman L, Frazier AL, et al. Germ cell tumors. In: Principles and practice of pediatric oncology. Philadelphia: Wolters Kluwer; 2016. p. 899–918.
23. Altman RP, Tandolph JG, Lillry JR. Sacrococcygeal teratomas: American Academy of Pediatrics surgical section survey—1973. J Pediatr Surg. 1973;4:389–98.
24. Herman TE, Siegel MJ. Cystic type IV sacrococcygeal teratoma. J Perinatol. 2002;22(4):331–2. https://doi.org/10.1038/sj.jp.7210706.
25. Wilson RE, Oleszek JL, Clayton GH. Pediatric spinal cord tumors and masses. J Spinal Cord Med. 2007;30(Suppl. 1):15–20. https://doi.org/10.1080/10790268.2007.11753963.
26. Wang PI, Wang AC, Naidu JO, DiPietro MA, Sundgren PC, Quint DJ, et al. Sonographically guided lumbar puncture in pediatric patients. J Ultrasound Med. 2013;32(12):2191–7. https://doi.org/10.7863/ultra.32.12.2191.
27. Fotter R, Sorantin E, Schneider U, Ranner G, Fast C, Schober P. Ultrasound diagnosis of birth-related spinal cord trauma: neonatal diagnosis and follow-up and correlation with MRI. Pediatr Radiol. 1994;24(4):241–4. https://doi.org/10.1007/bf02015444.

Neonatal Musculoskeletal System

12

Kanimozhi Vendhan and Nick Owen

12.1 Introduction

Ultrasound is a particularly useful imaging modality in neonates and children due to its wide availability, high-spatial resolution and ease of performance at the bedside without the need for sedation. It is the only imaging modality that allows a diagnostic study in an active or unsettled baby.

Neonates have little subcutaneous fat and this combined with the unossified skeleton allows the interrogation of deeper structures using ultrasound. A high frequency (9–15 MHz) linear array transducer is ideal for the evaluation of joint and soft tissue anatomy and pathology. Lesion characterization, including solid vs cystic, vascularity, etc. is possible with ultrasound along with assessment of relationship to adjacent structures.

12.2 Developmental Dysplasia of the Hip

Developmental dysplasia of the hip (DDH) encompasses a spectrum of abnormalities of hip development that vary in severity. These may range from mild acetabular dysplasia with a stable joint to an unstable joint and frank dislocation. If DDH is left untreated, progressive dysplasia of the joint can occur in infancy and in early ambulation and functional impairment is common, but not universal. The recognized long-term complications include hip pain, gait disturbances, and hip joint osteoarthritis [1].

The incidence of DDH is about 1.5 per 1000 births, with female infants two to seven times more likely to be affected than male infants [2]. The increased incidence in females may be due to the ligamentous laxity caused by maternal relaxin and foetal oestrogens. In certain geographic populations, a higher incidence of DDH is seen due to a cultural tradition of swaddling newborns with hips in extension and adduction [3]. Two of the strongest risk factors for DDH are a family history of a first-degree relative with DDH and breech position in utero. Extreme hip flexion and knee extension associated with a breech position can lead to hip instability and acetabular dysplasia. Increased risk of DDH has also been reported in infants with congenital deformities such as metatarsus adductus, calcaneovalgus, arthrogryposis, torticollis, and in conditions associated with mechanical constriction of the foetus such as oligohydramnios and large for gestational age [2].

K. Vendhan (✉)
Kanchi Kamakoti CHILDS Trust Hospital, Chennai, Tamil Nadu, India

N. Owen
Whittington Health NHS Trust, London, UK

K. S. Sodhi (ed.), *Neonatal Ultrasound*, https://doi.org/10.1007/978-981-97-8576-6_12

12.2.1 Clinical Examination and Imaging

Clinical examination of the hips is performed at birth by the attending neonatologist and subsequently by the pediatrician. Physical signs of DDH include limited abduction of the hip, asymmetry of inguinal or thigh skin folds, leg length discrepancy, and an abnormal Ortolani or Barlow manoeuvre. However, abnormal physical findings on clinical examination can be absent in acetabular dysplasia without instability. This can be detected only by imaging.

In neonates, pelvic radiographs are not sensitive to assess DDH as the femoral head is unossified. Ultrasound is the modality of choice to demonstrate the cartilaginous femoral head, cartilaginous roof, and the labrum. In addition, joint instability can be detected only on ultrasound and not on radiographs. Ultrasound evaluation can be performed until about 6 months of age, around which time the femoral head ossifies thereby impairing visualization of the acetabulum in its entirety.

12.2.2 Sonographic Evaluation

12.2.2.1 Screening

Ultrasound screening for DDH is important as the disease can be initially occult and early diagnosis is key to reducing complications and associated morbidity. A universal screening programme is advocated in some countries such as Austria and Germany, where neonatal hip sonography was developed, and is used to screen all newborns for hip dysplasia. In most countries, this is not feasible due to the cost and manpower that would be required for such a screening programme. Instead, selective screening is done in infants with the aforementioned risk factors or in those with abnormal neonatal clinical examinations. Sonographic examination is generally performed around 6 weeks of age in order to avoid false positive results that can occur secondary to anatomical immaturity or 'physiological' laxity of hips in neonates. However, the scan may be performed earlier if clinical examination reveals unstable hips.

12.2.2.2 Graf Technique

The Graf technique is a static method of assessing the hip joint based on coronal imaging of the hip. This technique is widely used in most European countries for the evaluation of DDH. The advantage with the Graf technique is that it utilizes a standardized and reproducible technique to obtain images [4]. The scan is performed with a high frequency linear array transducer with the baby in lateral decubitus position and hip in physiologic neutral position (15–20° flexion). Graf recommends the use of a specialized cradle to immobilize the baby on its side, thus ensuring standardized positioning for the scan. In the absence of such a fixation device, the parent can assist in positioning the baby on the examination couch. It has been shown that such manual fixation is effective and image quality is equivalent to that obtained using a Graf immobilization device [5].

The first step in the Graf technique is identification of the anatomical landmarks (Fig. 12.1). With the baby in lateral decubitus position, images of the hip are obtained in the coronal plane. Once the chondro-osseous junction is identified on the coronal image, the transducer is moved forward and backward in small movements to identify the lower limb of the iliac bone—this is the undersurface of the medial

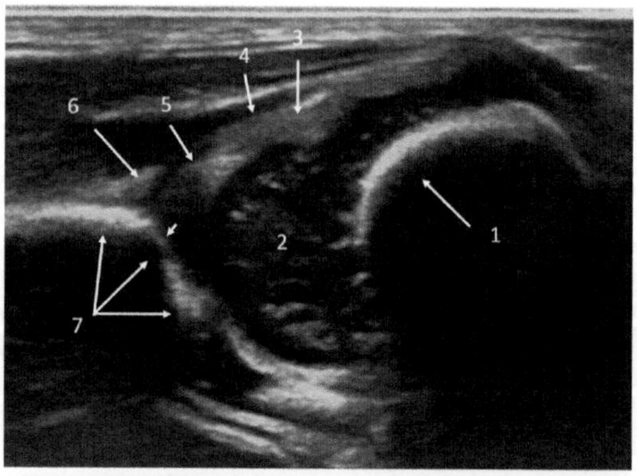

Fig. 12.1 Anatomical identification. Coronal image of the hip. (*1*) Chondro-osseous border, (*2*) Femoral head, (*3*) Synovial fold, (*4*) Hip joint capsule, (*5*) Labrum, (*6*) Cartilaginous roof and proximal perichondrium, (*7*) Bony roof. Bony rim (short arrow) is the turning point from concavity to convexity in the bony socket. A small acoustic shadow is seen just medial to the turning point

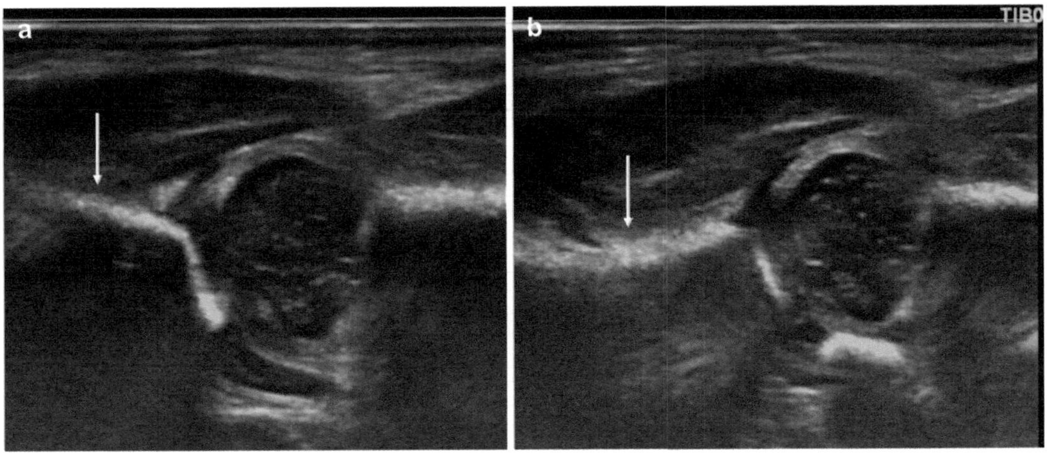

Fig. 12.2 Rotational errors. (**a**) The iliac bone (arrow) bends anteriorly towards the transducer indicating anterior sectional plane. (**b**) The iliac bone (arrow) curves posteriorly away from the transducer indicating posterior sectional plane

border of the acetabulum where the ilium meets the triradiate cartilage. It is the centre of the joint and is seen as a strong echo in the middle of the acetabulum, caudal to which the triradiate cartilage is seen as a largely echo-free zone. Once the lower limb of the ilium is identified the transducer is rotated, with the lower limb as the pivot point, so that the silhouette of the iliac bone above the acetabulum appears straight and parallel to the transducer indicating the mid sectional plane. Rotational errors should be recognized and corrected at this stage by appropriate movement of the transducer—in the posterior sectional plane the iliac bone bends posteriorly away from the transducer and in the anterior sectional plane the iliac bone bends anteriorly towards the transducer (Fig. 12.2). When the lower limb of the ilium is seen and the silhouette of the iliac bone is straight, the labrum is always visible (Fig. 12.3). These three landmarks typify the standard reference plane which is the true coronal plane of the hip joint on which all measurements are made. Two angles—alpha and beta—are measured by way of drawing three lines on the standard reference plane (Fig. 12.4).

The three lines are:

1. Base line—a horizontal line passing through the plane of the ilium.

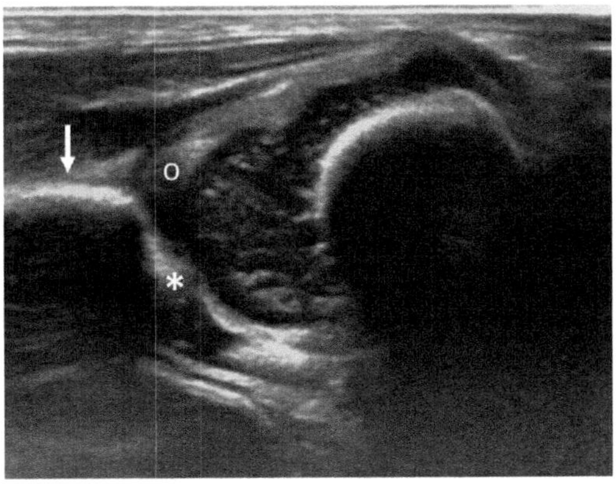

Fig. 12.3 Standard reference plane. Coronal image of hip demonstrating the 3 key structures on the standard reference plane: lower limb of iliac bone (*), the iliac bone (arrow) straight and parallel to surface of transducer and labrum (o). Beneath the lower limb of the os ilium, the hypoechoic triradiate cartilage is seen

2. Bony roof line—a line passing laterally from the lower limb of ilium and just touching the bony roof.
3. Cartilage roof line/inclination line—a line that is drawn from the bony rim through the middle of the labrum. The bony rim is the most lateral point of the concave bony socket and is identified as the turning point from concavity to convexity. Often a small acoustic shadow is seen just medial to this turning point.

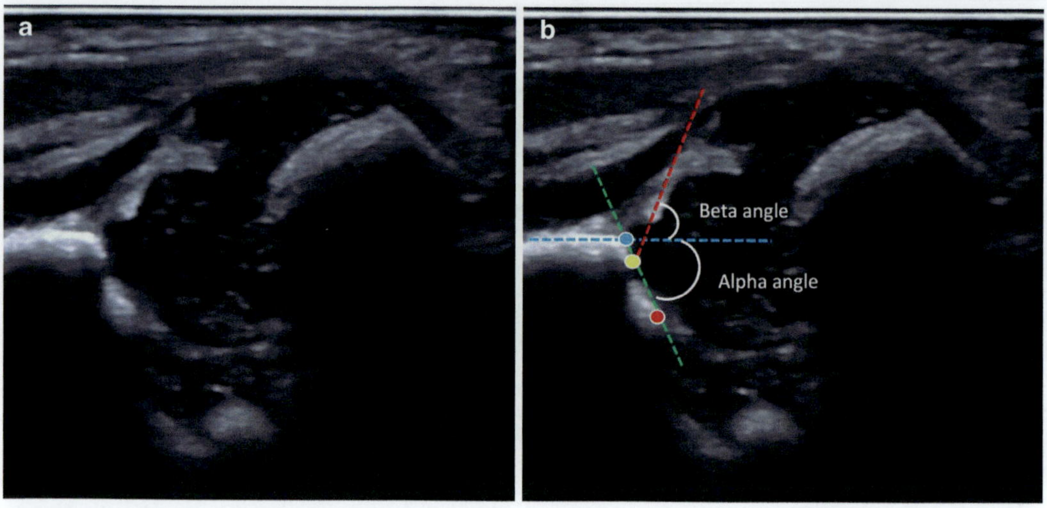

Fig. 12.4 Lines and angles. (**a**) Standard reference plane (**b**) Measurements demonstrated on the standard reference plane. Base line (blue dash line) is drawn along the echo of the ilium. Bony roof line (green dash line) is a tangent drawn from the lower limb of os ilium (red dot) just touching the bony roof (blue dot). Cartilaginous roof line (red dashed line) is drawn from the bony rim (yellow dot) passing through the middle of the labrum. Note the small acoustic shadow just medial to the bony rim

Table 12.1 Classification of DDH (adapted from Graf hip classification [6])

Hip type	Alpha angle (degrees)	Cartilaginous roof/Beta angle (degrees)	Description
Type 1	≥60	Cartilaginous roof covers femoral head	Mature hip
Type 2a	50–59	Cartilaginous roof covers femoral head	Physiologically immature (age 0–12 weeks)
Type 2b	50–59	Cartilaginous roof covers femoral head	Delayed ossification (age > 12 weeks)
Type 2c	43–49	Beta angle <77	Critical hip
Type D	43–49	Beta angle >77	At risk of dislocation
Type 3	<43	Proximal perichondrium pressed upwards	Dislocated
Type 4	<43	Proximal perichondrium pressed downwards between femoral head and bony acetabulum	Dislocated

The alpha angle quantifies the bony acetabular roof and is measured as the angle between the base line and the bony roof line. An alpha angle of 60° or greater is normal. The beta angle quantifies the cartilaginous acetabular roof and is measured as the angle between the baseline and the cartilage roof line. A beta angle of <55° is normal. The Graf hip classification (Table 12.1) is mainly based on the alpha angle (Fig. 12.5). The beta angle is used to differentiate between Type 2C and Type D hips. In Type 3 and Type 4 hips, the femoral head is dislocated. In a Type 3 hip, the perichondrium of the cartilage roof goes upwards and cranially, whereas in a Type 4 hip the perichondrium is displaced downwards and is interposed between the dislocated femoral head and the bony acetabulum (Fig. 12.6).

12.2.2.3 Dynamic Technique

The dynamic sonographic technique incorporates stress manoeuvres to assess for joint stability, in addition to static evaluation of the hip joint anatomy. This is the most widely used technique in North America and consists of evaluation of the hip in coronal and transverse planes. A minimum of five images are obtained—coronal and transverse images of the hip joint in neutral position and in hip flexion, followed by a transverse flexion image with stress manoeuvre (Fig. 12.7). The infant lies supine on the examination couch and the trans-

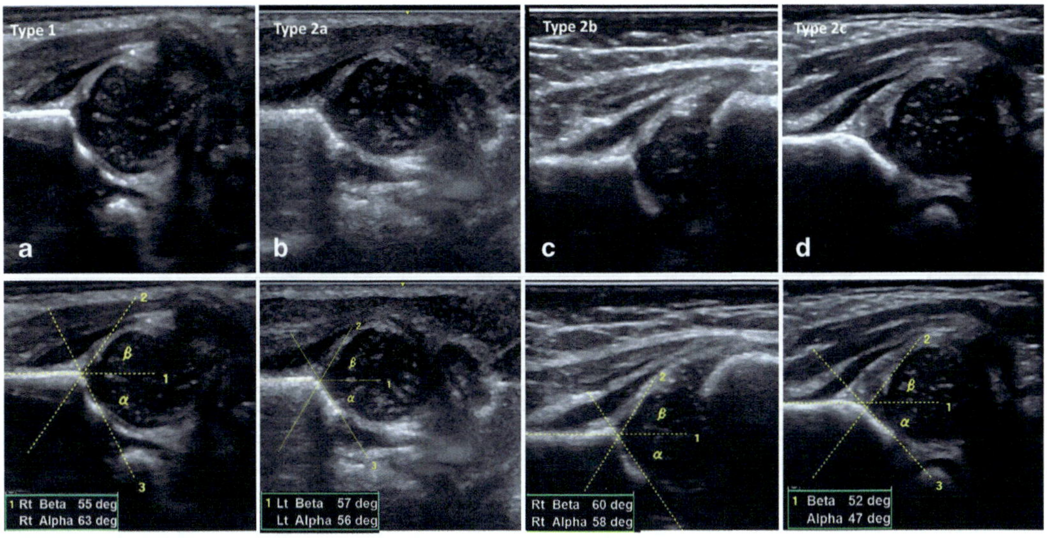

Fig. 12.5 Top row shows Graf type 1 to Graf type 2c hips. Bottom rows shows the angle measurements on the corresponding images. (**a**) Shows normal Graf Type 1 hip in a 7 weeks old infant. The alpha angle is normal and measures 63°. (**b**) Shows Graf type 2a hip in a 6 weeks old infant with breech presentation at birth. The alpha angle measures 56°. (**c**) Shows Graf 2b hip in a 14 weeks old infant with a family history of DDH. Alpha angle measures 58°. (**d**) Shows Type 2c hip in a 6 weeks old female baby with breech presentation at birth. The joint is centred, but the acetabulum is shallow. Alpha angle measures 47° and beta angle measures 52°. The beta angle is used to differentiate between a type 2c hip and type D hip. Since the beta angle here is <77° this is a type 2c hip

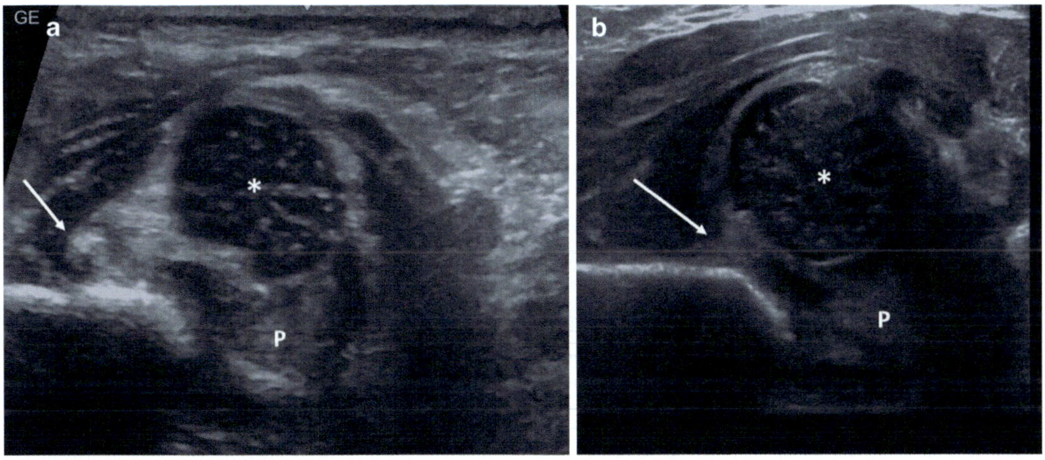

Fig. 12.6 Graf Type 3 and Type 4 hips (dislocated hips). (**a**) Graf type 3 hip. The femoral head (*) is dislocated and is seen out of the bony socket. The proximal perichondrium (arrow) is displaced upward. Increased amounts of echogenic fibrofatty tissue, termed as pulvinar (P), is seen in the bony socket. (**b**) Graf type 4 hip. The femoral head (*) is dislocated. The proximal perichondrium (arrow) is interposed between the dislocated head and the bony acetabulum. *P* pulvinar

ducer is placed on the lateral part of the hip. On the coronal view, the femoral head is seen within the acetabular fossa with >50% of the femoral head covered by the bony acetabulum. In a normal hip, a 'ball on spoon' appearance is seen—the femoral head represents the ball, acetabulum is the bowl of the spoon, and the straight line of the iliac bone is the handle [7]. On the transverse view, the femoral head is seen in the centre of a V-shaped acetabulum formed by the triradiate cartilage centrally, the

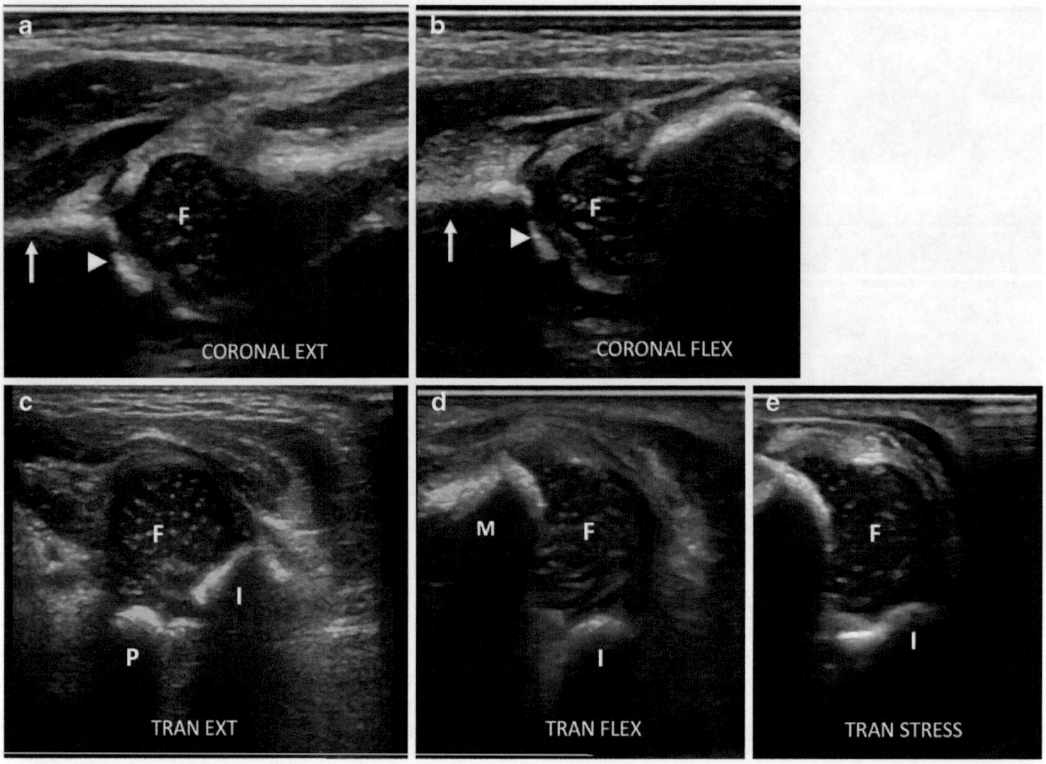

Fig. 12.7 Dynamic technique. (**a**) Coronal extension view (**b**) Coronal flexion view. On the coronal views the femoral head is seen within the acetabulum with approximately half of the femoral head being covered by the bony acetabulum. (**c**) Transverse extension view (**d**). Transverse flexion view. (**e**) Transverse flexion with stress manoeuvre. On the transverse flexion views the pubic bone (P) is obscured by the femoral shaft. The femoral head remains seated within the acetabulum with the stress manoeuvre (Image E). *F* femoral head, *I* ischium, *M* femoral metaphysis, *P* pubic bone, arrow—ilium, arrowhead—bony acetabulum

pubic bone anteriorly and the ischium posteriorly. Stress test is done during transverse imaging, with the baby in supine position, by performing the Barlow manoeuvre. With the hip in flexion and adduction, pressure is applied on the knee to push it posteriorly and superiorly while imaging the femoral head. If the joint is unstable, the femoral head will be seen to move out of the acetabulum with this manoeuvre. In a stable joint, the femoral head will remain seated within the acetabulum.

Hip sonography can be used to evaluate position of the hip during treatment with a Pavlik harness in situ to ensure satisfactory relocation of the femoral head and to assess maturation of the bony acetabular roof. Dynamic manoeuvres and instability tests should not be performed during Pavlik harness therapy.

12.3 Joints

12.3.1 Normal Anatomy

The sonographic appearances of joints vary depending on the type of joint and the maturity of the neonate (viz. term vs preterm). Most epiphyses are generally completely cartilaginous at birth; an ossific nucleus can be seen in some epiphyses, such as in the distal femur or the proximal humerus depending on the gestational age. Due to its high water content, the cartilaginous epiphysis appears hypoechoic relative to adjacent soft tissues. Additionally, it usually contains internal echoes producing a speckled pattern, which helps to differentiate cartilage from intra-articular fluid (Fig. 12.8).

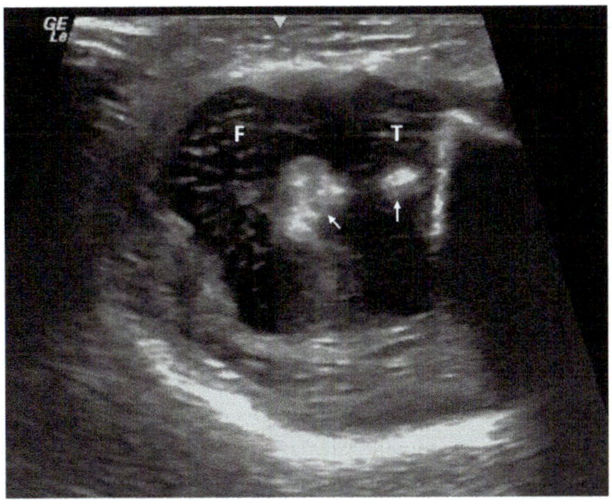

Fig. 12.8 Normal cartilaginous epiphysis. Coronal oblique view of the knee joint in a term neonate shows the hypoechoic cartilaginous epiphysis of the distal femur (F) and proximal tibia (T). An ossific nucleus (arrows) is evident in both. A typical speckled pattern of the cartilage is seen

12.3.2 Bone and Joint Infection

Osteomyelitis in neonates is more common than septic arthritis, but in this age group they usually co-exist. They are usually due to haematogenous spread of infection to the metaphysis with early secondary involvement of the adjacent joint. The most common organism is *Staphylococcus aureus*; other organisms include group *B strepto-cocci*, *Klebsiella*, *Escherichia coli*, and *Enterobacter* sp.

12.3.2.1 Osteomyelitis

Osteomyelitis in the neonate is usually via the haematogenous route to the metaphysis. Due to the sluggish flow in the terminal vessels of the metaphysis, bacteria lodge here and establish an infection [8]. Osteomyelitis and septic arthritis often co-exist (in up to a third of cases) due to the unique vascular anatomy of the epiphysis in this age group. In neonates and infants, transphyseal vessels connect the epiphyseal and metaphyseal circulation (Fig. 12.9). An infective focus in the metaphysis can spread retrograde via these transphyseal vessels, into the epiphysis, and subsequently into the joint cavity [9]. In older children, above the age of 18–24 months, these transphyseal vessels involute and the physis then serves as barrier to the spread of infection from the metaphysis to the joint.

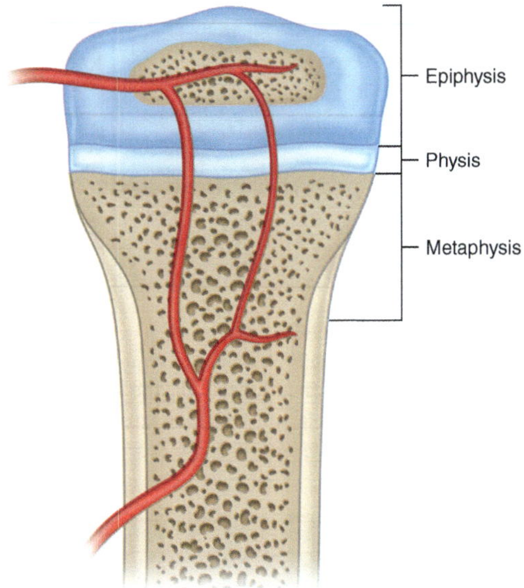

Fig. 12.9 Vascular anatomy of epiphysis. In neonates and infants transphyseal vessels connect the epiphyseal and metaphyseal circulation. These transphyseal vessels provide a route for spread of infection from the metaphysis to the epiphysis

The femur is the most common site of osteomyelitis followed by the tibia and humerus [10].

Radiographs are often normal at presentation. Bony changes are apparent on radiographs only later in the disease course when significant bone destruction has occurred [11]. Ultrasound can aid early detection of osteomyelitis. Ultrasound findings include altered echogenicity of the deep soft tissues adjacent to the bone, subperiosteal collections (Fig. 12.10) and extra-periosteal abscess [12]. However, a normal ultrasound does not rule out osteomyelitis. A limitation of ultrasound is that it cannot demonstrate changes in the intramedullary cavity. With disease progression ultrasound can demonstrate cortical erosions (Fig. 12.11).

MRI is superior to ultrasound in the detection of bone changes of osteomyelitis and can be performed if readily available. However, the logistics of obtaining an urgent MRI scan and the consequent potential delay in initiation of treat-

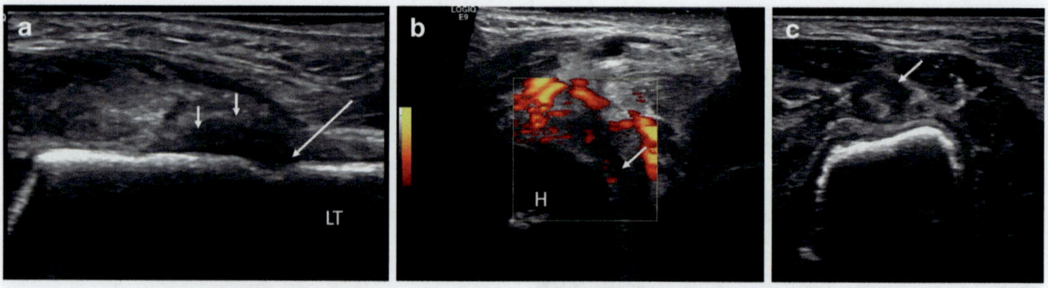

Fig. 12.10 Osteomyelitis with septic arthritis. Three weeks old neonate with h/o not moving left arm for 2 days. (**a**) Longitudinal image of the left proximal humerus shows a cortical erosion (long arrow) with a subperiosteal abscess (short arrows). (**b**) A small joint effusion (arrow)) with synovial thickening is seen in the glenohumeral joint. H—proximal humeral epiphysis. (**c**) Axial image of the upper humerus. An effusion is seen in the biceps tendon sheath (arrow) since it communicates with the glenohumeral joint

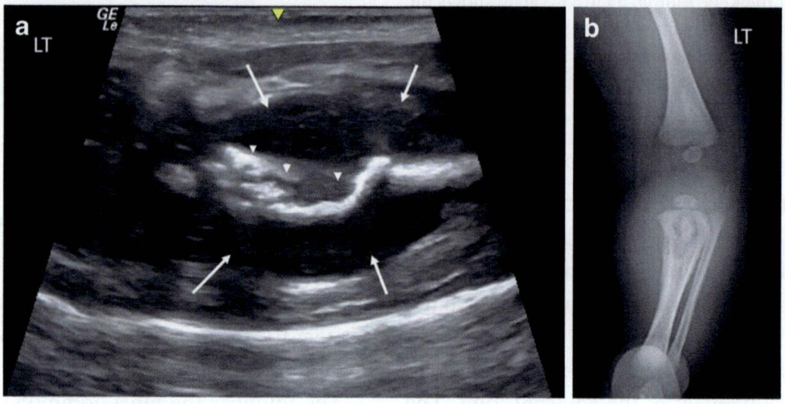

Fig. 12.11 Osteomyelitis. Three weeks old term baby with h/o swelling in the left calf and not moving the left lower limb for 1 week. (**a**) Longitudinal ultrasound image of the proximal tibia shows a large collection (arrows) adjacent to the tibial metaphysis with bone irregularity and destruction (arrowheads). (**b**) X-ray done subsequent to the ultrasound shows a lytic lesion in the proximal metaphysis of tibia

ment needs to be considered and decided accordingly.

12.3.2.2 Septic Arthritis

Many cases of septic arthritis are due to direct spread from adjacent osteomyelitis in the metaphysis (Fig. 12.10), but it can also occur by direct haematogenous spread of infection to the joint leading to inflammation of the synovium and a purulent joint effusion. Infection may also spread to the joint from an adjacent infective focus such as cellulitis or abscess.

The most commonly affected joints are the hip, knee, and ankle. Early clinical diagnosis of septic arthritis can be difficult as the initial symptoms may be vague and non-specific with an absence of systemic signs. There is usually decreased movement of the affected limb (pseudoparalysis). Joint swelling and erythema occur later in the disease course. Moreover, neonates and young children often do not have raised inflammatory markers in osteomyelitis or septic arthritis.

Septic arthritis is a surgical emergency that if left untreated can lead to destruction of the articular cartilage and the ossification centres in the epiphysis. Radiographs have poor sensitivity to detect joint effusions and are usually normal early in the course of the disease. Ultrasound plays a key role in the early diagnosis of septic arthritis. Even small effusions are well demonstrated by ultrasound. The scan needs to be done with a light hand, as excessive pressure with the transducer may compress the joint capsule and displace the fluid. The echogenicity of the fluid is not a reliable indicator of infection and cannot be used to distinguish from non-infective reactive synovitis. Absence of internal echoes in the fluid does not rule out septic arthritis.

In neonates, the hip is the most frequently involved joint. In the hip, joint fluid is easiest to detect anterior to the femoral neck on a parasagittal view with hip in neutral position. In the early stages, when the effusion is small to moderate in size, ultrasound shows loss of normal concavity of the anterior joint capsule with the fluid causing an outward convex bulge of the capsule (Fig. 12.12). Comparison with the contralateral normal joint can be beneficial to detect subtle abnormalities. When the effusion is large, fluid is seen surrounding the femoral head. A large effusion can lead to subluxation or even dislocation of the joint due to the lax nature of the muscles and soft tissues surrounding the joints in neonates (Fig. 12.13). Other findings that may be present include synovial thickening within the joint and thickening of the joint capsule. An adjacent soft tissue abscess may also be present.

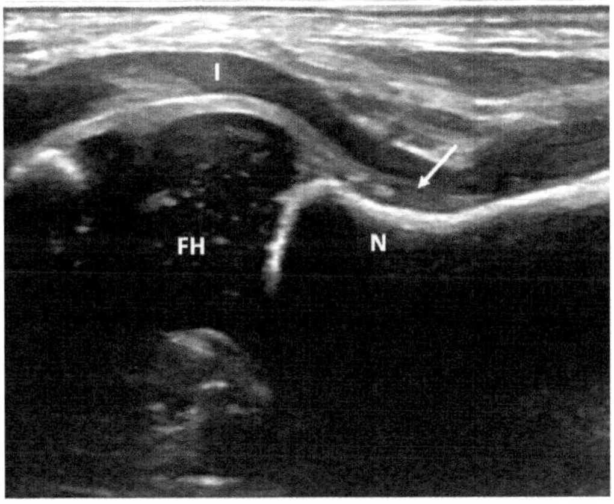

Fig. 12.12 Normal hip joint anatomy. The anterior hip joint capsule (arrow), consisting of anterior and posterior layers, is hyperechoic relative to muscle. The anterior surface of the joint capsule has a normal concave contour. *FH* cartilaginous femoral head, *N* femoral neck, *I* iliopsoas muscle

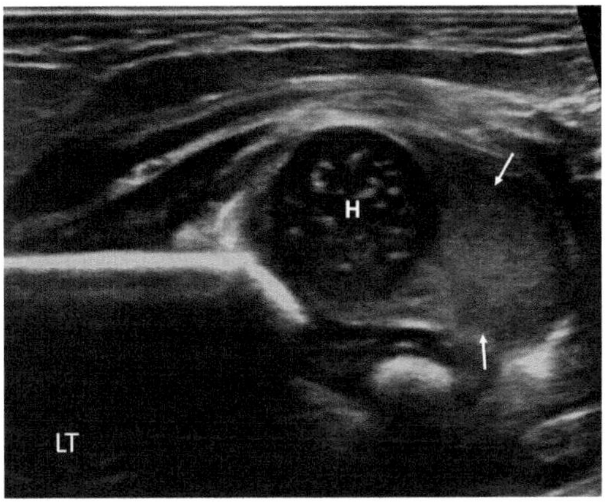

Fig. 12.13 Septic arthritis of hip joint. Sixteen day old term baby with h/o not moving the left leg for 1 day. Coronal ultrasound image of the left hip joint shows a large joint effusion with echogenic fluid (arrows) surrounding the femoral head (H) and distending the joint capsule. The femoral head appears subluxed

Early arthrotomy and joint drainage is necessary to prevent joint destruction and permanent damage.

12.3.3 Physeal Separation

Distal humerus physeal separation is a transphyseal fracture that occurs secondary to birth trauma, after both vaginal and caesarean deliveries, if considerable traction was applied to extract the baby. It is essentially a Salter-Harris type 1 physeal injury (Fig. 12.14).

Biomechanically, the physis is the weakest location in the distal humerus and a rotational shear force can lead to fracture at this site [13]. These babies present within a few days after birth with elbow swelling and decreased movements of the affected upper limb.

The normal epiphysis-metaphysis relationship cannot be ascertained on radiographs as the distal humeral epiphysis is entirely cartilaginous in neonates. Radiographs may show posteromedial displacement of the proximal radius and ulna with respect to the distal humerus. This can be

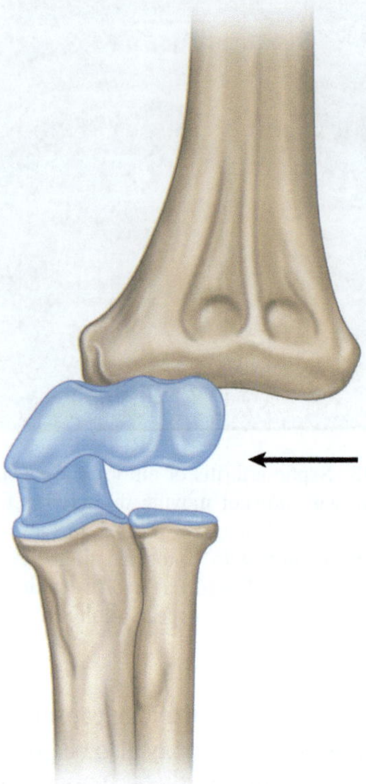

Fig. 12.14 Illustration shows distal humeral epiphyseal separation. A fracture through the physis leads to medial and posterior displacement of the humeral epiphysis

misinterpreted as an elbow joint dislocation on radiographs. Ultrasound is the preferred modality to assess physeal separation injuries as the cartilaginous epiphysis and its relationship to the ossified metaphysis can be readily visualized. On ultrasound, the cardinal finding is the altered relationship between the distal humeral epiphysis and metaphysis. The cartilaginous epiphysis appears separated from the bony distal humerus. As a result, a bare surface of the distal humeral metaphysis is seen that is not covered by epiphyseal cartilage (Fig. 12.15).

Separation of the proximal humeral epiphysis following birth trauma has also been reported [14]. The presentation is with joint swelling and paucity of movement of the upper extremity. Clinically this may be misdiagnosed as clavicular fracture, Erb's palsy or septic arthritis. A plain radiograph of the shoulder joint may show increased glenohumeral distance on the affected side. Ultrasound of the shoulder joint will demonstrate separation of the epiphysis from the metaphysis with the proximal humeral epiphysis located within the confines of the glenoid labrum.

Growth plate injuries elsewhere are rare in neonates although in older infants non-accidental metaphyseal fractures are a form of Salter-Harris type 1 or 2 fractures.

12.3.4 Congenital Knee Anomalies

12.3.4.1 Congenital Anomalies of the Patella

The patella normally ossifies between 3 and 4 years of age and therefore radiographs of the knee are not helpful to assess patellar anomalies in young children. Ultrasound can readily demonstrate the size and position of the cartilaginous patella and is useful for the diagnosis of congenital anomalies of the patella such as absence, hypoplasia, and dislocation. These anomalies can occur as an isolated entity or may occur in association with syndromes such as nail-patella syndrome, Meier-Gorlin syndrome, and ischiopatellar dysplasia.

Congenital dislocation of the patella is usually bilateral and presents soon after birth with knee flexion contracture. In some cases, there may be delayed diagnosis in early childhood. Dislocation of the patella can occur as part of syndromes with increased joint and connective tissue laxity such as Down syndrome, Larsen syndrome, and arthrogryposis. On ultrasound, the patella is displaced laterally and is located at the lateral aspect of the femur. On dynamic sonographic assessment, it is seen that the patella does not return to its normal position at the trochlear surface of femur on flexion or extension of the knee joint [15].

12.3.4.2 Genu Recurvatum

The term genu recurvatum denotes hyperextension of the knee which can be classified into three types as: (1) simple hyperextension without dislo-

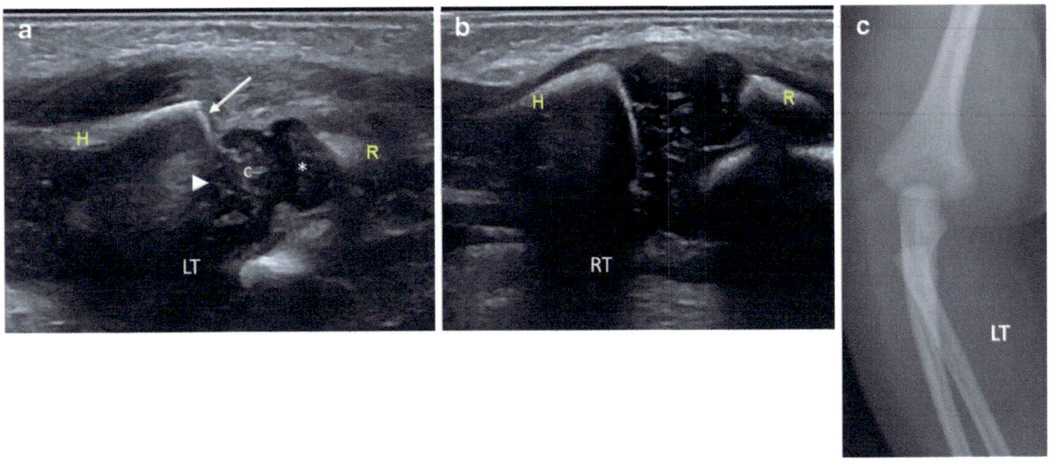

Fig. 12.15 Distal humerus epiphyseal separation. Seven day old baby with h/o birth trauma and not moving left upper limb since birth. (**a**) Lateral coronal ultrasound image shows a step-off at the distal humeral metaphysis on the left. There is posterior displacement of the distal humeral epiphysis (arrowhead) leading to a bare area (arrow) in the humeral metaphysis. The relationship of the capitellum (c) and head of radius (*) remains unchanged. (**b**) Normal appearances are seen in the right elbow joint. *H* humeral shaft. *R* shaft of radius. (**c**) Frontal radiograph of the left elbow shows medial displacement of the distal radius with respect to the distal humeral metaphysis

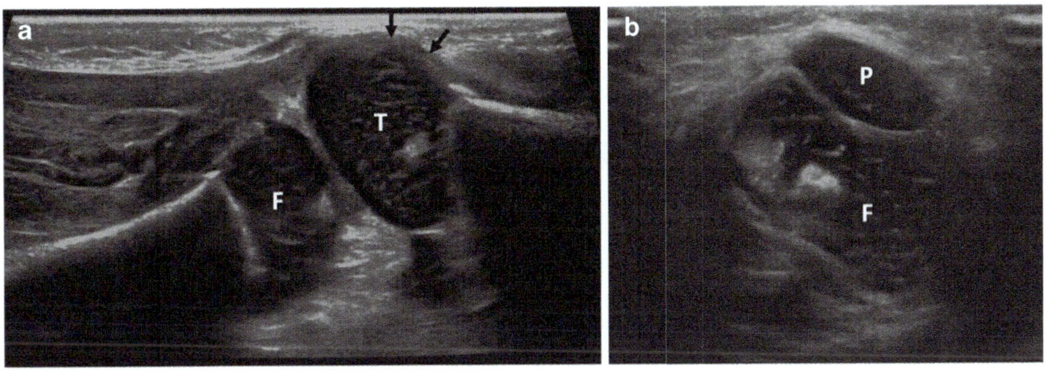

Fig. 12.16 Genu recurvatum in a newborn. (**a**) Longitudinal ultrasound image shows that there is anterior subluxation (arrows) of the tibia on the femur. (**b**) Transverse ultrasound image shows a normally enlocated patella sited in the trochlear groove of the distal femur. *F* distal femoral epiphysis, *T* proximal tibial epiphysis, *P* patella

cation, (2) hyperextension with anterior subluxation of tibia on the femur, (3) hyperextension with anterior dislocation of tibia on the femur [16]. This can occur as an isolated deformity, in association with other musculoskeletal anomalies such as club foot or in association with syndromes (*such as that described in the section on congenital dislocation of patella*). Ultrasound is useful in evaluating genu recurvatum as it shows the femoro-tibial relationship and allows assessment of the quadriceps tendon and distal quadriceps muscle (Fig. 12.16). Focal fibrosis and increased echogenicity of the quadriceps muscle has been reported in congenital dislocation of knee [17]. Ultrasound is also useful for evaluating reduction of the knee joint after manipulation or surgery.

12.4 Brachial Plexus Injury

Neonatal brachial plexus injury (NBPI), is the most common peripheral nerve injury in infants, with an estimated global incidence between 0.4 and 5 per 1000 live births [18].

Several maternal and foetal risk factors have been implicated, but two of the strongest risk factors are shoulder dystocia and high birth weight [19]. NBPI results in flaccid palsy of the upper extremity with neurological deficit ranging from mild weakness to complete paralysis. Classically, the brachial plexus is formed by the ventral rami of C5–T1 spinal nerves. The most common injuries are those involving C5–C6 nerve roots (Erb's palsy); however, the entire plexus (C5–T1) can be involved. MRI is the preferred imaging modality to assess the anatomic location and severity of NBPI. Recently, ultrasound has been increasingly used to evaluate these injuries due to ease of availability and high-spatial resolution. Ultrasound can reliably image the proximal roots of C5, C6, and C7. However, a limitation is the difficulty in visualizing C8 and T1 nerve roots on ultrasound [20, 21].

12.4.1 Sonographic Technique

A high frequency linear transducer (10–18 MHz) is used to perform the scan.

With the baby in supine position, the head is slightly extended and rotated to the contralateral side. Images are obtained at the three locations described below (Fig. 12.17).

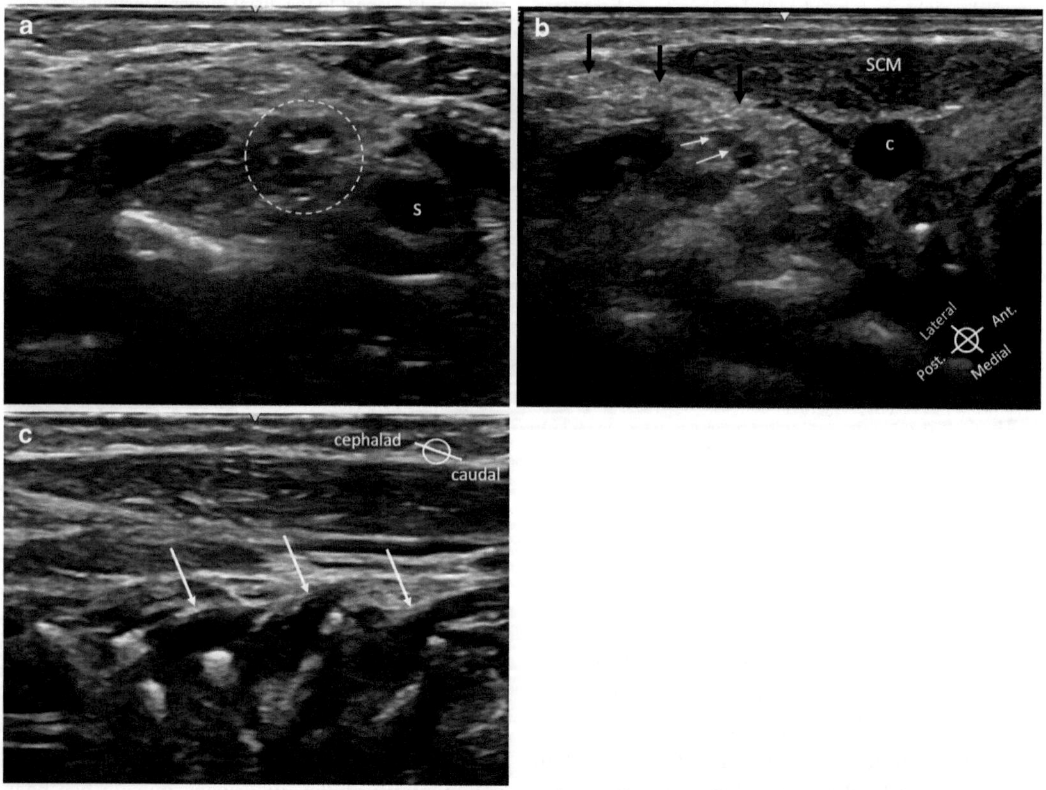

Fig. 12.17 Brachial plexus. (**a**) Supraclavicular level. The divisions of the brachial plexus in the supraclavicular fossa appear as a 'cluster-of-grapes' (circle) in close proximity to the subclavian artery. (**b**) Interscalene triangle. The trunks (white arrows) appear as a series of tubular structures. The brachial plexus and the muscles are surrounded by brown fat (black arrows) seen as granular hyperechoic tissue. The large amounts of brown fat along with a paucity of connective tissue results in a poor delineation of structures. (**c**) Extraforaminal region. Long axis view shows the roots (arrows) exiting the neural foramina and then curving out and downward. *c* carotid, *s* subclavian artery, *SCM* sternocleidomastoid

Supraclavicular region—The transducer is placed immediately above and parallel to the clavicle. The divisions of the brachial plexus and the proximal cords are seen in close proximity to the subclavian artery, immediately cranial to the first rib. The nerves here appear as a cluster of round hypoechoic structures described as 'bunch of grapes' appearance.

Interscalene triangle—From the supraclavicular level the transducer is moved cranially to identify the interscalene triangle. Here the nerves appear as oval hypoechoic structures between the anterior and middle scalene muscles. C5–C7 roots are seen superior to subclavian artery, while the C8 and T1 roots are posterior to the artery [22].

Paravertebral extra-foraminal region—The roots exit cephalad to the respective pedicle and transverse process, except the C8 and T1 nerve roots which exit inferior to the transverse process. The roots are visualized as hypoechoic tubular structures as they leave the foramina in a downward and outward direction.

In pre-ganglionic injury, i.e. nerve root avulsion, there is non-visualization of the affected nerve root and a pseudomeningocele may be seen. The imaging sign of post-ganglionic injury is periscalene soft tissue [19]. This appears as asymmetric thickening of the nerves in the interscalene space. A post-traumatic neuroma is seen as segmental fusiform thickening of the affected nerve.

Ultrasound has a limited role in the demonstration of the full extent of pre-ganglionic brachial plexus injuries. The main use of ultrasound is the assessment of extra-foraminal nerve root integrity and the demonstration of post-ganglionic nerve injuries.

12.5 Soft Tissues

12.5.1 Vascular Anomalies

Vascular anomalies result from abnormal embryologic development or cellular proliferation of blood vessels and lymphatic channels. They may be detected at birth or may present shortly thereafter.

The International Society for Study of Vascular Anomalies (ISSVA) classification is widely used in clinical practice for the diagnosis and management vascular anomalies. The ISSVA classifies vascular anomalies into two categories as vascular neoplasms and vascular malformations (Fig. 12.18).

Vascular anomalies are generally evaluated with ultrasound initially followed by MRI to evaluate the extent of larger lesions and to plan treatment. The advantage with ultrasound is that in addition to grey-scale imaging, colour, and spectral Doppler can be used to assess real-time flow dynamics within the lesion. It is vital that the patient history and findings of the clinical examination should be considered when interpreting the imaging features.

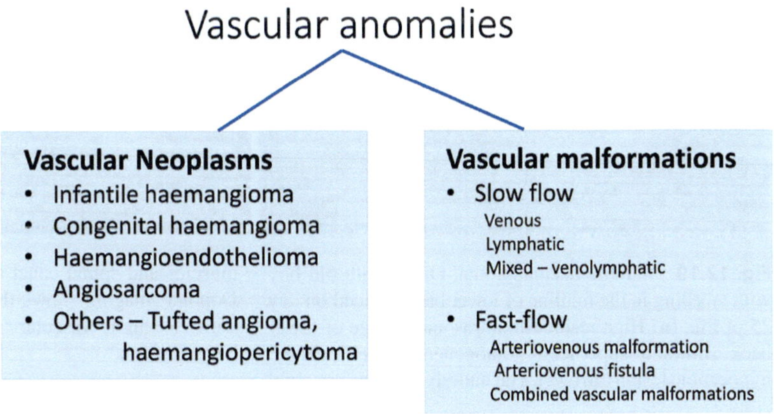

Fig. 12.18 ISSVA classification of vascular anomalies

12.5.1.1 Vascular Neoplasms

Infantile haemangioma: Infantile haemangioma is a benign neoplasm of endothelial cells and is the most common vascular tumour of infancy. At birth a mass is not present, but there may be a skin nodule or an elevated red papule. It proliferates in the first few months of life and then undergoes involution from about the age of 1 year. Infantile haemangiomas are positive for glucose 1 transporter protein (GLUT 1 +ve) [23]. Liver lesions may be found in about a third of infants with cutaneous haemangiomas [24]. On ultrasound, an infantile haemangioma appears as a well-defined solid lesion of variable echogenicity in the subcutaneous plane (Fig. 12.19). The lesions are hypervascular, demonstrating both arterial and venous waveforms on Doppler imaging [25]. During the phase of regression, the echogenicity of the lesion increases as the lesion is replaced by fibrofatty tissue, and this is associated with a decrease in internal flow.

Congenital haemangioma: Congenital haemangiomas are a biologically different entity to an infantile haemangioma. Congenital haemangiomas are GLUT 1 −ve [23]. A congenital haemangioma is fully developed at birth and appears as a bluish-red nodule or plaque with a peripheral pale rim [26]. Three types of congenital haemangioma have been described: rapidly involuting congenital haemangioma (RICH), partially involuting congenital haemangioma (PICH) and non-involuting congenital haemangioma (NICH). The imaging features of congenital haemangiomas are similar to those of infantile haemangiomas. Occasionally, calcification can be present in congenital haemangiomas [27].

Kaposiform haemangioendothelioma: Kaposiform haemangioendothelioma (KH) is a locally aggressive vascular neoplasm. It presents shortly after birth and is most often seen on the trunk and proximal portion of the limbs as an enlarging red to purple plaque. There may be spread to the adjacent soft tissues and regional lymph nodes. KH can be associated with Kasabach-Merritt phenomenon which consists of thrombocytopenia and consumptive coagulopathy. Ultrasound shows a poorly defined infiltrative lesion with increased internal vascularity.

12.5.1.2 Slow-Flow Vascular Malformations

Lymphatic malformation: Lymphatic malformations are slow-flow lesions present at birth and usually become apparent in the first few years of life as a soft fluctuant mass. Based on

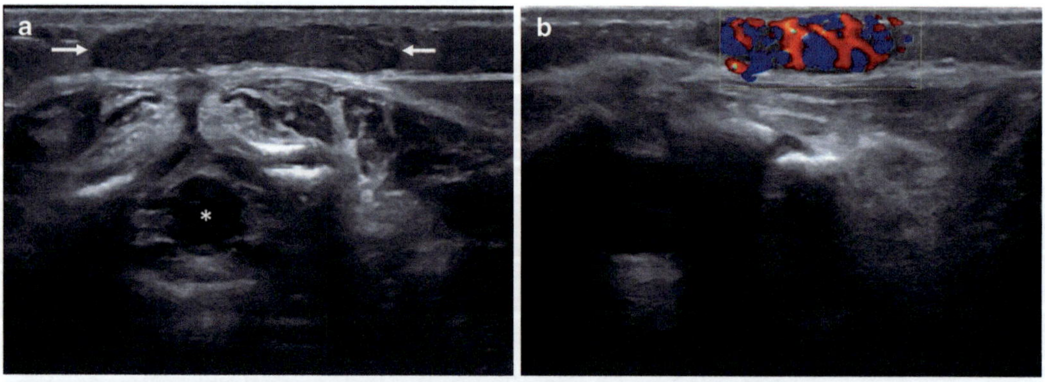

Fig. 12.19 Infantile haemangioma. One month old boy with swelling in the midline of lower back noticed on day 25 of life. (**a**) High resolution ultrasound image of lower back shows a superficial homogeneous, well-defined, hypoechoic lesion (arrows). The underlying para-vertebral muscles and spinal canal (*) appear normal. (**b**) Colour Doppler imaging shows that the lesion is hypervascular with a high vascular density characteristic of a haemangioma

the size of the locules on imaging, it can be divided into macrocystic, microcystic, and mixed types. In the macrocystic type, the cystic spaces are larger than 1–2 cm, while the microcystic type contains subcentimetre cysts.

On ultrasound, lymphatic malformations are seen most often in the subcutaneous tissues as multiloculated cystic lesions with posterior acoustic enhancement (Fig. 12.20). As the cysts can be easily obliterated, copious amounts of gel with light pressure is to be used when performing the ultrasound scan. The cysts are generally anechoic but may appear echogenic in the presence of haemorrhage or infection. Fluid-fluid levels may also be noted if there is haemorrhage within the cysts. Doppler imaging shows flow in the septae with lack of flow in the fluid-filled locules. Microcystic lymphatic malformation can appear as a solid hyperechoic lesion as the tiny cysts are too small to be resolved on imaging as discrete structures.

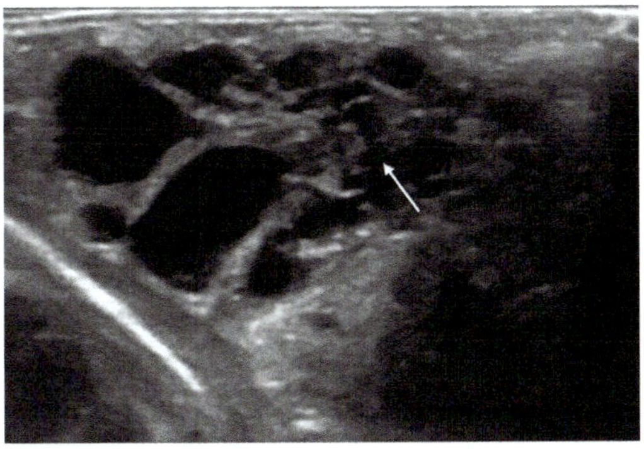

Fig. 12.20 Lymphatic malformation. Five weeks old girl with swelling in left axilla. A multiloculated cystic lesion is seen in the subcutaneous layer. Macrocysts and microcystic components (arrow) are present. The cysts contain anechoic fluid and are separated by fibrous septae

Venous malformation: Venous malformations are slow-flow lesions that present as a soft compressible lesion. The overlying skin may show a bluish colour change. On ultrasound, the lesion shows multiple tubular anechoic to hypoechoic channels and spongiform venous spaces with heterogeneous surrounding stroma [28]. On Doppler imaging, the tubular channels show low velocity monophasic flow. The presence of phleboliths within the lesion is a diagnostic marker of venous malformation. These are seen as echogenic foci with posterior acoustic shadowing (Fig. 12.21).

12.5.1.3 High-Flow Vascular Malformations

High-flow malformations include arteriovenous malformations (AVMs) and fistulas. They present as a pink to red skin patch that is warm on palpation with a thrill and bruit. Ultrasound shows multiple hypoechoic channels without a solid mass. The lack of a solid mass differentiates these lesions from a haemangioma. Doppler shows high velocity arterial flow and arterialized venous waveforms due to AV shunting.

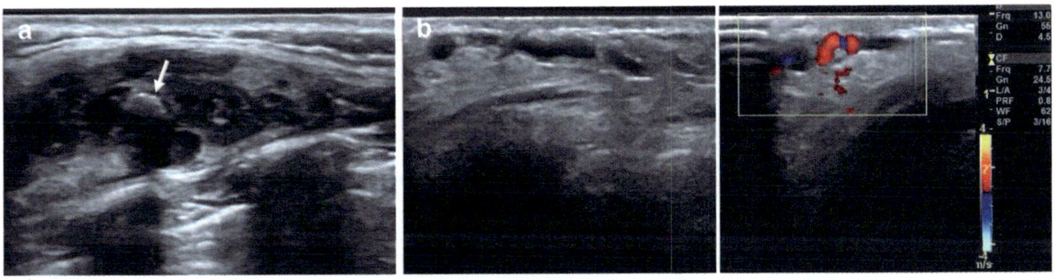

Fig. 12.21 Venous malformation. (**a**) Infant with h/o swelling over the right scapula since birth. Transverse ultrasound image of the soft tissues overlying the right scapula shows multiple anechoic tubular channels and cystic spaces in the superficial plane. A phlebolith (arrow) with posterior acoustic shadowing is seen. (**b**) Images from another infant with swelling over the left elbow show tubular anechoic channels immediately deep to the dermis. The colour Doppler image shows low flow within the lesion. Note the low PRF settings on the Doppler image

12.5.2 Soft Tissue Lesions

Ultrasound is useful in evaluating superficial soft tissue masses to describe the size and internal characteristics of the lesion and its position in relation to other anatomic structures. It can is determine whether a lesion is solid or cystic.

Subcutaneous fat necrosis of the newborn: Subcutaneous fat necrosis of the newborn (SCFN) can occur as a transient complication of birth asphyxia or trauma in full-term or post-term neonates. It is a self-limiting condition characterized by superficial firm nodules that typically develop over bony prominences in the back, cheeks, proximal extremities, and buttocks. These resolve spontaneously over a period of several weeks. A rare, but dangerous complication that has been reported is the development of hypercalcemia which can occur as late as 6 months after birth. Hence long-term follow-up of serum calcium levels is warranted in these babies [29]. Ultrasound appearances range from poorly marginated thickening of the subcutaneous tissues to discrete superficial hyperechoic nodular lesions without any fluid collection (Fig. 12.22). A localized variant of this condition is caused by forceps delivery with lesions around the jaw and occiput (Fig. 12.23). These typically appear as a tubular swelling in the subcutaneous tissues.

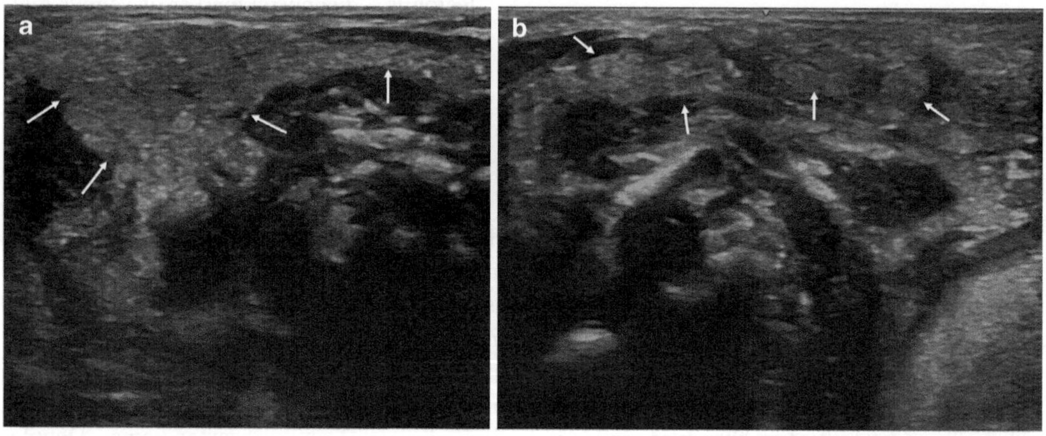

Fig. 12.22 Subcutaneous fat necrosis of newborn. Fifteen day old term baby with h/o birth asphyxia and new onset of indurated nodules in the left supraclavicular region & shoulder. (**a** and **b**) High frequency ultrasound images of the left supraclavicular fossa show a lobulated hyperechoic lesion (**a**) along with multiple nodular lesions in the subcutaneous tissues (**b**)

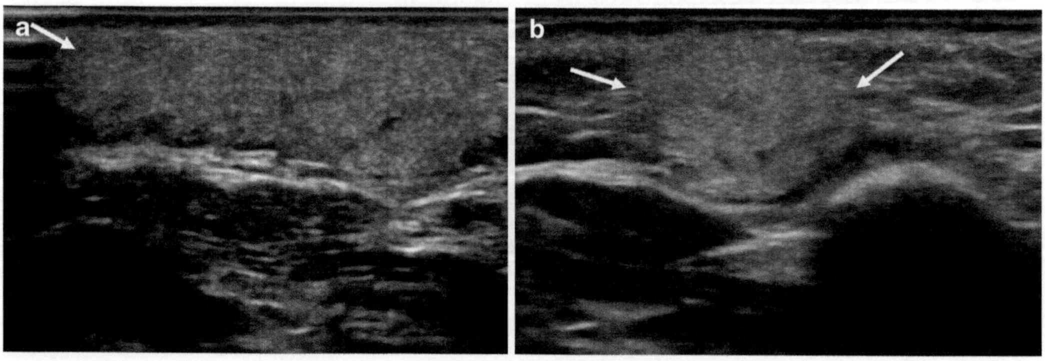

Fig. 12.23 Forceps related fat necrosis. Three weeks old female baby with history of forceps delivery, presenting with a lump at the angle of left mandible. Longitudinal (**a**) and transverse (**b**) ultrasound images show a fairly well-defined echogenic lesion (arrows) in the subcutaneous tissues

12.5.2.1 Soft Tissue Neoplasms

In general, soft tissue neoplasms are uncommon in neonates. Ultrasound features may not be pathognomonic but are useful in the initial evaluation of soft tissue neoplasms to identify the plane and extent of involvement. Colour Doppler imaging can be used to demonstrate tumour vascularity. It may not always be possible to definitively differentiate between benign and malignant masses based on their ultrasound appearances. Following ultrasound, MRI is the imaging modality of choice to further characterize the tumour and for local and distant staging.

Infantile fibrosarcoma: Infantile fibrosarcoma is a mesenchymal malignant tumour that is usually found in children under 2 years of age and frequently involves the extremities. Less commonly involved sites include the trunk and head and neck regions. It is the most common soft tissue sarcoma in children <1 year of age. About 30–50% of these tumours are present at birth [30]. Ultrasound shows a solid fairly homogeneous lesion of variable echogenicity with increased vascularity (Fig. 12.24). When internal necrosis is present anechoic cystic spaces may be seen.

Infantile fibrosarcoma and other highly vascularized soft tissue sarcomas can have clinical and imaging appearances similar to that of a congenital haemangioma and risk being misdiagnosed as a vascular anomaly. Certain ultrasound and Doppler characteristics can help to differentiate between the two. On grey scale imaging, both a haemangioma and a sarcoma can appear as a homogenous solid lesion, but a mixed solid-cystic architecture is a common finding in sarcomas. On Doppler imaging a haemangioma demonstrates both high vessel density throughout the lesion and a high peak arterial Doppler shift. Using a high frequency linear transducer, a vessel count of >5 per cm^2 on colour Doppler imaging and a peak arterial Doppler shift > 2 kHz on spectral Doppler imaging can be used to distinguish a haemangioma from a sarcoma [31]. Very rarely do soft tissue sarcomas fulfil both these Doppler criteria. In clinical practice, using a 9 MHz transducer, 2 kHz Doppler shift equates to a peak velocity of >50 cm/s, when the insonation angle is 70° or less (the Doppler formula can be used to calculate the peak velocity when parameters are varied). In some cases, if findings are equivocal and there is difficulty in distinguishing between a soft tissue sarcoma and a haemangioma, a biopsy is required for definitive diagnosis.

Rhabdomyosarcoma: Rhabdomyosarcoma (RMS) is a malignant mesenchymal neoplasm that is usually of the embryonal type in neonates. It frequently occurs in the head and neck region but may be seen anywhere in the body. On ultrasound, it appears as a solid iso- to hypoechoic mass with increased internal vascularity. Cystic areas may be seen owing to necrosis. The margins are ill-defined when there is local invasion. Compared to older

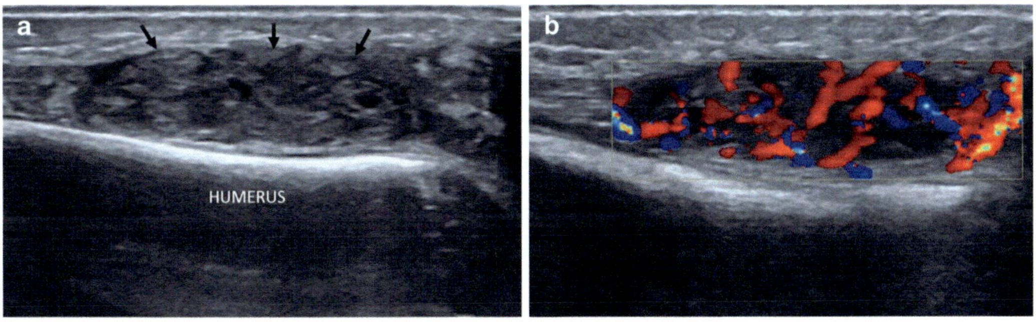

Fig. 12.24 Infantile fibrosarcoma. Two weeks old boy with swelling in right arm, noticed on day 10 of life. (**a**) There is a moderately well-defined iso to hypoechoic intramuscular mass (arrows). The underlying humerus appears normal. (**b**) Colour Doppler image shows increased vascularity within the mass

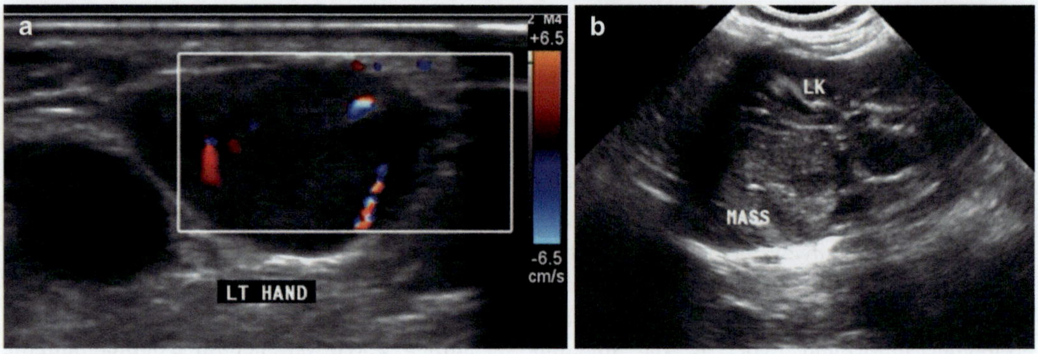

Fig. 12.25 Neuroblastoma metastases. Six weeks old boy presenting with multiple small lumps in left hand, face and back. (**a**) High frequency ultrasound image of a soft tissue lump in the left hand shows a well-defined hypoechoic solid mass with some internal vascularity. The low vessel density rules out the diagnosis of an infantile haemangioma. (**b**) An ultrasound of the abdomen was then performed which showed a left supra-renal mass (arrows). *LK* left kidney

children with RMS, neonates usually have a worse prognosis.

Neuroblastoma metastases: Neuroblastoma may present in the neonatal period with multiple metastatic superficial soft tissue nodules. On ultrasound, these appear as iso- to hypoechoic solid lesions with variable internal vascularity (Fig. 12.25). It is prudent to obtain an ultrasound of the abdomen to locate the primary lesion. Neonatal neuroblastoma has a very good prognosis due its favourable biologic behaviour. Spontaneous regression can be seen and survival rate is >90%.

Other diseases that can cause multiple subcutaneous metastatic nodules in the neonate include congenital leukemia, Langerhans cell histiocytosis, and metastatic rhabdomyosarcoma.

Lipoblastoma: Lipoblastoma is a benign well-encapsulated mesenchymal tumour consisting of immature fatty tissue that arises most frequently in the subcutaneous tissues of the extremities and trunk followed by the head and neck region. When the lesion is poorly circumscribed and infiltrative it is referred to as lipoblastomatosis. On ultrasound, lipoblastoma appears as a homogeneous hyperechoic mass. Areas of mixed echogenicity and fluid-filled spaces may be seen [32].

Infantile myofibromatosis: Infantile myofibromatosis is a benign tumour localized to the extremities of newborns and infants. It appears as a reddish dermal or subcutaneous mass. These tumours may be solitary or multicentric; visceral involvement may be seen in the multicentric type which is associated with a poor prognosis. On ultrasound, infantile myofibromatosis appears as an isoechoic to hypoechoic soft tissue mass with low-grade internal vascularity.

12.5.3 Soft Tissue Infection

Soft tissue infections in neonates are most often caused by Staphylococcal or Streptococcal species. A focus of infection in the deep soft tissues may be difficult to detect on physical examination. Ultrasound is useful to identify if the infection is confined to the superficial tissues or if there are signs of infection in the deeper tissues (Fig. 12.26) and thus facilitates the initiation of appropriate treatment.

Cellulitis: Cellulitis is an acute infection of the dermis and subcutaneous tissues without involvement of the underlying muscles. In neonates, Group B streptococcus is the organ-

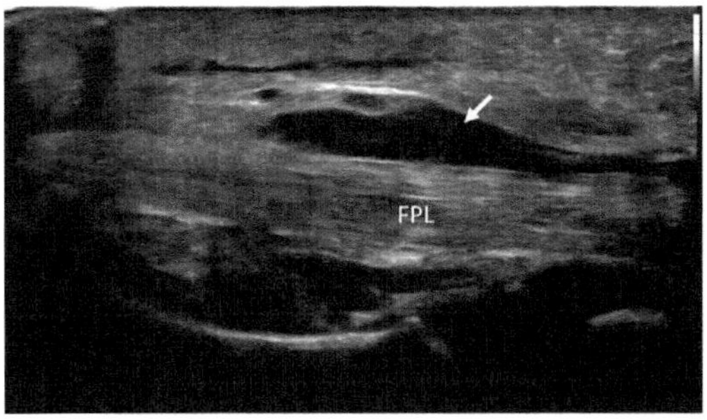

Fig. 12.26 Deep palmar infection. Infant with fever and swelling of the right palm. Longitudinal ultrasound image of the base of thumb shows fluid in the tendon sheath (arrow) of the flexor pollicis longus (FPL) denoting tenosynovitis. The overlying superficial tissues show thickening and increased echogenicity indicative of infective/inflammatory changes

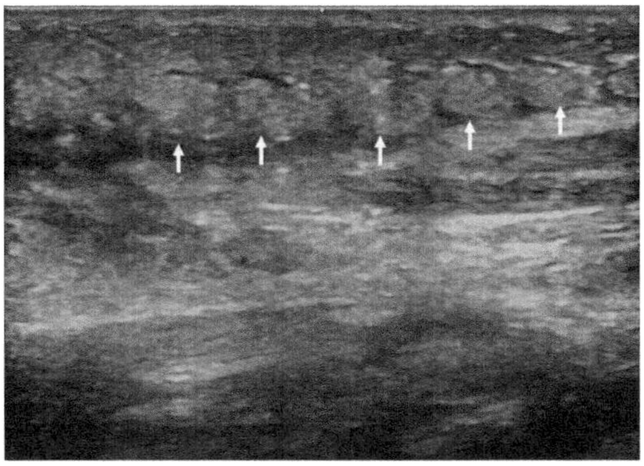

Fig. 12.27 Cellulitis. Three weeks old neonate with swelling of left upper thigh. Ultrasound image shows increased echogenicity of the subcutaneous tissues with cobblestoning (arrows). Linear areas of hypoechoic fluid are seen separating the fat lobules. Also note loss of definition in the deeper tissues

ism implicated in most cases. On ultrasound, there is thickening and increased echogenicity of the subcutaneous tissues (Fig. 12.27). Small pockets of fluid may be seen along with striations in the superficial tissues. Doppler shows hyperaemia in the affected region.

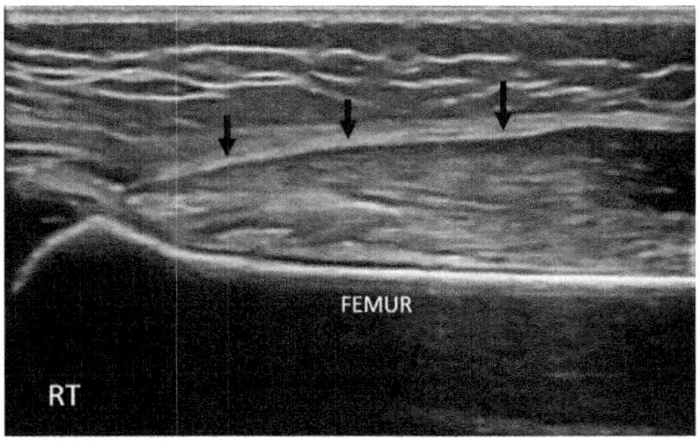

Fig. 12.28 Myositis. One month old girl with h/o fever and right thigh swelling for 2 days. Longitudinal ultrasound image of right anterior thigh shows oedematous vastus muscles with increased echogenicity (arrows)

Myositis: In the early stages, intramuscular infection is seen as increased echogenicity of the affected muscle along with muscle enlargement (Fig. 12.28). Ongoing infection leads to suppurative pyomyositis; at this stage, intramuscular fluid collections can be seen.

Abscess: Detecting an abscess is important as it may warrant surgical intervention. In neonates, since the route of spread of infection is usually haematogenous, multifocal infection can be present and a superficial abscess may be seen with concurrent joint infection at a distant site (Fig. 12.29). Abscesses may be thin or thick walled depending on the chronicity. They are usually present in the subcutaneous plane and are of variable echogenicity with increased through transmission. Internal echoes are usually seen within the fluid (Fig. 12.30). On Doppler imaging, the wall of the abscess exhibits hyperaemia with lack of flow within the abscess cavity. Ultrasound can be used to guide aspiration and drainage of the fluid.

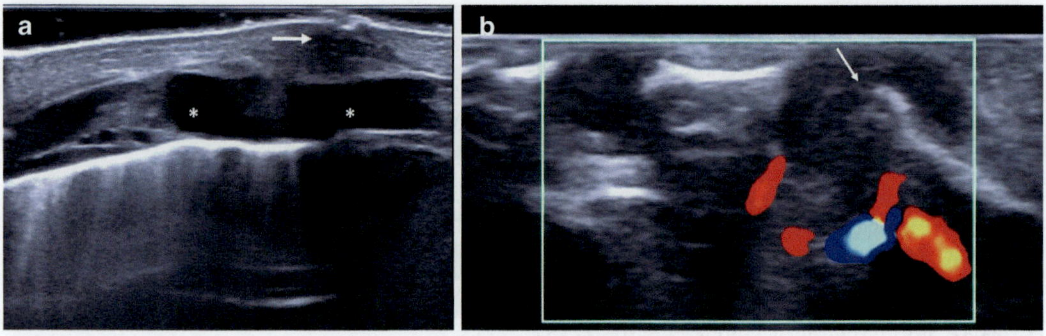

Fig. 12.29 Multifocal infection. Three weeks old preterm neonate presenting with irritability, swelling over lower sternum and a swollen right thumb. *S. aureus* growth was seen in blood cultures. (**a**) Longitudinal ultrasound image of the anterior chest wall shows an intraosseous abscess (*) in the sternum along with a subcutaneous abscess (arrow). (**b**) Oblique coronal image of the MCP joint of right thumb shows erosion of the head of the metacarpal (arrow) with synovial thickening and a small joint effusion

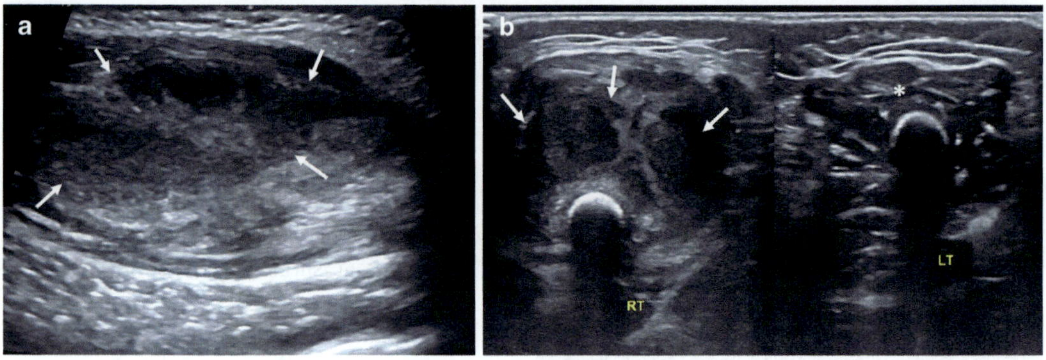

Fig. 12.30 Thigh abscess. Three weeks old girl with h/o right thigh swelling for 2 days. (**a**) Longitudinal ultrasound image of right upper thigh shows an intramuscular abscess (arrows). (**b**) Split screen transverse ultrasound image of upper thighs shows normal appearances of the vastus muscles on the left (*). A large intramuscular abscess containing echogenic fluid is seen on the right (arrows). The femur, showing strong echoes characteristic of normal cortex, is seen posterior to the abscess

12.6 Conclusion

Ultrasound is an excellent first-line imaging modality for the evaluation of musculoskeletal lesions in the neonate. It plays a key role in the early diagnosis of septic arthritis in neonates.

Ultrasound can be readily performed at the bedside and can also be used to guide aspiration of joint fluid or biopsy of lesions.

Despite its multiple advantages, ultrasound has its own limitations. In instances where it is not possible to arrive at a precise diagnosis with ultrasound examination, further evaluation with MRI is prudent.

References

1. Dezateux C, Rosendahl K. Developmental dysplasia of the hip. Lancet. 2007;369(9572):1541–52.
2. Kilsdonk I, Witbreuk M, Van Der Woude HJ. Ultrasound of the neonatal hip as a screening tool for DDH: how to screen and differences in screening programs between European countries. J Ultrasonogr Polish Ultrasound Soc. 2021;21:e147–53.
3. Kutlu A, Memik R, Mutlu M, Kutlu R, Arslan A. Congenital dislocation of the hip and its relation to swaddling used in Turkey. J Pediatr Orthop. 1992;12(2):598–602.
4. Graf R, Scott S, Lercher K, Baumgartner F, Benaroya A. Hip sonography: diagnosis and management of infant hip dysplasia. Springer; 2006.

5. Voitl P, Sebelefsky C, Hosner S, Woditschka A, Diesner S, Böck A. Ultrasound of the infant hip: manual fixation is equivalent to Graf's technique regarding image quality—a randomized trial. BMC Pediatr. 2019;19(1):14.
6. Graf R. Classification of hip joint dysplasia by means of sonography. Arch Orthop Trauma Surg. 1984;102(4):248–55.
7. Harcke T, Grissom L. Performing dynamic sonography of the infant hip. Am J Roentgenol. 1990;155:837–44.
8. Trueta J. The three types of acute hematogenous osteomyelitis. J Bone Joint Surg Br. 1959;41-B(4):671–80.
9. Ogden J. Pediatric osteomyelitis and septic arthritis: the pathology of neonatal disease. Biol Med. 1979;52(5):423–48.
10. Faden H, Grossi M. Acute osteomyelitis in children. Reassessment of etiologic agents and their clinical characteristics. Am J Dis Child. 1991;145(1):65–9.
11. Offiah AC. Acute osteomyelitis, septic arthritis and discitis: differences between neonates and older children. Eur J Radiol. 2006;60:221–32.
12. Bureau NJ, Ali SS, Chhem RK, Cardinal E. Ultrasound of musculoskeletal infections. In: Seminars in musculoskeletal radiology, vol. 2; 1998.
13. Peterson HA. Physeal fractures. In: Morrey F, editor. The elbow and its disorders. Philadephia: W.B Saunders; 1985. p. 222–36.
14. Goldfisher R, Amodio J. Separation of the proximal humeral epiphysis in the Newborn: rapid diagnosis with ultrasonography. Case Rep Pediatr. 2015;2015:1–3.
15. Yan Z, Yao Y, Yang Q, Ma B, Li T, Wang Y. Application of ultrasound in the early diagnosis of congenital patellar dislocation: a case description. Quant Imaging Med Surg. 2023;13(10):7362–6.
16. Carlson D, O'Connor J. Congenital dislocation of the knee. Am J Roentgenol. 1976;127(3):465–8.
17. Kamata N, Takahashi T, Nakatani K, Yamamoto H. Ultrasonographic evaluation of congenital dislocation of the knee. Skeletal Radiol. 2002;31(9):539–42.
18. Shah V, Coroneos CJ, Ng E. The evaluation and management of neonatal brachial plexus palsy. Paediatr Child Health. 2021;26(8):493–7.
19. Gunes A, Bulut E, Uzumcugil A, Oguz KK. Brachial plexus ultrasound and MRI in children with brachial plexus birth injury. Am J Neuroradiol. 2018;39(9):1745–50.
20. Smith EC, Xixis KI, Grant GA, Grant SA. Assessment of obstetric brachial plexus injury with preoperative ultrasound. Muscle Nerve. 2016;53(6):946–50.
21. Pillen S, Semmekrot B, Meulstee J, Verrips A, Van Alfen N. Ultrasound of the cervical roots and brachial plexus in neonates. Muscle Nerve. 2015;51(1):35–41.
22. Gilcrease-Garcia BM, Deshmukh SD, Parsons MS. Anatomy, imaging, and pathologic conditions of the brachial plexus. Radiographics. 2020;40(6):1686–714.
23. Hand JL, Frieden IJ. Vascular birthmarks of infancy: resolving nosologic confusion. Am J Med Genet. 2002;108(4):257–64.
24. Nord KM, Kandel J, Lefkowitch JH, Lobritto SJ, Morel KD, North PE, et al. Multiple cutaneous infantile hemangiomas associated with hepatic angiosarcoma: case report and review of the literature. Pediatrics. 2006;118(3):e907–13.
25. Wildgruber M, Sadick M, Müller-Wille R, Wohlgemuth WA. Vascular tumors in infants and adolescents. Insights Imaging. 2019;10(1):30.
26. Bruder E, Alaggio R, Kozakewich HPW, Jundt G, Dehner LP, Coffin CM. Vascular and perivascular lesions of skin and soft tissues in children and adolescents. Pediatr Dev Pathol. 2012;15(Suppl. 1):26–61.
27. Gorincour G, Kokta V, Rypens F, Garel L, Powell J, Dubois J. Imaging characteristics of two subtypes of congenital hemangiomas: rapidly involuting congenital hemangiomas and non-involuting congenital hemangiomas. Pediatr Radiol. 2005;35(12):1178–85.
28. Reis J, Koo KSH, Monroe EJ, Shivaram GM, Otjen JP, Tang ER, et al. Ultrasound evaluation of Pediatric slow-flow vascular malformations: practical diagnostic reporting to guide interventional management. Am J Roentgenol. 2021;216(2):494–506.
29. Akcay A, Akar M, Oncel MY, Kızılelma A, Erdeve O, Oguz SS, et al. Hypercalcemia due to subcutaneous fat necrosis in a newborn after total body cooling. Pediatr Dermatol. 2013;30(1):120–3.
30. Soule EH, Pritchard DJ. Fibrosarcoma in infants and children. A review of 110 cases. Cancer. 1977;40(4):1711–21.
31. Dubois J, Patriquin HB, Garel L, Powell J, Filiatrault D, David M, et al. Soft-tissue hemangiomas in infants and children: diagnosis using Doppler sonography. Am J Roentgenol. 1998;171(1):247–52.
32. Moholkar S, Sebire NJ, Roebuck DJ. Radiological–pathological correlation in lipoblastoma and lipoblastomatosis. Pediatr Radiol. 2006;36(8):851–6.

Correction to: Neonatal Spine

Noah Seymore, Krystle Barhaghi, and Maja Herco

Correction to:
Chapter 11 in: K. S. Sodhi (ed.), *Neonatal Ultrasound*,
https://doi.org/10.1007/978-981-97-8576-6_11

The original version of Chap. 11 was inadvertently published with an incorrect author name, Krystle Barhaghi, instead of Krystal Barhagi. The chapter has now been updated with the correct author name.

The updated version of this chapter can be found at
https://doi.org/10.1007/978-981-97-8576-6_11

K. S. Sodhi (ed.), *Neonatal Ultrasound*, https://doi.org/10.1007/978-981-97-8576-6_13

